T0354369

Sleep Problems:
FOOD SOLUTIONS

Also by Dr. Diane Holloway Cheney

American History in Song
American Law Enforcement
American Police Dilemma
Analyzing Leaders, Presidents and Terrorists
Authors' Famous Recipes and Reflections on Food
Autobiography of Lee Harvey Oswald, Ed.
Before You Say 'I Quit'
Brushes with Greatness:
A Chronicle of Five Generations of American Life

Confessions of an American Sheriff
Dallas and the Jack Ruby Trial
I Did Not Burn the Church Down:
I Only Started the Fire

Interrupted Lives: Hood's Texas Brigade
Jacuzzi: A Father's Invention to Ease a Son's Pain
Legendary Lawman: Johannes F. Spreen
The Mind of Oswald
Stampin' Out Ignorance
Tragedy in Black and White
Who Killed Detroit?
Who Killed New Orleans?

Sleep Problems:
FOOD SOLUTIONS

The Impact of Sleep Problems on Society

Diane Holloway Cheney, Ph.D.

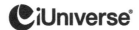

SLEEP PROBLEMS: FOOD SOLUTIONS
THE IMPACT OF SLEEP PROBLEMS ON SOCIETY

Copyright © 2017 Diane Holloway.

Scripture quotations taken from the New American Standard Bible® (NASB), Copyright © 1960, 1962, 1963, 1968, 1971, 1972, 1973, 1975, 1977, 1995 by The Lockman Foundation Used by permission. www.lockman.org

iUniverse books may be ordered through booksellers or by contacting:

iUniverse
1663 Liberty Drive
Bloomington, IN 47403
www.iuniverse.com
1-800-Authors (1-800-288-4677)

ISBN: 978-1-5320-2505-1 (sc)
ISBN: 978-1-5320-2506-8 (e)

Library of Congress Control Number: 2017908801

Print information available on the last page.

iUniverse rev. date: 07/31/2017

This book is dedicated to my grandson,
Keith William Wagoner, R.N.

TABLE OF CONTENTS

LIST OF RECIPES IN THIS BOOK

Chapter Two
Shakespearean Gooseberry or Blueberry Fool
Grape Dumplings (Tsalagi)
German Glowing Wine (Gluhwein)
Civil War Fried Apples

Chapter Three
Vincent Price Zabaglione
Pease Porridge (15th century English recipe)
Hasty Pudding or Mush
Alexandre Dumas Apricot Compote
Fairy Bread for Children

Chapter Four
Austrian Walnut Balls
Alexandre Dumas Strawberry Omelette
Baked Cherry Batter Pudding
Thomas Jefferson Sweet Potato Pie
English Lemon Soufflé Pudding Cake

Chapter Five
Henry Ford Model-T Crackers
NASA Fruit/Veggie Space Food Sticks
NASA Sunflower Seed Space Food Sticks
Astronaut Breakfast Cereal

FOREWORD

Dr. Kenneth Z. Altshuler encouraged me to write in the field of medicine. He kindly allowed me to be his co-author for my first medical article when he was the Chairman of the Department of Psychiatry at Southwestern Medical School, now University of Texas Health Science Center. He was the chair from 1977-2000 and now occupies the Stanton Sharp Chair of Psychiatry.

Ken published a book entitled *Managing Sleep Complaints*, which he co-authored with William C. Orr and Monte L. Stahl. Some of his many articles about sleep are "Comments on Recent Sleep Research Related to Psychoanalytic Theory" and the most recent was "Body Movement Artifact as a Contaminant in Psychophysiological Studies of Sleep" in the *Journal of Psychophysiology* in 2007.

Ken once said, "The work of Dement and Kleitman in 1957 and the rapidly increasing number of their colleagues confirmed beyond question the coincidence of rapid eye movements (REM) and visual dreams, and led to the recognition of dreams as a universally occurring cyclical phenomena, biologically rooted in man's genetic neurophysiological endowment. Thus, a physiological necessity for dreaming is suggested." Just as Sigmund Freud encouraged research on dreams and sleep through biological investigation, so has Ken encouraged those of us who sought more clarity about sleep and dreams.

Before I turned to the study of sleep, I researched and wrote about the assassination of President John F. Kennedy because I worked at Parkland Hospital November 22, 1963, when he was taken there. I conducted psychological testing of Major General Edwin Walker, whom Lee Harvey Oswald had tried to shoot on April 10th of 1963. I wrote about that terrible event in *The Mind of Oswald* and *Dallas and the Jack Ruby Trial* and in some of my earliest books.

Ken's wife, Ruth Altshuler, was selected to organize the 50th anniversary of Kennedy's assassination. Ruth was one of many who awaited the President at the Dallas Trade Mart the day of the assassination. When it was learned that Oswald murdered Dallas policeman, J. D. Tippet before his arrest, Ruth and others immediately arranged a fundraiser of $650,000 for Tippit's family. When Jack Ruby killed Oswald, she was selected to be on the jury panel who handed down the indictment against Ruby. Ruth was the ideal choice for the sensitive treatment of the assassination 50th anniversary.

For that event, she summoned famous historian David McCullough to deliver the memorial notes. Ruth asked ex-Cowboy quarterback, Roger Staubach, to arrange a fly-over since he had served in the Navy as did John Kennedy. She also invited the Navy choir to sing for the occasion.

Ken and Ruth's support for medicine and medical investigators has been long-standing and profound. I wish to thank Ken for encouraging me in my work and my writing beginning so very long ago.

PREFACE

Let me explain why I wrote this book.

It was a cold day in 1941 when I lost my crib to my newborn brother. I had always slept well next to my mother's side of the bed. It was good to be warm and safe, with mother attending my every need until I was four. But when I was displaced by my baby brother, I was not comfortable in my rickety old cot at the foot of my parents' bed. Whenever I moved much, the bottom of the cot fell down with a clatter awakening everyone. I probably awoke when my parents' made love or mom fed my baby brother. I hated those early awakenings and I hated that little cot with a passion.

I solved the problem of so many clatters by getting up before everyone. I crept into the living room to read by a little furnace fire in early mornings. That experience made me empathize with Western actor/singer Gene Autry who sang *Did You Ever Hafta Sleep at the Foot of the Bed?* around 1951.

Those early awakenings became a lifelong pattern. Only recently did I decide to research sleep problems. My new husband and his comments when I vacated our bed made me decide to look into my sleep patterns in more depth.

I learned about scientific sleuths who uncovered the causes of sleep problems and who offer cures so that we can all sleep better. The bad sleepers are not alone. In fact, a poor sleeper can become a hero for himself and his family and all those he puts at risk by sleepiness. Solving sleep problems will prevent accidents, ill health, chronic fatigue, and possibly even accidental death. I learned many wondrous things about the human condition that I'll pass along.

One discovery was that certain foods produce the sleep hormone (melatonin). During my research, I began to understand age-old traditions like why we have dessert, and how different cultures organize their meals, days, and nights and what happens when people sleep together. I learned how our sleep traditions vary widely from other countries and how we could improve sleep by learning a few lessons from them.

When I began researching sleep problems in various professions, I was shocked! I had no idea that sleep problems cost the lives of so many who serve daily as we go about our business. I wrote this book because I uncovered staggering evidence about the high price we pay for accidents involving sleep problems. The price of sleep deprivation is immense and we must change things.

Thankfully, I also learned many ways to improve my own sleep and will share those findings.

ACKNOWLEDGEMENTS

Nobody can write a book like this without lots of help from many people. I am very much indebted to all those who looked over pertinent sections of this book and improved this work by their comments and recommendations.

Alan B. Cheney, Ph.D., graciously and admirably served as the chief editor of this book. He is a psychology professor for Liberty University online, and was an associate professor of psychology (tenured) and student counselor for Saba University School of Medicine in the Netherlands Antilles. Previously Alan was a vice president of consulting for Psychological Associates in St. Louis, Missouri. He obtained his organizational psychology doctorate at the University of North Texas.

Chief Rob Biscoe of the North County Fire and Medical District of Arizona, has led his department to become the first Arizona fire district to acquire an Insurance Services Office (ISO) rating of One (out of ten), which places them at the top one per cent of the nation's 49,000 fire departments. They have also achieved CFAI accredited agency status, and are notable as a Heart Safe Community and a Premier EMS Agency. Biscoe has also organized the Arizona Fire and Medical Authority combining some fire districts. This will result in lower insurance costs, bulk purchasing discounts, reduced firefighter overtime hours, lower annual physical examination rates, better service, and lower tax rates for citizens.

Mark Gotfried, M.D., is the Medical Director for Pulmonary Associates. As a pulmonologist, he has handled and written about numerous lung issues and sleep disorders. He also conducts research on sleep disorders and is affiliated with Banner Medical Center and HonorHealth John C. Lincoln Medical Center.

Hal Lind, with B.S.E.E. and M.S.E.E. degrees, was a (Howard) Hughes fellow, a communications officer for the U.S. Army in the Korean War, and a designer of military radios and satellite communications with five patents for inventions. He was chief scientist for Hughes Communications Division, a team member of the GM SunRaycer solar car project in Australia, and consultant for the GM-Chevy Racing Team.

Aaron Staryak is the Associate Director of Security Intelligence at K&L Gates LLP. He is responsible for the firm's cyber threat detection and monitoring, threat intelligence, and counterintelligence programs. Previously, Aaron served as a Military Intelligence and Information Operations Officer in the United States Army where he attained the rank of Major. Over the course of his 13 years of service, he held leadership positions in an organization that conducted Cyber Counterintelligence, Document and Media Exploitation, and Information Operations. He recommended that a book include the exploration of WWII German substances created to keep military forces awake for days at a time.

Chief Deputy (retired) A. Jay Six, Jr. served as a police officer for two years at the University of Texas in Arlington, 24 years as a police officer and lieutenant at the Arlington Police Department, and 14 years as Chief Deputy of Patrol at the Tarrant County Sheriff's Office. He currently teaches police supervision and ethics at The Center for American and International Law in Plano, Texas. He also serves on their advisory board as well as the Institute of Law Enforcement Administration.

James A. Abbott (8/26/27 -5/19/2017) was a quintessential FBI Special Agent, in Charge of the North Texas FBI from 1977-1980, when he retired. A friend of forty years, Jim explained how sleep issues were a bigger problem in the past when agents had to be vigilant for hours on end as they were frequently re-assigned just when coming off duty. Agents rarely saw their families except on weekends and could be gone for months or years at a time, depending upon assignments. He wanted me to help others grasp the depth of errors continually made by all law enforcement agents and by politicians, due to the life they lived, with the lack of sleep and the absence of usual life routines when people serve the public.

Lieutenant Colonel (retired) Ed Carr was an Air Force pilot who joined the military in 1955 and retired in 1978 as a highly-decorated Vietnam veteran and pilot. He flew the C-133 for six years, and was charged with investigating helicopter and aircraft accidents in which fatigue was often a factor, despite the wording required for such military conclusions. More recently he was the Executive Vice President of School Specialty providing educational products to schools across the U.S.

Alexandra French, R.N., worked in Canada, Great Britain, and the United States. Her areas of practice included obstetrics, psychiatry, public health and included teaching other nurses and nursing assistants.

Jack Hawn is a retired *Los Angeles Times* Sports and Entertainment writer and author of *Blind Journey: A Journalist's Memoirs*. "Lovable Jack" rubbed noses with premier sports figures and entertainment idols through his life. He has served as an outstanding guru for those who took up newspaper reporting in the Valley of the Sun in Arizona.

Keith Wagoner, R.N., is a charge nurse at the Park Highland Nursing and Rehabilitation Center in Athens, Texas. His years of nursing from 2008 have included several employers and he has found that the shortage of nurses has caused employers to ask nurses to work overly long hours.

Diane Patrick is the Vitamin Director of Vitamin Cottage located in Dallas, Texas. Diane has worked for this chain of researched vitamin wholesalers for over 20 years. She has taken the time to supply the author with a variety of vitamins and substance which have been recommended to help people sleep. In this way, I have been able to learn about alternative items that insomniacs may want to know about.

Stuart Cheney, Ph.D., is the Associate Professor of Musicology at Texas Christian University in Fort Worth, Texas. He has taught music, specializing in ancient instruments, at Goucher College in Baltimore, University of Maryland, Vanderbilt University, and Southern Methodist University before coming to T.C.U. He has published numerous articles about music and is the editor of the *Journal of the Viola da Gamba Society of America* from 1999 to 2007. He was helpful in uncovering the relationship between musicians and dreams.

Ed Van Cott ably assisted this project with his background in business as president and vice president of engineering, operations, planning and program management. He was a "rocket scientist" for Raytheon. He has experience in managing, planning, forecasting, negotiating, cost estimating and presentations. He also served as a consultant on factory layout and construction. Van Cott has a B.S. degree in mechanical engineering and an M.S. in communications. His knowledge of the English language and word use is excellent. He also happens to be my beloved husband and soul mate.

INTRODUCTION

My parents introduced me to skepticism and wonder in my young life. They explained the fossils I brought home from the gravel in my school yard. They discussed the stars as we lay on blankets at night looking up. They taught me how to figure things out for myself. This made me seek the scientific explanation of all things, even sleep problems.

Early in life I wanted to learn about the human body and how to help people with medical problems. I began work at Southwestern Medical School while it was being built in Dallas, Texas. I was lucky enough to work for their first open-heart surgeon, Hugh Wilson, M.D.; first oral surgeon, Robert Walker, M.D., D.D.S; and first neurosurgeon, Kemp Clark, M.D. Dr. Clark pronounced President John F. Kennedy dead on November 22, 1963.

As I began training to become a nurse, psychiatric nursing was most fascinating. I undertook training to be a psychologist while supporting myself in psychiatric nursing. My psychoanalytic focus came from my Hungarian relative (who hired me in 1957 to run his travel agency in the British Isles). He described his classes in Vienna with psychoanalysis founder—Dr. Sigmund Freud. I will refer to Freud later when we discuss dreams.

In my psychoanalytic counseling, many interesting people came to deal with problems and improve their lives. Knowing them so intimately has improved me. Most of my patients were ordinary people like you and me. But there were a few notable actors/actresses, archaeologists, artists, astronomers, ballerinas, band leaders, bee-keepers, cartoonists, chefs, comedians, designers, disabled people, executives, firefighters, geologists, government officials, law enforcement officers, millionaires, musicians, nurses, politicians, physicians, preachers, psychiatrists, senators, teachers/ professors, war heroes, writers, and some holding positions that cannot be disclosed. Psychological careers like mine are quite educational and absorbing, even though we could not come home and share confidentialities with our mates.

There were some who could neither read, write, nor calculate, and some who were sent to be evaluated for brain dysfunction, dementia, or Alzheimer's. There were few psychologists in Dallas who understood the locations in the brain for various abilities —an area later undertaken by neuropsychologists in the U.S., but some of those referrals came my way. Over all of my career, most patients came to improve themselves. My conclusion was that most people want to be a better person.

Over the many years of counseling and consulting with individuals, couples, government agencies, and companies, my small company was hired to develop a morale survey for the Dallas Fire Department Union. Their entire department participated and the results were given their Fire Chief, whom they believed was unsympathetic to their needs. Those results improved the relationship between firefighters and their chief.

I was working at Parkland Hospital as a psychiatric nurse when the assassination of President Kennedy occurred. It was intensely interesting because, in preparation to be a psychologist, I was asked to do the psychological evaluation of another of Lee Harvey Oswald's targets, Major General Edwin Walker, for Attorney General Bobby Kennedy. Several books about the Kennedy assassination, Lee Harvey Oswald, and Jack Ruby came from that experience. My books became sources for Bill O'Reilly's book *Killing Kennedy* and Vincent Bugliosi's book *Reclaiming History: The Assassination of President John F. Kennedy.*

Later, my crew was hired to develop the first assessment centers of the uniformed services (police and fire) for the City of Dallas. This involved close observations of various ranks performing their duties, preparation of tests and exercises for candidates to perform those duties, selection and training of police and fire officials flown in and housed for the center, and training of those who would perform the ratings. This set the assessment model for the uniformed services to select good people to fill upper level jobs.

I was later appointed the first Drug Czar (or was it Czarina) of Dallas under Mayor Annette Strauss. After setting up an anti-drug coalition with 53 agencies and writing grants to bring millions of federal dollars into Dallas, it has since been carried on in various forms. It became time to retire and I chose Sun City West, Arizona where community service, lecturing, and writing books is how typical weeks are filled.

This will not be a technical book about the details of sleep problems, diagnoses, treatments for each, and associated medical problems. Those problems require a physician or psychologist qualified as a sleep specialist, and often sleep laboratory personnel are required for evaluation and treatment. The answers to sleep problems always come from science these days.

Since I'm a psychologist, many things were explored such as how people have slept through the ages and the influence sleep mates have upon sleep patterns. It was sobering to examine our responsibilities to others and to ourselves in staying alert.

Using the latest research about sleep-inducing ingredients, I thought why not include old recipes, some from famous people, just to make the book more interesting. Any of us can take a person's main recipe ideas and make our own evening concoctions.

When considering the consequences of pilots, surgeons, firefighters, police officers, ship captains, truck drivers, and world leaders who can't sleep any better than us, it was scary. The consequences are enormous--they cost lives and create injuries. Mistakes are becoming too expensive. Sleep is the new enemy of life and productivity. The advances in transportation, communications, and security have transformed and unified the world but we are letting everyone down when we make drowsy mistakes.

Sleep was not a popular subject in early medical circles. We all attended William Dement's talks when he visited the new Dallas medical school. He can be called the "Father of Sleep Medicine." Most of us learned only enough about the sleep of our patients to make diagnostic and pharmacological decisions. Some of us helped people look into their dreams when they so desired, examining dreams from the Freudian standpoint as patients tackled personal problems and tried improve their behavior and their lives.

Often, patients were helped with sleep problems through the medicines they took for their depression or other disorders. My hospital privileges in the Dallas area enabled me to treat psychological cases and prescribe only psychoactive medications. However, my recent research into the field of sleep has yielded much important information which should be available to those who seek it. This book will summarize my studies about the importance of sleep and sleep problems in our lives.

Chapter One

COMMON SENSE AND RECOMMENDATIONS ABOUT SLEEP

Are you reading this book because you didn't sleep a wink last night? Chances are that you've already heard many typical sleep recommendations. You want to know more or you wouldn't read this book. You probably want to know whether anybody has something more to offer so you can finally get some good sleep.

Can Food Choices Help Us Sleep Better?

What about food solutions? There are special diets for acid reflux, ADD, ADHD, allergies, Alzheimer's disease prevention, anemia, asthma, autism, cancer, cardiovascular disease, celiac disease, cirrhosis, colds, colitis, Crohn's disease, depression, diabetes, fatty liver, fibromyalgia, flu, gall stones, gluten intolerance, gout, Graves' disease, headaches, hemorrhoids, hepatitis C, hiatal hernia, high cholesterol, hypertension, hyperthyroidism, irritable bowel syndrome, kidney disease, lactose intolerance, leukemia, low potassium, lupus, multiple sclerosis, osteoarthritis, osteoporosis, psoriasis, rheumatoid arthritis, rosacea, seizure disorders, wound healing, and a host of others. You may wonder if there is a diet to help one sleep.

Obviously, what we eat has some impact on our body just as a little tiny pill or half or a quarter of it can make such a difference throughout our body. The latest research shows that the best supper to induce sleep includes protein (which contains tryptophan) combined with or followed by something sweet to convert the tryptophan into melatonin—the sleep hormone.

Melatonin is mainly produced by complete darkness but can be activated to a limited extent from the foods we eat. While food choices may make some difference, they have less to do with sleep than the recommendations for sleep at the end of this chapter.

Hormones are chemicals secreted into the blood from glands. Hormonal chemicals are carried to organs and tissues to do their jobs for the body. There are about seventeen main hormones and here are the most familiar: adrenaline, cortisol, insulin, melatonin, testosterone, progesterone, thyroxine, Vitamin D, oxytocin, leptin, erythropoietin, glucagon, and prolactin.

Melatonin—Sleep Hormone

Melatonin, almost absent at birth, increases rapidly through puberty and then steadily decreases during adulthood. Melatonin controls body temperature, sleep-wake cycles and glucose. Light creates melatonin in animals to regulate sleep-wake cycles, time of reproduction, sexual behavior, coat growth, skin camouflage, and color. Melatonin was discovered in 1917 and so named because the Greek word for dark is "melano".

The endocrine glands that produce hormones like melatonin are ovaries (female sex), testes (male sex), pancreas (sugar), adrenal (stress), pituitary (growth), thyroid (heart rate and energy), parathyroid (calcium), thymus (immune system), hypothalamus (temperature, thirst, sex, sleep) and pineal (sleep).

The tiny pineal gland up close to eyes in the forebrain contains photosensitive cells which contain a luminance detector. The pineal gland makes melatonin by taking tryptophan from protein which is circulating in our bloodstream. It converts tryptophan into serotonin which produces melatonin when the eyes see only darkness.

Fluorescent light bulbs and LED lights may greatly suppress melatonin production. Red light is not as intense so dim red lights could serve as night lights. If one must work with electronic devices at night, consider wearing blue-blocking glasses or installing an application on computers that filters the blue/green wavelength at night. Many people are unable to turn off light so it is hard for their brain to trigger the sleep hormone. But remember this!

This L-tryptophan that comes from proteins (mainly meat) can only enter your brain to produce melatonin by eating something sweet (a strawberry or half a banana) with or after your protein meal. Was this why desserts after evening meals were created so very long ago?

Common Sense Sleep Recommendations

What does common sense tell you about sleep? The following sleep recommendations are no mystery. They come from a variety of sources that have accumulated over the ages.

1. Most people with insomnia say they can't sleep because they have too much on their mind. Clear your mind by jotting down what's bothering you and what you must do the next day. What problems must you solve? Call it your "worry journal" and write down two or three things to do tomorrow to deal with at least one worry. Hey, you may dream up answers to your questions!

2. Keep a pen and paper by your bed so if you wake up with an idea, note it (even in the dark). You'll be reading later about how many famous people had an answer to a problem or an inspiration from a dream that helped them figure something out.

3. Don't go to bed until you're tired! Wait until your eyelids are getting heavy and your mind is drifting off. Hopefully, sleepiness occurs at nearly the same time every evening so

you can establish a sleep pattern and wake up at a similar time every day.

4. Don't use bed for anything other than sleep, fooling around, and cuddling. Watch television or read somewhere else. Associate your bed only with sleep.
5. Don't listen to music or TV when you go to bed. They interrupt sleep.
6. Don't have a light in your bedroom. The tiniest night light is all you need. Melatonin, the sleep hormone, is triggered by dark. Let your eyes (cover them if needed) see no light when you want to sleep.
7. Make your bed comfortable by being warm enough with covers in a cool room—don't let it get too hot for comfort.
8. If you are a snorer, put on and adjust a chin strap or CPAP device.
9. If you sleep with a snorer, put in your earplugs or some white noise in the background.
10. Sleep on your side in a fetal position with knees bent slightly toward the chest area, if you want to cuddle with somebody. Kiss, cuddle, and then stretch out for the night sleeping on your back if possible or whatever is most comfortable.
11. Don't nap during the day. If you fall asleep, let it be only a short refresher nap.
12. Exercise nearly a half hour a day even if it's only walking in or out of your house. Don't exercise just before bedtime because it speeds up heart rate and creates adrenaline.
13. Don't eat for three hours before bedtime unless it is a very small snack or night beverage. Digesting food uses energy. After eating, gravity takes food down your digestive tract. If you are horizontal (lying down), you may get heartburn, acid reflux, and insomnia if you eat close to bedtime. Use foods in this book to help you sleep but eat them long before you lie down.
14. Avoid caffeine six or more hours before sleep. If you drink alcohol in the evening, remember that it sends glucose

into your system, which can awaken you later, so indulge carefully.

15. Don't do anything exciting an hour before bedtime. Don't watch violent or spooky movies or sports or news. A comedy or love story or musical might calm you before sleep as will reading and chatting.

16. If desired, eat a half banana, a bit of cereal in milk, cheese on crackers or walnuts after your supper.

17. Drink some tart cherry juice (perhaps mixed with a drop or two of vanilla for taste) a half hour before bedtime.

18. If desired, drink an herbal tea (chamomile, lavender, valerian or your favorite) about a half hour before bedtime.

19. Bathe or shower with essential oils of herbs described in this book before bed.

20. If you can't sleep, set your bedtime one hour later than usual (for a couple of weeks) so that you are really sleepy when you go to bed. Do some quiet relaxing activities and/or a warm bath before bed.

21. Once you go to bed, don't watch the clock. If you sense that you are awake after 30 minutes or so, get up. Go in another room. Write down ideas to deal with whatever is on your mind—plans for tomorrow or it might be something else. Then watch or read something dull like a book about sleep or an old Turner Classic Movie. Don't read a book on a lighted panel like a Kindle, just read a regular print book by lamplight.

22. If your home is in an unsafe area, invest in a security alarm. If you can't afford one, place a notice of security protection in your house or yard. Every night, lock all doors, windows and garage.

23. When traveling, book hotel rooms on the third floor or higher. Traffic and street noises are louder nearer the street. Plus, criminals choose rooms to vandalize on the first or second floor to get away faster. Lock all locks on your hotel door. Don't open your door unless you have called someone.

Are these good ideas for you? Would you like to change what you've been doing for years? You may feel a little like Humphrey Bogart in *Key Largo* who commented: "When your head says one thing and your whole life says another, your head always loses." It's so hard to change.

Well, quick as a wink, you have all the main recommendations for sleep. But let's throw in one more, just for the fun of it. Writers like Dorothy Parker (1893-1967) could turn anything into a laugh. I always liked her take-off on the old line "You can lead a horse to water but you can't make him drink.: She said "You can lead a horticulture, but you can't make her think!" Oh, well! Parker wrote several books converted into movies such as these: *A Star Is Born, Saboteur, The Little Foxes.* About sleep, she said,

> How do people go to sleep? I'm afraid I've lost the knack. I might try busting myself smartly over the temple with the night light. I might repeat to myself, slowly and soothingly, a list of quotations from minds profound; if I can remember any of the damn things!

All kidding aside, sleep is more critical than most people realize so we'll explore it in many revolutionary ways. We'll examine sleep through history, literature, songs, movies, sports, popular quotations, and the lives of famous individuals. We'll delve into how sleep might differ on other planets as compared to ours. We'll include rather unique recipes with ingredients to produce sleep. But meanwhile, here is a short description of the various kinds of sleep problems that trouble people.

Insomnia

If you think you have insomnia, ask yourself these questions:

1. Does it take you more than thirty minutes to fall asleep or do you wake up during the night and have trouble returning to sleep, or do you wake up earlier than desired?

2. Do you have daytime symptoms such as fatigue, moodiness, sleepiness or reduced energy?
3. Do you give yourself enough time in bed to get at least seven hours of sleep each night but still don't get that much sleep?
4. Do you go to bed in a safe, dark and quiet environment that should allow you to sleep well but still can't get to sleep?

If you answered "yes" to all of these questions, you may have insomnia. If you've had insomnia for at least three months (chronic insomnia) consider booking an appointment with a board-certified sleep physician. If you've had insomnia for fewer than three months, you may have short-term insomnia. Try to follow good sleep hygiene and the preceding recommendations. If the problem does not go away in three months, talk to a sleep physician.

A board-certified sleep physician can diagnose insomnia and work with a sleep team to treat it. Before your appointment, the doctor will possibly ask you to keep a sleep diary for two weeks. By recording when you go to sleep and when you wake up, along with how long you were awake during the night, your physician can see your habits. This may give your physician clues about the cause of your insomnia and the course of treatment to take.

This physician will need to know your medical history, prescribed medicines, and over-the-counter drugs. He will want to know whether anything has happened such as an accident or major event that is causing stress or trauma. He may give you a written test to analyze your mental and emotional well-being. You may have blood tests if the physician suspects a medical problem is causing insomnia.

You may not need an overnight sleep study unless the sleep medicine physician suspects you have sleep apnea or another sleep disorder.

Hypersomnias

Hypersomnias are a group of sleep disorders that cause a person to be excessively sleepy. They may fall asleep at times that are inconvenient or dangerous, such as at work or while driving. They may cause a lack of energy and trouble thinking clearly.

Narcolepsy is a lifelong sleep disorder that makes you feel overwhelmingly tired, with the potential for sudden uncontrollable sleep attacks. It can impact your entire life. There are two main types of narcolepsy. Idiopathic Hypersomnia involves daily periods of an irrepressible need to sleep. A total sleep time of 12 plus hours is typical over a 24-hour period. The other main type of narcolepsy is the Kleine-Levin Syndrome which involves recurrent episodes of excessive sleepiness and sleep durations. Each episode may last for two days to five weeks. These episodes tend to recur more than once a year. Narcolepsy with cataplexy involves excessive sleepiness in the daytime and a sudden loss of muscle tone, or slurred speech, or buckling knees—usually occurring with strong emotions such as joy, surprise, laughter or anger.

Insufficient Sleep Syndrome occurs when you regularly fail to get enough sleep at night. The result is sleep deprivation. This keeps you from feeling alert and well rested during the day.

Long Sleeper is when you regularly sleep much longer than other members of your age group. Your sleep is normal and of good quality, but because of the demands of work or school, long sleepers may not get the amount of sleep that they need.

Parasomnias

Parasomnias are sleep disorders that involve unwanted events or experiences, which may occur while you fall asleep, are sleeping, or are waking up. You remain asleep during them although others may see you do strange things.

Confusional Arousals cause you to act in a strange and confused way as you wake up or just after waking up and it may appear that you don't know where you are or what you are doing.

Sleepwalking involves getting up and walking around when you are asleep and not remembering how you got to some other place.

Sleep Terrors cause you to wake up in intense fear with barely any memory of a terrifying dream. These episodes may cause you to wake up with the look of great fear, kicking, thrashing, or your heart racing.

Sleep Eating Disorder causes you to binge while you are only partially awake. You may have only a slight memory of the binge and the food may be highly caloric or strange.

REM Sleep Behavior Disorder during Rapid Eye Movement sleep causes you to act out vivid dreams as you sleep. You may kick, punch, or flail in response to a dream and episodes may get worse over time.

Sleep Paralysis causes you to be unable to move your body when falling asleep or waking up. These episodes usually last only seconds or minutes.

Nightmares. If these prevent you from getting a good night's sleep or if you fear going to sleep or have difficulty falling back asleep because of intense nightmares, you may have this disorder.

Bedwetting can occur in children and adults. Primary bedwetting is a failure to wake up when the bladder is full. Secondary bedwetting happens in children who face stress or as a sign of other medical problems such as diabetes or a urinary tract infection.

Sleep Hallucinations are imagined events that seem very real. They may involve sound, touch, taste, and smell and you may not be sure if you are awake or asleep.

Exploding Head Syndrome is when you hear a loud imaginary noise just before you fall asleep or awaken. It can sound like a bomb exploding, cymbals crashing, or a loud bang. It can be distressing and people often think they are having a stroke or a brain problem.

Sleep Talking is common and harmless. The words may be loud and nonsensical. It can occur by itself or be part of another sleep disorder.

Sleep Movement Disorders

Restless Legs Syndrome causes a burning or itching inside your legs when you lie down, making it difficult to get comfortable enough to fall asleep. Symptoms leave when awake.

Periodic Limb Movements involve uncontrollable repetitive muscle movements that severely disrupt your sleep. They most often occur in the lower legs.

Sleep Leg Cramps occur with sudden and intense feelings of pain in the leg or foot. They may occur when awake or asleep and the pain is caused by muscle contractions.

Sleep Rhythmic Movement involves repeated body movements when drowsy or asleep. Children may rock their body or bang their head or roll over in repetitive fashion.

Bruxism involves the grinding or clenching of teeth during sleep. When these contractions are strong, sometimes they produce the sound of teeth grinding.

Circadian Rhythm Sleep-Wake Disorders

Delayed Sleep-Wake Phase is a sleep pattern delayed by two or more hours so you go to sleep later at night and sleep later in the morning.

Advanced Sleep-Wake Phase causes people to fall asleep several hours before a normal bedtime and wake up hours earlier than most people wake in the morning.

Irregular Sleep-Wake Rhythm causes people's rhythms to be so disorganized that there is no clear sleep or wake pattern. People sleep off and on in a series of naps over 24 hours.

Non-24-Hour Sleep-Wake Rhythm causes a person's sleep time to shift a little later every day. Sleep times may go in and out of alignment with other people over time.

Shift Work that involves shifts when most people are asleep can cause a shift work disorder. It causes your sleep to be poor and you feel fatigue or exhaustion.

Jet Lag occurs when you travel across multiple time zones and have difficulty adjusting to the new time schedule upon arrival at your destination.

Sleep Related Breathing Disorders

Snoring occurs in 37 million Americans according to the National Sleep Foundation. This loud noise occurs as you sleep when the flow of air from breathing makes the tissues in the back of your throat vibrate. It can be a nuisance for your partner or anyone nearby but it may not disturb you. Snoring is often seen in sleep apnea and you should be checked to see if you suffer from this serious disorder in which you stop breathing hundreds of times each night.

If you do not have that problem, you might consider buying a chin strap so your mouth does not hang open in sleep. Lose weight because research has proven that weight loss interventions improve daytime sleepiness and reduce snoring. The more weight lost, the less daytime sleepiness. Some 42 studies in many countries have reached these conclusions.

Snorers may wish to do without a strap and change snoring behavior. These exercises may strengthen your mouth and tongue. Do each of these 20 times a day:

1. Push the tip of the tongue against the roof of the mouth and slide the tongue backward
2. Suck the tongue upward against the roof of the mouth and press the entire tongue against the roof of the mouth.
3. Force the back of the tongue against the floor of the mouth while keeping the tip of the tongue in contact with the bottom front teeth.
4. Elevate the soft palate and the uvula that hangs from the soft palate while making the vowel sound "A" for a long time.

Sleep Related Groaning, also called catathrenia, is a prolonged sound usually during REM (when dreaming) sleep that resembles groaning while you exhale. It is rare, more common in men, and is bothersome to your bed partner. Some sufferers also had sleep talking as a child.

Infant Sleep Apnea may result from a birth defect and breathing problems may cause severe complications for infants. Physicians will discuss this with the parents to see what is needed.

Child Sleep Apnea occurs in about 2% of children. This trouble breathing often occurs when tonsils and adenoids are large compared to the throat space and requires treatment by physicians.

Central Sleep Apnea causes your body to reduce or stop breathing during sleep and it is caused by a problem in the brain or heart rather than a blockage of the airway.

Obstructive Sleep Apnea causes you to stop breathing during sleep because of obstruction in the airway. People with this disorder often snore loudly or make choking noises as they try to sleep. When you become oxygen-deprived every night, you can develop high blood pressure, heart disease, stroke, diabetes, and/or depression. If you snore, stop breathing when you sleep, wake up gasping or choking, have frequent awakenings, wake up to go to the bathroom, are overweight, have high blood pressure, have a neck size of 17 inches for men and 16 inches for women, have heart disease or heart problems or a stroke, have diabetes, or are sleepy during the day, ask your doctor if you should be evaluated for sleep apnea or another sleep disorder.

Is Insomnia Fatal?

Usually insomnia is not fatal. However, there is one rare disorder that is fatal. It is called Fatal Familial Insomnia and is inherited. There is no known cure and it has only been found in about 100 people in just 40 families world-wide. If only one parent has the mutated gene, offspring have a 50% chance of inheriting it. If both parents have the gene, it is a death sentence for their children. The age of onset is variable, ranging from 18 to 60, with an average age of 50. Death usually occurs between 7 and 36 months from onset.

Fatal Familial Insomnia has four stages:

1. The person has increasing insomnia, gradually resulting in panic attacks, paranoia and phobias. This stage lasts for about four months.
2. Hallucinations and panic attacks become noticeable, continuing for about five months.

3. Complete inability to sleep is following by rapid loss of weight. This lasts about three months.
4. Dementia, during which the patient becomes unresponsive or mute over the course of six months, after which death follows.

This dreadful disorder simply wears the person out more each day with inability to repair body processes during sleep. How must those with this disorder feel? "This is your life and it's ending one minute at a time." Sleeping pills and barbiturates simply worsen the symptoms and hasten the course of the disease. When videotaped, these patients look as if they are about to nod off and then every few seconds, suddenly open their eyes and stiffen up from a slouch. They are literally dying to go to sleep. Fortunately, this is extremely rare.

Chapter Two
SLEEP THROUGH THE AGES

My early memories about bedtime when I was nine are wonderful. Mom and Dad used to have couples over and they would talk and dance and sing while my mother played the piano. They got ready for these evenings by dressing up, putting on perfume, powders, and various scents. I lay in bed with the daughter of one of the visiting couples and we would go to sleep listening to these beautiful sounds of music and people having fun. I expected to grow up, go dancing, and adorn myself with magical aromas and dine with men. It took a few husbands before I found a dancer and it's a very nice way to celebrate togetherness. I always felt safe in the arms of my man in bed or out of it. Safety is a relatively new feature of human life, and found only in some places.

Night and Day in Prehistoric Times

From the beginning of our earth some 4.5 billion years ago, it has been exposed to a cycle of light and dark based on the light of the sun as the earth spins. It now takes us 24 hours for each spin of the Earth and 365 days for a year. This is slower than Earth's earlier rotation of about 22 hours long ago.

We're getting slower as we spin out farther. When the earth was formed, the moon was originally 14,000 miles from earth and it is now 238,900 miles away, slipping farther from us at about 1½ inches per year. We are farther from the sun and our moon is even farther from us as space keeps expanding. What does this have to do with sleep?

Plants and animals have developed not only a daily life cycle based on light and dark, but a seasonal cycle based on reduced activity (hibernation, drought, etc.) versus increased activity (hunting, migration, flowering, reproduction, etc.). It is possible that some animals never sleep but research is scant on such creatures. Most animals sleep with part of their brain awake to scan for threats or obstacles. Half-awake, half-asleep systems are needed by all creatures to balance breathing, sleep, and safety from predators.

Aquatic mammals originated on land but returned to the sea so they are different than other mammals. In the water, there is no place to hide so they must always be on the alert. They must keep swimming with little rest because of predators. Thus, when they come out of the water onto land and find a snug hiding spot, they sleep and have rapid eye movement suggesting that they dream. Whales and dolphins have little REM sleep and yet they are exceedingly smart creatures. Perhaps they dream with a different kind of eye or brain wave pattern than humans, animals, and birds.

Some animals and plants have learned to live in the light and some in the dark. Some sleep in one main phase of several hours. Others sleep in two phases, waking for a while in between sleeps, like apes, humans, and monkeys. Obviously, sleep is of use to all life, or nature has made a huge blunder. People usually sleep one-third of the time. Animal species vary from the owl monkey sleeping 17 hours, to the chimpanzee at 9-10 hours, and some animals sleep only 3-4 hours in a 24-hour period.

Human Sleep in Prehistoric Times

In hunter-gatherer, pre-agricultural times, life expectancy was only about 20 to 30 years. It didn't rise to 40 years until the late 1800s, (due to high infant mortality) except for occasional extraordinarily fit people like John Adams and Thomas Jefferson. Only recently has life expectancy risen to the ripe old ages of the 70s and sometimes more despite long ages mentioned in the Bible.

In prehistoric times, people slept closely together for heat and security, rising occasionally to check for predators or unfavorable conditions. Gradually, couples and their progeny began to sleep separately from the whole group. Some tribes, however, had separate sleeping quarters for men and women and some even had quarters for women who were menstruating or women with small children. Early sleeping sites consisted of nests made from grass or straw, leaves, animal hides, mats, or inside caves. The basic sleeping requirements were safe, warm, dry places.

We learn about ancient traditions from investigators who visit or live with people who were recently discovered living under primitive conditions. Researchers who have lived with Aborigines in Central Australia describe how they slept together outside in the open on the ground or on mats. Certain people were responsible for staying awake on the lookout for problems. People felt protected by these sentinels. Sometimes, events would occur and the group was awakened to discuss it. Or they were awakened by loud events or when climatic conditions changed.

The tradition of some people staying awake was mentioned in Shakespeare's *Hamlet*, Act III, Scene 2, where we find the phrase: "For some must watch while some must sleep."

In Shakespeare's time, sweets such as pancakes, marzipan called marchpane, and gooseberry fool were popular and may have helped people sleep as a sweet dessert. Gooseberries are hard to find but blueberries will do for this dessert which will help transport the evening protein into the brain to form the sleep hormone. This recipe comes from a combination of several ancient recipes, but this is their general theme.

Shakespearean Gooseberry or Blueberry Fool

1 lb. gooseberries or blueberries (save a few berries for a swirl)
4 tablespoons sugar
Cordial such as Triple sec, Frangelico, or Kahlua
2 cups whipping cream

Boil sugar and berries 10 minutes. Cool *completely* in refrigerator. Whip cream slowly until stiff. Blend berry-sugar mixture with whipped cream. Pour in a teaspoon or so of a cordial and mix. Mash a few berries and stir them through the Fool leaving a sort of swirl. Serve in wine glasses if desired. Serves 6-8.

Early Bedrooms and Beds

One-room houses and/or a shared bedroom were common during a large part of history. What did a couple do when they wanted to have sex? They just did it despite having their children or relatives in the same bed or the same room. When did sex become private? Well, some rather detailed books have been written about that. But the real answer has much to do with the wealth of a family and the ability to have more than one room and more than one bed. A bed was a very expensive and important piece of furniture down through the ages.

Humans, unlike many animals, can have sex at any time, whether the female is in a fertile period or not. It gradually became a bonding activity between couples rather than just a reproductive force in human society. Also, unlike most animals, it can be done face to face which invites more conversation, emotion, and attention to the interaction. The conjugal bed is the site for the most intimacy between humans, unless it is shared by others.

My Bed

When my father was away on business trips, it was common for my mother to take me and my brother into her bed. It was our opportunity to enjoy closeness with her, other than those days gone by when she breast-fed us. We siblings enjoyed the intimacy to chat and be secure for the night with our mother. We felt special. I don't know why my mother did that. Perhaps she was afraid to sleep alone. Many people feel more vulnerable when they retire at night. Bedmates of any sort afford a stronger sense of security from thieves, arsonists, ghosts, and bad people.

My real sleep problems began when I had rheumatic fever at age eight in 1945 and had to spend my days in bed for several months. Rheumatic fever developed a couple of weeks after a streptococcal throat infection with fever, a rash, and soreness or inflammation in my legs, especially my knees. I also felt unable to catch my breath but that may have partly been my childhood asthma. The doctor found an elevated sedimentation rate in my blood and started me on some medicine—sulfa. Penicillin had just been invented but was only being used with infections of GIs during World War II.

The word "rheumatic" was unfamiliar to me and I thought the doctor was telling me about a "romantic" fever. After all, when the doctor said I wasn't supposed to walk, it was my father who swooped me up and carried me places the most. I was in bed most of the day. A teacher came to my house weekly to bring my lessons to complete. The idea was to control rheumatic pain and spare damage to the heart. Well, the latter failed because I later had open heart surgery to repair the damaged mitral valve caused by the rheumatic fever.

When my family learned that I would be in bed for many months, my grandfather, a carpenter, built a larger than usual bed for me. It was our most special and prized possession because of the hand-carved headboard and footboard. My bed was a little higher than my cot was. In my day and earlier, children were usually confined to trundle beds or cots or bunk beds or the floor on mats of some sort. Anthony Burgess wrote about this in his 1982 book, *On Going to Bed.*

Illness and Beds

When lying in bed day after day, night after night, sleep ran together with what bit of life could be enjoyed. This illness created my interest in the field of medicine. How to keep track of my sleep? How to develop a plan for returning to school and friends? My illness was during the war so my parents gave me little toy soldiers, airplanes and ships. I plotted clever attacks on German and Japanese enemies playing with these little figures on my bed covers.

My mother gave me the book *A Child's Garden of Verses* published in 1913 written by Robert Louis Stevenson (1850-1894). Here is some of my favorite of his poems--"The Land of Counterpane."

> When I was sick and lay a-bed,
> I had two pillows at my head,
> And all my toys beside me lay,
> To keep me happy all the day.
>
> And sometimes for an hour or so
> I watched my leaden soldiers go,
> With different uniforms and drills,
> Among the bed-clothes, through the hills;
>
> And sometimes sent my ships in fleets
> All up and down among the sheets;
> Or brought my trees and houses out,
> And planted cities all about.

Fear of Harm at Night Caused Sleep Rituals

Recovery and normal life returned and my parents moved to Dallas, Texas. When I was 12, a man (nicknamed by the press as the "Love Burglar") came into our house one night. We thought we were in a safe place and did not lock doors and windows at night. This man stole some money from purses and then proceeded to my parents' bedroom whereupon my mother awoke. She saw someone standing under the hall light near her bed and said "Can I help you?" Then she screamed to my father, "Lawrence, there is a man in our house."

My father, who slept nude, grabbed blankets about him and said "Get out of here!" The man left, but as he turned around my mother saw the name of his employer on his shirt. My parents called the police and the man was arrested. Eventually, Fred Felix Adair was electrocuted for his former rapes and murders of women. We learned that dark nights presented dangers and we began a nightly ritual to lock our doors and hide our purses to make it harder for criminals to harm us at night.

In the past when people could see little at night, they depended more heavily upon hearing, vibrations, touching, smelling, and other senses. Candles were costly so many tried to keep some bit of fire in the hearth until bedtime. Most people had nighttime duties to prepare for the dark because there was considerable fear of the time when people were most vulnerable.

To calm their anxieties, some took a bit of wine or brandy or laudanum (a form of opium). Some spent the evening spinning, mending, socializing, enjoying the tales of storytellers, or slipping off to the local taverns or brothel. After a certain dark hour, people bolted doors and windows to deter thieves and let out the dog for the night. Dogs were valuable as can be seen in this little poem of 13th century England when ne'er do well troubadours, gypsies, and beggars came amongst the people looking for anything they could filch. Strangers were never trusted. So, this became a popular ditty.

> Hark! Hark! The dogs do bark
> The beggars are coming to town.
> Some in rags, some in tags,
> Some in velvet gowns.

The Italians had a different slant on strangers when they said: "Trust everyone—just don't trust the devil inside them." To be safe, swords, firearms, sticks or weapons were kept nearby at night. Many would sleep in the same bed for safety and warmth. Bug hunts of furniture and bedding for fleas and bedbugs were common. Bodies were examined to remove lice and tend to sores. Viruses and epidemics were rife and someone sick was commonly tended by family members. Parts of the body might be washed or hair combed or pillows fluffed or chamber pots set for those who had such luxuries. Curtains were drawn.

Hot stones might be wrapped in rags and placed in bedding to maintain warmth. This was still the custom in certain English and Scottish hotels when I traveled there in 1957. The warmth of a wrapped hot stone at the foot of one's bed was most satisfying on a cold night. "Bed is a medicine" according to an Italian proverb.

Fires were banked to prevent sparks from creating fires. Nightcaps were worn to shield heads from cool air. Smocks or regular day clothes might be worn to save the expense of special clothing and blankets. Devotions and prayers were said, such as this one.

> Now I lay me down to sleep
> I pray the Lord my soul to keep
> If I should die before I wake
> I pray the Lord my soul to take.

To keep demons from entering chimneys, or other imagined creatures from entering their dwelling, amulets might be hung. The heart of a pig over the hearth was a common ritual in England. Sayings were invoked and sometimes a cross was drawn in the evening ashes by the hearth.

Sometimes, people boarded with animals for warmth and protection. Cattle might be kept below a house and the family slept above the animals on the second floor. Such living quarters were quite messy and stinky but supplied what the families thought they needed. I have been a guest in such houses in Turkey, Morocco and Jordan. The widespread problems of night dangers that frightened people in the past have gradually subsided but our ancestors experienced many dangers in Medieval Times.

Sleeping Partners in Early Times

During the past 500 years, some economically destitute women living in European cities confessed to Catholic priests that they murdered their unwanted infants by laying on them in order to control family size. This caused priests to threaten ex-communication, fines, and removal of infants from parental beds. This made some people worry more about sleeping with their infants than about the benefits of co-sleeping with their babies.

Around the same time, the idea of "romantic love" spread through Europe replacing some arranged marriages. The more important the husband-wife relationship became, the more it strengthened the movement to separate an infant from its parents soon after birth. This separation sometimes meant not only putting an infant in his own crib but removing him from the marital bedroom. This physical separation, especially of the father from his children, made him a more distant and imposing leader of the family. But he may have wanted this separation so he could have a lustier relationship with his wife.

Nightly Fears in Early America

Meanwhile in the Americas where several European countries began to explore, new dangers awaited. The Mayans were known for human sacrifices and terrorism. These characteristics were present in the Pueblo Indians later called Anasazis, who settled Chaco Canyon, New Mexico, and surrounding areas. As long as abundant rain for corn crops promised abundance, residents had no particular fears. Occasional omens such as Halley's comet and the supernova of 1054 (depicted in petroglyphs at Chaco) were seen by night sentinels. These were thought to be omens predicting either good or bad times.

The Indians in Chaco Canyon had few provisions but made sweets such as the following dumplings. These cookies from an Indian tribe near Chaco have many variations but are all called Tsalagi (pronounced Sahl-Ah-Ghee). Most of their recipes are something like this.

Grape Dumplings (Tsalagi)

2 ½ cups flour
1 bottle grape juice such as Welch's
¼ cup sugar

Knead flour with about ½ cup juice as if you were making bread dough. Roll the dough out on a floured board until very thin. Drop teaspoonful's into hot boiling grape juice and let boil a short time. Remove and let cool.

However, residents at Chaco began to distrust and fear their rulers when the droughts of 1090 and 1130 destroyed their crops. Then Chaco Canyon disintegrated rapidly. Some of them resettled nearby in Cowboy Wash in southwestern Colorado. But terrorism and cannibalism were found there among the ruins. Seven individuals (adults and children) were killed, their bodies smashed, and they were cooked in pots where human residues were found. Human proteins were also found in the feces of other humans who ate them. Fears of attacks by such tribes must have disrupted life and sleep in adjoining communities of those ancient Puebloans.

The shocking fact was that no attempt was made to hide the evidence of killing, skinning, cutting up and cooking human beings. Thus a message of terrorism was sent to all. So, local inhabitants prior to the arrival of Europeans already had fears which might keep them awake at night.

British Criminals Were Sent to America

The Europeans and the British settlers arrived in America in the 1400s and 1500s. England began shipping their criminals to the

United States in 1718 to save money and to keep their people safer. This was in addition to the transportation of slaves to the United States by Great Britain.

The largest group to be transported were from around London, England. The next largest group were the Irish, and third largest were the Scots. Most were young single males. Women were sometimes sent but did not provide much labor. Trips took six to eight weeks and many died on route to their destination. Virginia and Maryland demanded white labor for their plantations. Gradually, black slaves became the cheaper cost of labor.

Benjamin Franklin likened British criminals to rattlesnakes who rattle a warning before they attack, but convicts don't. The transportation of convicts to the British colonies continued until the American Revolution in 1776, at which time England began to ship criminals to Australia. However, the shipment of slaves from various other countries continued because slave sales in the states were very profitable.

The Pathetic Early Law Enforcement System

No police system was established in England until 1839 when London set up "bobbies" named after Prime Minister Robert (Bobbie) Peel. Before that time, constables, volunteers, and those who were being punished did night watches for no pay. Those men often poorly manned their posts and many of them drank heavily while on watch. This left villages to still protect themselves from criminals and to alter their sleep routines so that some might maintain watches.

There were three penalties for criminals short of execution in England: whipping, burning and torture. England wanted to be rid of criminals and prisons. Execution was used when the criminal seemed to have no redeeming value. Usually, those sent to America longed to return to family and friends. They were assigned to work on plantations, businesses, and households. Many escaped back to the British Isles where they were executed if caught.

Americans felt very unsafe in early times and took turns looking after their neighborhoods. It took years before the earliest police services were formed in the United States, and they were mainly slave patrols. These were intended to terrorize slaves so that they would not run away for fear of recapture and terrible punishments. Patrols were sometimes offered to Indians as well as Caucasians in the 1750s and later. It is no wonder that people had trouble sleeping, since they needed to be wary.

After the American Revolution, the United Kingdom sent their criminals to Botany Bay on the eastern coast of Australia. The high shipping cost was offset by the fact that establishing a colony for prisoners there was less likely to disturb local natives, and escape would be very difficult.

Nighttime gas lighting on the main streets of London and Paris was set up to deter criminals in the 1500s. By the 1800s, it had spread to some smaller towns. Gas lights declined in the 1890s due to new electric street lights. There was little of gas or electric lighting systems in early America.

Mankind Was Built for Midnight/Morning Sex

These days, few of us realize that before Thomas Edison's electric light bulb and 24-hour electrification, we used to sleep more than we do now. We slept in two main sessions. Before electric lights, people went to bed at dark. They awoke after 3 or 4 hours, were awake 1 or 2 hours, and went back down for another 3 or 4 hours until dawn. Sleeping straight through the night has happened only in the last 150 years in most places in the world.

Some ancient scholars wrote that sex during the middle of the night would improve fecundity. The intriguing idea that fertility increased with early morning intercourse attracts our attention. Many studies have found that men have the highest levels of testosterone in early mornings and the least at night. That does not necessarily suit women who may prefer sex following a romantic evening.

Among the reasons journalists tout morning sex are: It makes you feel upbeat for the rest of the day. You don't have to get dressed up for the event. It allows you to stay in bed a little longer. You won't feel bad about being too tired for sex at the end of the day. It won't make you late for work. You can shower together. It strengthens your immune system. A man has more energy for morning sex and can last longer. None of that is very scientific but it is popular in our culture.

Mother Nature has built into mammals a sexual feature that seems peculiar to many—nightly penile erections. Virtually every dream with rapid eye movement (REM) is accompanied by a male erection from the beginning of life. It does not depend upon erotic desire. Many times, a couple may convert the morning "woody" into an early hour sexual surprise, but it usually just seems like a bother to the man who wakes up in this condition.

The blood flow to the penis increases during REM and this produces a hard penis without many sexy thoughts but occasionally one shows up. Ain't that fun? This blood circulation keeps the genitals functioning properly whether one has sex or not. While nobody knows why this was valuable in the evolution of male mammals, an erection during sleep may display fitness to predators and, therefore, protect the sleeper from attack. Many male animals display erections during aggressive interactions with other males to assert dominance or to protect territory.

Other researchers have studied the sleep-wake cycle and melatonin. Thomas Wehr, a scientist at the National Institute of Mental Health, studied how exposure to light affects sleep. He placed 14 volunteers in total darkness for 14 hours a day every day for a month. He instructed them to sleep as long as they wanted.

For the first two weeks, they slept an average of 11 hours. By the third week they settled into a pattern of sleeping about eight hours a night in two segments, separated by an hour or two of wakefulness. He concluded that *biphasic* sleep broken by a waking phase was the prehistoric sleep pattern for human beings. The amazing result was that it took less than a month to return to this ancient pattern.

Out of his research, a Polyphasic Sleep Society emerged where people tried to live with biphasic sleeping patterns. However, it dissolved a few years later because people must live and sleep in a world of 24-hour business and electricity.

He and other scientists found that melatonin secretion triggered breeding and other seasonal phenomena. What? Melatonin triggers breeding? Well, it turned out that melatonin enhanced sexual behavior in the male rat. Some ladies always thought some men were rats! But now rats were being used to create medicines to enhance human erectile function.

So, you are asking yourself, how does a sexually receptive female rat behave? She wiggles her ears, she humps, she runs around full of energy and stops to present her rump at the right place to the right rat. In addition, any rat owner will tell you about the odors. Both sexes hump and mark (with a drop of urine) a place in their cage or their environment. Those scents contain information about age, sex, amount of testosterone and progestin, how long ago they marked, and have lots of information for those who are looking for a mate.

Psychologists studying rats and other mammals learn lots of interesting things about sex. Their rat subjects may be stinky, but so are we when you think about it!

However, if you happen to find yourself feeling amorous and having some melatonin tablets around a human female in heat- -forget it! The melatonin amounts in that study were some 190 times the typical dose used as a sleep aid. You're not likely to be as effective as those rats! Raw oysters might help you, according to recent scientific studies.

But what about raw oysters? Are they aphrodisiacs? Scientists have found that oysters have much zinc. High levels of zinc are found in sperm. Of course, the Venetian adventurer, Giacomo Casanova (1725-1798,) knew something about this. He described eating 50 oysters for breakfast and claimed that helped him seduce the 122 women he described in his book. In chapter six of *The Memoirs of Jacques Casanova*, he described the sensual process with the slippery silky oyster, then a scene which we will bleep out, and then a good night's rest with his lover. He wrote:

I placed the shell on the edge of her lips and after a good deal of laughing, she sucked in the oyster, which she held between her lips. I instantly recovered it by placing my lips on hers.

Being Awake at Night Has Been Described for Centuries

I looked into "biphasic sleep" and found that midnight prayer was not unusual in Biblical times. *The Holy Bible*, American Standard Version published by International Council of Religious Education in 1929 is used for these quotations. *Psalms 119*:62 stated: "At midnight I will rise to give thanks unto thee." *Acts 16:25* said: "But about midnight Paul and Silas were praying and singing hymns unto God..."

Sleep was a subject of concern to Jesus when his apostles continually fell asleep in the Garden of Gethsemane. They had just indulged in a heavy Last Supper that included wine. But when Jesus asked them to stay an hour keeping watch over him while he prayed, they fell asleep. Despite his reprimands and warnings, they allowed themselves to fall asleep three times. *Matthew: 26: 40* "Peter, what, could ye not watch with me one hour?" *Mark 14:37* "Peter, Simon, sleepest thou? Couldest thou not watch one hour?" *Luke 22: 46* "Why sleep ye? Rise and pray that ye enter not into temptation." Jesus was finally able to wake them when he said his betrayer was approaching. Their sleeping suggested a lack of responsibility and faith. But we understand human imperfection and the natural processes of the body.

Venetian sailor Marco Polo (1254-1324) who traveled by the Silk Road from Italy to China from 1271 to 1295 was interested in sleep. He wrote about his 24-year expedition:

> When a man is riding through this desert by night and for some reason—falling asleep or anything else—he gets separated from his companions and wants to rejoin them, he hears spirit voices talking to him as if they were his companions, sometimes even calling

him by name. Often these voices lure him away from the path and he never finds it again... For this reason bands of travelers make a point of keeping very close together. Before they go to sleep they set up a sign pointing in the direction in which they have to travel, and round the necks of all their beasts they fasten little bells, so that by listening to the sound they may prevent them from straying off the path.

Sleep was of interest to Christopher Columbus (1450-1506) who had read Polo's travel documents. When he arrived in the Caribbean in 1492, he found that people slept in hammocks that were easy to carry from place to place. Sleeping on the ground was undesirable as tiny creatures might crawl into one's ear. Of course, Columbus' sailors also found it hard to sleep because they feared being overwhelmed by local Natives. It was usually the other way around. His men could overpower the helpless people who had no horses, nor steel, nor immunities to the illnesses brought in by these Europeans.

There was an old saying among sailors who ravished women in other countries as they sailed about the world: "A night with Venus, a lifetime with Mercury." Mercuric chloride did not cure syphilis (as did penicillin later), but it helped one sleep better for a while. Venereal (from the root word of Venus) disease was the one curse that Natives had against the onslaught of illnesses (small pox, flu, colds, tuberculosis, cholera, measles, chicken pox, etc.) brought in by foreigners.

English poet Geoffrey Chaucer (1340-1400) in *Canterbury Tales* and Homer in *The Odyssey* described various awakenings during the night. So did Sir William Killegrew (1606-1695) of London who wrote *Mid-Night Thoughts* in 1682. He said:

The author...grew to such a habit of Nightly Meditations (at his first waking) as proved more pleasant than sleep, and in a short time became more delightful than any other thought could entertain his mind with...

A regenerate man's frequent devout meditations do raise in him a delight to converse so with God, and doth increase that delight, unto the most immense joys that the soul of man can reach on earth.

Insomniacs are in good company with authors because writers have been complaining about the lack of sleep forever. "I have not slept one wink" was in William Shakespeare's (1564-1616) *Cymbeline* in 1609. A "wink" is a short time—the time of an eyelid to blink. Miguel de Cervantes (1547-1616) wrote *Don Quixote de la Mancha* about 1605 and used the phrase "without a wink of sleep." English essayist Alexander Pope (1688-1744) wrote "I cannot sleep a wink" in his 1733 *Imitations of Horace*.

We have few accounts of women writing about fatigue and sleep. But Alexandre Dumas' son (1824-1895) wrote *The Lady of the Camellias* (later simply called *Camille*), of a signal sent by the prostitutes of France. They indicated by wearing a red camellia that they were menstruating or too fatigued for an encounter, but they were rested and available when wearing a white one.

How things have changed since we began keeping more track of time. We have developed so many ways of counting time but originally there were only a few methods. Pointing at the highest point of the sun in a day (called "day marks"), sundials, obelisks, water clocks and hour glasses were used. They did not change our sleep patterns. Our first big sleep enemies were clocks and wrist watches in the last two centuries to "keep track of time." Next came gas-lights and then electrification of streets. Finally, lighted establishments and lighting in homes became common. During the last 150 years of trying to sleep all night long, sleep problems have been escalated notoriously.

The Curse of 24-Hour Light

Rudyard Kipling, a British author and poet born in India, wrote a poem called *The City of Sleep* in 1895. He wrote this just before he and his wife moved from Vermont to Great Britain. They were very unhappy with life in the United States and this poem explains some of their disappointment. Kipling had insomnia. He referred to daytime as Policeman Day where pitiless rules must be followed and sleep is elusive.

> Over the edge of the purple down,
> Where the single lamplight gleams,
> Know ye the road to the Merciful Town
> That is hard by the Sea of Dreams—
> Where the poor may lay their wrongs away,
> And the sick may forget to weep?
> But we—pity us! Oh, pity us!
> We wakeful; ah, pity us!—
> We must go back with Policeman Day—
> Back from the City of Sleep!

Another person who paid attention to sleep and nighttime lights was Russian Communist ruler Joseph Stalin. He duped his people by leaving lights on in the Kremlin all night. Then he could say, "Look up at my office in the Kremlin. Even in the middle of the night you will see a light on because I am at my desk working for Russia."

The abrupt changes in sleeping that occurred between the late 1800s and the early 1900s were a problem for many people in the United States, where electrification became more noticeable. Suddenly, habits of centuries had to be changed so that parents could stay awake with light, radio, television, evening dances, and games. They had to figure out how to put their children to sleep for a whole night. What could they possibly do to help children sleep despite their noise and entertainments? They had to get very creative with poems, songs, and stories to overcome a child's wish to stay up with parents. How could they lull a child to sleep?

What Does Herring Have to Do with the Sleep Hormone?

A popular poem that parents read to children at bedtime was *Wynken, Blynken and Nod.* Those words allude to a wink of sleep, blinking the eye, and nodding off to sleep. This poem was penned by Eugene Field of St. Louis, Missouri, in the 1800s. How do three fishermen using a Dutch shoe for a boat put children to sleep? A parent reads these rhythmical words:

Wynken, Blynken, and Nod one night
Sailed off in a wooden shoe—
Sailed on a river of crystal light
Into a sea of dew.
"Where are you going, and what do you wish?"
The old moon asked the three.
"We have come to fish for the herring fish
That live in this beautiful sea;
Nets of silver and gold have we!"
Said Wynken, Blynken, and Nod.

All night long their nets they threw
To the stars in the twinkling foam—
Then down from the skies came the wooden shoe,
Bringing the fishermen home:
'Twas all so pretty a sail, it seemed
As if it could not be;
And some folk thought 'twas a dream they'd dreamed
Of sailing that beautiful sea;
But I shall name you the fishermen three:
Wynken, Blynken, and Nod.

Wynken, Blynken and Nod were fishing at night with fading light. Fish come up for insects at night. Perhaps the author knew that. Why did they want herring fish? Was it common knowledge so long ago that herring helped people sleep? It is an excellent source of tryptophan--an amino acid used to form serotonin, which produces our sleep hormone—melatonin. How does this work?

Researchers have found that people can go to sleep more easily four or five hours after eating a protein meal containing, or followed by, carbohydrates. This has caused researchers to look into meals that combine protein with carbohydrates. Examples of such meals are chicken salad with strawberries, or ham with candied yams, etc.

There is a journal devoted to tryptophan research and they have articles showing that a tryptophan-enriched food might help raise the serotonin and melatonin levels in the brain and blood. That is just what we need for sleep. The Neurobehavioral Research Laboratory and Clinic in San Antonio, Texas, found that the problem is getting protein into the brain to increase melatonin production, due to the competition of the other 14 amino acids. The secret was that transport of proteins can be done by carbohydrates included or following the evening meal.

The body's "master clock" is located in the pineal gland of the brain as we mentioned earlier. That clock just keeps ticking away without regard for the world we live in. What turns on the sleep hormone in that pineal gland master clock? Total darkness! That pineal gland relays information from the eyes to the brain. When we see no light, the master clock tells the brain to start making melatonin so you get sleepy. Eating foods containing tryptophan, accompanied or followed by glucose carries that amino acid right into the brain. So now you know it's okay to have a sweet tooth in the evening.

Foods That Can Make Us Sleepy

What are some good sources of tryptophan? Foods to eat in the evening are apples, bananas, barley, beef, bran, bread, cabbage, carrots, cheese (cheddar), cherry juice (tart), chicken breast or dark without skin, chick peas, chocolate (sweet or semi-sweet), cocoa, colorful beans, corn flour, corn, cottage cheese if low-fat, cow's milk (whole or 2%), cruciferous vegetables, crustaceans, dates, eggs, fish, ginger, fish, ham, kiwi, leafy greens, oats, onions, nuts (almonds, cashews, peanuts, pistachios, and walnuts), oats, peas, pepitas, pineapple, pomegranate, pork, prune(dried), quinoa, radish, rice, salmon, scallops, seeds (chia, flax, hemp, pumpkin, sesame), soybeans, soy milk, spinach, spirulina, squash, strawberries, tahini, tomatoes, tuna (canned), turkey (dark or light skinless). whole grain and wheat bread and cereals, wheat germ, and whole milk. Check Appendix I for a list of the amount of tryptophan in most foods. Check the appendices for foods with melatonin, tryptophan and carbohydrates.

The amount of tryptophan, as mentioned earlier, is not the whole story. For example, one piece of prune or one banana make more tryptophan available to the brain for melatonin than a piece of turkey alone. Proteins need carbohydrates to achieve sleepiness in the human brain. Other sweets and a little wine are perfect ways to end your evening and help you create some melatonin to help you sleep. Ignore winemaker Paul Masson's mission that he will sell no wine before its time, and indulge in any kind you have on hand.

Sometimes when you cook out the alcohol, a wine treat gives you the perfect send-off for a good night's sleep. There's an example of such a treat from Austrian and German brews for a winter drink. I have made changes to fit in with an evening sleep inducer.

Glowing Wine (Gluhwein)

5 ounces red wine
Juice of ½ lemon
3 teaspoons of sugar
Dash Angostura bitters
Dash cinnamon
Dash nutmeg

Heat all ingredients in a saucepan over low heat just to boiling. Then pour into glass coffee mugs and serve with a stick of cinnamon for stirring

Hemingway, Sinatra, and Stevenson Couldn't Sleep!

Ernest Hemingway, who wrote *For Whom the Bell Tolls, The Sun Also Rises* and *To Have and Have Not,* had a lot of trouble with sleep. He wrote of this to the mother of his second wife in 1936, according to biographer A. E. Hotchner. He described working hard, waking up at or two in the morning with his mind racing on book ideas and in the morning he was pooped.

Sleep has many purposes. One is solving our problems and figuring out how to make our wishes come true. Frank Sinatra (1915-1998) sang *I Couldn't Sleep a Wink Last Night.* This 1943 number by Jimmy McHugh and Harold Adamson won an Oscar for the best song of 1944 in the movie *Higher and Higher.*

> I couldn't sleep a wink last night because we had that silly fight
> I thought my heart would break the whole night through
> I knew that you'd be sorry and I am sorry too.

This Fried Apples Civil War recipe is a nice sweet that might have helped Hemingway or Sinatra. You can adapt it according to the apples available.

Civil War Fried Apples

5 tart cooking apples
4 tablespoons butter
1 cup brown sugar
½ teaspoon nutmeg

Wash, core and slice the apples but do not peel. Melt the butter in a skillet and add the apples. Cover the skillet and cook for five minutes over medium heat. Stir the brown sugar and nutmeg into the apples. Continue cooking the apples covered for 10 to 12 minutes or until the apples are tender. Check every few minutes. Additional butter or water may be needed to keep apples from sticking.

Robert Louis Stevenson had another charming poem in his 1913 *Verses* called "The Land of Nod." He comforted a child going to sleep by showing sleep as a trek through wondrous places to find interesting things to eat in these lines.

> From breakfast on through all the day
> At home among my friends I stay.
> But every night I go abroad
> Afar into the land of Nod.
>
> All by myself I have to go,
> With none to tell me what to do—
> All alone beside the streams
> And up the mountain-sides of dreams.
>
> The strangest things are there for me,
> Both things to eat and things to see,
> And many frightening sights abroad
> Till morning in the land of Nod.

Food and sleep go together. We're animals and need both to survive. How and when does a natural act like sleep get complicated? Sleep problems began long before electrification and made parents develop creative stories and songs to put children to bed while they stayed awake.

Chapter Three

SLEEP IN SONGS AND FAIRY TALES

How have we helped children sleep for past centuries? Parents traditionally use soothing lullabies or cradle songs as a sleep aid for infants. The music is simple and repetitive. Lullabies usually have a rhythm giving them a characteristic swinging or rocking motion. This mimics movements a baby experiences in the womb. Parents also read fairy tales or children's books to invite sleep and dreams as well as teaching something to the child. In addition, something sweet before bedtime facilitates the conversion of food into melatonin—the sleep hormone.

My mother played piano and sometimes sang some little soft rhyming songs at bedtime. But I really loved it when she read fairy tales at night. It made me want to go to bed sooner to hear them. She did "Scheherazade" for the *Arabian Nights*, who kept the king from killing her because she never finished her stories. My mother read me a chapter or a part at the time, so I would go to sleep thinking and wondering what would happen next. I'm sure that contributed toward dreams and stimulated my imagination.

Nowadays, we tell children about Santa Claus, the Easter Bunny, the Tooth Fairy when they are little and then tell them the truth as they grow older. We believe their well-being depends upon them seeing the world as it really is. But why disabuse them of their imagination during their childhood?

P.T. Barnum ran shows to attract people to see unbelievable events. He said, "There's a sucker born every minute." Adults went and some believed that what they saw was true. Yes, there is something wrong with adults who believe in Santa Claus. But children must not grow up with rote learning and predicted yes and no responses to everything. They must search through dreams, feelings, myths, wishes, and media to learn about the world. Lullabies, songs, and fairy tales give them standards with which to cushion the hard realities of life.

Lullabies Make Children Sleepy

Lullabies slow heart and respiration rates. They also enhance parent-child bonding. Regardless of the words, lullabies possess a peaceful hypnotic quality. Combined with lament, lullabies even have a restorative property for hospice in-patients and their families.

Brahms's Lullaby (1868) is probably the most famous European lullaby by a classical composer. Chopin wrote a cradle song (*Opus 57*). A parlor song just before the Civil War, *Beautiful Dreamer,* was written by Stephen Foster. This song brings peaceful feelings to listeners by its monotony and repetition of the words "Beautiful dreamer, wake unto me".

The French lullaby *Frère Jacques* is well known even in America. "Brother John, are you sleeping? Morning bells are ringing, ding dang dong."

> Frère Jacques, Frère Jacques,
> Dormez-vous? Dormez vous?
> Sonnez les matines, sonnez les matines
> Ding dang dong, ding dang dong

Besides lullabies and poems, parents may read bedtime stories and fairy tales to children. Fairy tales can seem real to children and some classic tales were meant as a cautionary tale and may be scary. Parents used such stories and fairy tales as moral lessons for their children as well as sleep-inducers.

Fairy Tales Were Used Through the Ages

Sleeping Beauty

Sleeping Beauty is a children's tale by the Grimm Brothers based on old French and Italian stories dating back to the 1300s. How can this tale put children to sleep? It fulfills yearnings and wishes. A king and queen have a long-wished-for child. At the banquet to celebrate the birth of their infant princess, good and bad fairies arrive with gifts. One evil fairy cursed the child saying she would prick (drawing blood may refer to menstruation) her hand on a spinning wheel and die. The last good fairy reverses the "curse" (another word for menstruation) saying she would only sleep for 100 years and awaken with a kiss by a prince. Psychoanalyst Bruno Bettelheim (1903-1990) wrote *The Uses of Enchantment* about the origin and meaning of fairy tales. His interesting suggestions add much to our understanding of these fairy tales.

This tale most likely refers to a teenage girl who may not be of age to handle the consequences of reproduction. A worried king (who does not want his daughter's innocence to be lost) forbade spinning wheels in his kingdom. But when the princess was sixteen and about ready for marriage, she came upon an old woman spinning. The curious lass wanted to try the wheel but pricked her finger. She slept 100 years until a prince somehow discovered and kissed her. She awoke when she could respond to a kiss and was old enough to handle bearing and raising children. But that was not the end of the tale.

The two eloped because the prince did not want his parents to know about his new wife who would replace his mother, the Queen, one day. Sleeping Beauty bore two children, a daughter named Morning and a son named Day, both connected with awakening. The young man must replace his mother in his affection with his new bride. However, this prince knew his mother did not want to be replaced. After his father died, he had to tell his mother that he was replacing her with Sleeping Beauty as his queen. She was irate.

When the young king was off hunting, his mother plotted with the chef to kill Morning. The astute chef promised the old queen that he would bake little Morning in a fine sauce but substituted a lip-smacking good roasted lamb for the little girl. Next, the mother asked for Day to be baked but the savvy chef spared the son and prepared an excellent young goat. Finally, the old woman asked for Sleeping Beauty to be prepared in a Sauce Robert, popular in cookbooks since the 1600s. The clever cook prepared venison in the special sauce and the evil queen was pleased.

The moral of this story could have been—Anything tastes good when cooked in a French sauce! But instead, when the young king returned home, the chef explained what had transpired. The young man confronted his mother and she threw herself into a tub of snakes. The new young king, Sleeping Beauty, Morning and Day lived happily ever after. One of the many morals of fairy tales was that we must never hurt or kill anyone just because it suits us. However, the murder of an evil-doer to save innocent people is acceptable.

Snow White and the Seven Dwarfs

This German fairy tale by the Grimm Brothers was written in the mid-1800s but originated in many parts of Europe as variations on other similar fairy tales. A beautiful queen pricked her finger and drops of red blood fell upon white snow. The queen said: "I want to have a child with skin as white as snow, with hair as black as a raven, and lips as red as blood." She had the child but when she died, her husband took a new wife. The new vain wife looked in her magic mirror daily and said, "Magic mirror in my hand, who is the fairest in the land." For some years, the mirror reassured her that she was until Snow White grew about seven years old.

Instead of accepting that her step-daughter was becoming beautiful, she got angry and told a hunter to kill the girl and bring her lungs and liver as proof of death. He was sympathetic to the child, told her of the queen's plan, and bade her to run away. He brought the queen an animal's heart to cook and eat. She greedily ate it, perhaps to incorporate the young girl's beauty inside of her. Snow White found the cottage of the Seven Dwarfs. She entered it and ate some of their food, sipped some of their wine, tested their beds, and fell asleep in one.

They came home and found a mess. When they found Snow White, she awoke and explained her plight. Instead of casting her out, they agreed that if she would clean their house, cook their food, and be nice, she could stay. These little non-sexual miners worked seven days a week with no day off—hence the number seven. She learned to keep a neat house, cook food, and worked as a housewife for them.

One day the queen got out her magic mirror and it told her Snow White was "a thousand times prettier" than she and lived with the dwarfs. She disguised herself as a peddler and tempted Snow White offering some laces to give her a trim waist. She fainted because the laces were too tight to breathe and the little men awakened her. The queen returned with a comb to prettify her hair and the poison comb caused her to faint again. The dwarves came to her rescue. The third visit from the queen, whose mirror told her of Snow White's beauty, offered an apple cut in half. The queen ate the white part and Snow White ate the red part. Some say that perhaps red indicated the danger of menstrual development and sexual relations too early in life. The dwarves could not awaken her, so they placed her in a glass coffin.

One day a prince came along and opened the coffin. He raised her up so that the poison bite of apple was expelled from her mouth like a Heimlich maneuver. They went off to live happily ever after, but the queen became so irate she jumped up and down until she died. Perhaps the moral of this was to prepare for life as a busy housekeeper for a husband and family.

It kills a child's love of fairy tales and their imagination when we tell them what a fairy tale might mean. Let a fairy tale do its magic in a child's hopes and dreams.

Actor Vincent Price (1911-1993) was the son of a candy manufacturer so grew up with fine food and earned a college education. His father invented Price's Baking Powder and the family fortune was made. Vincent acted on stage and screen from 1938 to 1992 and became particularly famous for his villainous campy horror roles such as *The Fly*. He played a key role in the famous movie *Laura*. Another of his portrayals was the Magic Mirror in the 1984 production of a Faerie Tale Theatre series including *Snow White and the Seven Dwarfs*.

Scientific evidence shows that after a meal with proteins, tryptophan is produced. If tryptophan is followed by a sweet with glucose, it penetrates the blood-brain barrier to the pineal gland and produces melatonin—the sleep hormone. To finish a nice protein dinner, a tiny serving of the Italian dessert Zabaglione might carry you off to Dreamland.

Vincent Price Zabaglione

His idea was to beat 3 egg yolks gradually adding 1/3 cup sugar and 1/3 cup Marsala wine or sherry in the top of a double boiler over simmering water. Beat constantly until very thick and warm. The 15th century recipes I've seen recommend adding a dash of cinnamon and serving it in small cups.

Cinderella

Another bedtime story is *Cinderella*, the little girl whose father married another woman after his wife died. Her stepmother ordered her to sweep up cinders at the hearth while her own two daughters were given an easier life. When a prince threw a ball to help him find a bride, the taunting stepsisters made plans to attend. Some outside force like a fairy godmother helped Cinderella become beautifully attired. She was even given glass slippers to replace her slovenly shoeware. Little Cinderella wished to raise her poor opinion of herself by finding some man who valued her despite her low status.

Miraculously, a pumpkin was turned into a coach and mice were turned into horses and a lizard was their coach master to the ball. But Cinderella was required to leave the ball and return home by midnight. She and the prince danced, but she became sleepy and lost track of time. (If she had used some of our sleep remedies, her evening might have been different.)

She had a curfew time and like a naughty teenager, she abused it. She ran out of the palace just as she turned back into a cinder sweeper and lost one of her shoes in her rush. The prince vowed to find the person whose foot fit the shoe. The shoe test allowed the prince to recognize the heroine. Unlike a flexible leather shoe, she had worn a glass shoe, which does not give. The prince probably said something like "If the shoe fits, wear it!" So, she became his marriage choice, showing that a sweet fatigued girl with sleep deprivation is worthier to be princess than a conniving lazy vixen.

High heels were invented about 1590 and were worn by prostitutes in Venice. They transitioned through Madame de Pompadour, mistress to King Louis XV, into very attractive ways to show off the legs of ladies. As sexy movie actress Marilyn Monroe said, "I don't know who invented the high heel but women owe him a lot."

Who obtained the shoe Cinderella left behind and what was their goal? That person was on the side of the poor little girl. That person was like the parent who tells their child: "See there. Get enough sleep so you don't go losing something important." Without Cinderella's sleepiness, there is no story. The Prince and Cinderella would have gone off together after the ball. That is the McGuffin, as Alfred Hitchcock would have said—the key around which the entire story hangs.

This hard-working young lass, Cinderella, had experienced sleep deprivation in cleaning the hearth and house and could hardly stay awake to finish her dance with the prince. Sleep deprivation almost did her in!

A little girl might wait a long time for her Prince Charming but the old song "What's Keeping My Prince Charming?" is something that her mother might have sung in 1931. Once a lady's Prince

Charming comes, she expects to sleep a lot better. The lyrics were by Mann Holiner and the music by Alberta Nichols. The words went something like this:

> What's keeping my Prince Charming? I've been waiting patiently
> Needn't be so handsome, he needn't be so bold,
> But I wish he'd come and get me, before I get too old.

Goldilocks and the Three Bears

One bedtime story dating to the late 1700s is *Goldilocks and the Three Bears*. Sibling rivalry was at the heart of this story as an older girl tried to replace a small child/small bear in a family. One morning, a papa, mama, and baby bear went walking in the woods while their porridge cooled in three bowls. A snoopy little blonde girl rapped on their door and entered when no one answered. The naughty child was hungry and smelled the porridge. We may recall the children's song: "Pease porridge hot, Pease porridge cold; Pease porridge in the pot nine days old."

She tried one pot and said, "That's too hot." She tried the next and said, "That's too cold." She tried the last and said, "That's just right!" So, she ate it all up. After consuming that meal, she felt tired and sat down on a chair. She got up and said, "That's too big." She tried the next chair and said, "That's too wide." She tried the smallest chair and said, "That's just right." But she broke it because she was too big for the little chair. Being very sleepy after her porridge, she went upstairs and found three beds. She tried one and said, "That's too hard." She tried the next and said, "That's too soft." She tried the third and said, "That's just right!" and fell asleep, thanks to her porridge, a nice sleep-inducer.

The three bears returned home. Big bear said, "Somebody has been eating my porridge." Middle bear said, "Somebody has been eating my porridge." Little bear said, "Somebody has been eating my porridge and it's all gone." They discovered that somebody had been sitting in their chairs and little bear's chair was broken. Upstairs they found that someone had been sleeping in their beds. Little bear said, "Somebody has been sleeping in my bed, and here she is!" The scared Goldilocks awoke and ran out in fear of harm. She was peeping into secrets of bedrooms and trying to take the place of a sibling-like bear cub so she could remain a child instead of growing up and learning not to take the belongings of others. However, some children would hear the fairy tale and just get the message that a little girl or boy shouldn't use another's possessions because harm might come to them.

If this dish made Goldilocks fall asleep, it might do the same for you as your evening meal.

Pease Porridge (15th century English recipe)

1 pound yellow split peas
2 carrots cut in half
½ onion peeled
2 stalks celery cut in half
2 bay leaves
½ teaspoon salt
¼ teaspoon pepper

Place peas in a large bowl and cover with water to soak overnight. The next day, drain and place them in a large soup pan with 4 cups of water, carrots, onion, celery and bay leaves. Bring to a boil and simmer uncovered for 45 minutes. Turn off the heat. Mash. Stir in salt, pepper, and butter if desired.

Goodnight Moon

One of the more recent bedtime sleep books is *Goodnight Moon* by Margaret Wise Brown and Clement Hurd. The words in this charming 1947 book remind children of fairy tales they've heard. The art work is colorful in a soft quiet manner with some black and white drawings as well. The book is told as if a rabbit is telling everything in its room goodnight with drowsy rhyming phrases such as these, accompanied by charming pictures:

Goodnight comb and goodnight brush
Goodnight nobody goodnight mush

"Mush" was made from cornmeal and an evening treat might be a dish of warm mush to make one sleepy. The British and early Colonial Americans called mush Hasty Pudding because it could be made so quickly.

Hasty Pudding or Mush WWI Recipe

World War I American recipes for fried mush recommended a combination of 1 cup cornmeal, 1 cup cold water and 1 teaspoon of salt, gradually mixed into 3 cups of boiling water. Cooking about 15 minutes covered, with occasional stirring, yields a hot cornmeal mush. Cool it in a loaf pan and once firm, cut and fry slices of mush on both sides and sprinkle with sugar or pour syrup on to sweeten it.

The Princess and the Pea

A darling tale from Hans Christian Andersen of Denmark was *The Princess and the Pea*. This clever little tale was probably created to show that if one is really special, they are more sensitive than the average person. A prince wants to marry a sensitive princess but cannot find a suitable wife. Candidates have bad table manners, coarse talk, shabby personal hygiene, and so many flaws. He wants someone who is so sensitive to things that she would be sensitive to him.

One stormy night, a young woman drenched in rain sought shelter in the prince's castle. She claimed to be a princess so the prince's mother decided to test her. After a pea is placed under 20 mattresses, the princess thanked all for their hospitality the next morning. However, she said she could not sleep a wink because some hard object was in the bed. It was only the little pea. She was recognized as being very sensitive, so she married the prince and they lived happily ever after.

The Red Shoes

Many of us may recall the Hans Christian Anderson story of *The Red Shoes*. It was made into a ballet movie produced in England with Moira Shearer and other ballet dancers. This tale warned little girls about not getting too carried away with themselves.

A girl, whose poor mother died, found herself with a rich step-mother who provided everything the girl requested except motherly love. The youth loved music and wanted to dance because she received commendations from others. When she put on her expensive new red shoes and danced about, she began to receive more compliments than ever. Her feet began to respond automatically to compliments about her ability until they would not stop. Despite the amors of a young man, she preferred dance popularity. She danced day and night, unable to sleep. Finally, she danced herself to death. She was dancing to receive profound love but it did not come.

Red-headed Scottish ballet dancer Moira Shearer (1926-2006) perfectly portrayed the dancer in *The Red Shoes* movie of 1948. She was also in *The Tales of Hoffman (1951)* where she danced with Robert Helpmann, who portrayed the most dramatic Dracula ever. As a side note, I engaged Helpmann and English actor Michael Redgrave to address some of the tour groups that my company hosted in the British Isles in the late 1950s.

Alexandre Dumas who wrote *The Count of Monte Cristo* created this apricot dessert. It is even the same color as Moira Shearer's hair. A bit of this after your evening meal may send you right to sleep.

Alexandre Dumas Apricot Compote

½ cup water
1 cup sugar
8 ounces of apricot halves, fresh
1 orange juiced or 8 tablespoons orange juice

Halve and pit the apricots. In a heavy, medium saucepan, boil the water and sugar until thickened into syrup, about 5 minutes. Add the apricots to the hot syrup and cook over medium heat for 3 minutes.

Happily, most of us who dance do not die of it, because fatigue and the need for sleep stops us. A few characters in the 1969 movie called *They Shoot Horses Don't They?* did die of the fatigue and its consequences. In that movie about Depression-era marathon dances, a worn-out dancer played by Jane Fonda decided to kill herself but couldn't pull the trigger on her handgun. She asked her sleep-deprived dance partner to kill her and he obliged. He explained to policemen what happened by using the saying about ragged old horses that cannot go on. "They shoot horses, don't they?" Insomnia causes huge thinking problems that were displayed in the movie.

Girls Weren't the Only Ones Who Fell Asleep in Stories

Sleeping Beauty and other fairy tale heroines fell asleep. But there are many stories about men who slept for years. *The Seven Sleepers of Ephesus* was a story of some Christian boys who escaped persecution for believing in Jesus. They hid in a cave near Ephesus, Turkey, about 250 AD. They slept for 180 or 300 years, depending on which people told the tale. They awoke, delighted to find that the Roman Empire had become Christian. Among many who read about them was Washington Irving. He eventually wrote *Rip Van Winkle*, a book whose title evokes winking, blinking and sleep.

Puritans in England and America often accused each other of being idle, as people became increasingly conscious of time. Those who slept too much were criticized, just as those who were sluggish and seemingly unproductive. A popular 16th century adage about the needed hours of sleep was "Nature requires five, custom takes seven, laziness nine, and wickedness eleven." One Japanese adage says a man sleeps six hours, a woman seven hours, and a fool eight hours!

Washington Irving (1783-1859) was born in New York but went to England in later years to write. He was going bankrupt in Birmingham, England, when he decided to make money by writing short stories. He wrote about a Dutchman who lived in New York's Catskill Mountains. This henpecked husband left his wife when she nagged that he did nothing around their house and farm. He and his dog hiked off through the Catskills until they encountered a jolly little bearded fellow. The gent asked Rip for help to carry a keg of liquor to his mates. Rip obliged and they arrived at a boisterous gathering of little old fellows playing nine-pins—an early form of bowling. They all proceeded to drink and enjoy themselves and a drunken Rip fell asleep.

He awoke twenty years later to learn that his dog, wife, and many friends had died. He was shocked and pleased to learn that there had been an American Revolution (1775-1783). Now, instead of the British King George's picture everywhere, there was an American president named George Washington (for whom Washington Irving was named).

Rip's son had grown up and done well, so Rip was again able to resume his usual idleness. As he regaled others with his adventure, he found many henpecked men who envied what he did. These various tales revealed wishes to be included and loved rather than scorned, criticized, and lonely. Dreams often fulfill our wishes.

How to Help a Little One Go to Sleep

Let's consider the origin of sleep problems in childhood. Most infants sleep about two-thirds of the time. Children have even more dreams than adults. You could say they have a lot more to learn than adults. Periods of rapid eye movement (REM) sleep when the eye is moving about looking at scenes in a dream take place during about 60% of their sleep time in the first weeks of life. In adults, 20% of sleeping is spent in dreaming, usually about every 90 minutes during a typical night's sleep.

Sometimes, when a baby is crying, you want to soothe and help the poor infant get back to sleep. An old-time remedy used by mothers and grandmothers since time began is often effective within one minute. Take a handkerchief or even a Kleenex or napkin. Slowly drag it across the face of the infant, again and again and in most cases for about a minute. Usually, the child will slowly be calmed and begin to their shut eyes and drift off.

Here are some soothing remedies passed down over the ages. If an older crying child is in some distress rather than just sleepy, you can swaddle him snugly in a soft, cuddly blanket with his arms down. Sway him gently in a motion that resembles the womb. Sit holding him or her on a rocking chair. It will soothe both of you. Make shushing sounds or sing to the infant softly.

Turn on some white noise, a fan, or some quiet lullaby type of music. Give him or her something to suck on such as a pacifier or finger. Stroke the child in long slow strokes from the neck down the spine and from the hip down to the leg. Give the child a bath using lavender oil and rubbing gently over the body while smiling and looking into his or her eyes. The lavender aroma relaxes the baby and you. Keep trying things to see what works but land on two or three plans that become repeated so the baby knows how to respond.

Sleep-wake rhythms develop during the first two years of life. At the onset of sleep, serotonin is secreted in the brain and triggers sleep without dreams. Shortly after that process starts, secretion of acetylcholine is released into the brain. That switches to rapid eye movement sleep where dreams occur. That chemical also sends messages to the spinal cord that cause temporary paralysis of the body. Without that chemical, dreaming could be very dangerous as people might move about to act out a dream.

Sleep Terrors in Children

Two common sleep problems for children are sleep terrors and sleep walking. Sleep terrors or night terrors occur when the child is partially awake and crying or screaming and having bodily reactions of intense fear, such as a racing heartbeat or sweating. Children may have a terrified or glassy-eyed look. Some thrash around and kick during these episodes. It takes time to calm a child down after these episodes. Most often, children do not remember the night terror the next morning.

Sleep sleuths studied this and reported that the most common age for sleep terrors was 18 months of age, with about 35% of all children experiencing sleep terrors at that age. Since children are small compared to animals and adults, some may have scary dreams of large things or people. Accidents and surprises may bring pain, discomfort, and anxiety. Kids try to figure out in dreams how to cope with things they fear. Sleep terrors are common at least once in about 56% of all children and have been found to occur up to age thirteen or so.

By the age of five, most normal children have become detectives about themselves and realize that dreams are not real. By age seven, they usually know that they create their own dreams. At times, a child may resist going to sleep to avoid dreaming, if they've had nightmares. Parents can play a key role in keeping these fears at bay. That is where evening poems, fairy tales and reassuring comments from parents ease them into sleep. Since sleep restores the body at rest and dreams help consolidate things they learned during the day into their long-term memory, it is vital to growth.

Robert Louis Stevenson's *A Child's Garden of Verses* contains a charming little poem that parents read to children years ago. Here is part of that little poem.

Fairy Bread by Robert Louis Stevenson
Come up here, O dusty feet!
Here is fairy bread to eat.
Here in my retiring room,
Children, you may dine
On the gold smell of broom
And the shade of pine;
And when you have eaten well,
Fairy stories hear and tell.

Fairy Bread for Children

A children's treat called Fairy Bread is popular in Australia, New Zealand, and elsewhere. Spreading butter or Nutella (a paste of hazelnut, cocoa and milk) on one side of two slices of bread per child. Use a cookie cutter to cut out a shape from one of the two slices. Place the uncut slice, Nutella spread side up. Then place the cut slice on top. Sprinkle colored sparkling sugar in the space made on the bottom piece of bread. The two pieces of bread together show the beautifully colored design to the child who will delight in the treat. Butter is typically used but Nutella or peanut butter mixed with grape jelly makes it a tryptophan treat and is equally suitable for catching sweet-tasting sprinkles.

Sleepwalking in Young and Old

Sleepwalking is the other most common sleep condition in children. A sleepwalking child is often described as not knowing where he or she is, having slow speech during the episode, and slow in responding to questions or requests. Some children will get dressed, wander around their rooms, or go to the refrigerator. The most common age for sleepwalking is ten years of age. Overall, about 29% of children experience sleepwalking at least once during childhood. Since sleepwalkers often run in families, parents can be of comfort with their child's meanderings. Unfortunately, some parents worry too much about it and are not very reassuring to their perplexed child.

There are references to sleep problems throughout literature. One reference to sleepwalking is in William Shakespeare's famous play *Macbeth*. Lady Macbeth has played a part in killing her husband, the king, and is so haunted by her bad deed that she develops a sleep disorder. She walks about with a candle seeking solace or some other person to blame. Others in the play comment on her sleepwalking disorder. Shakespeare makes it is clear that she does not completely darken her sleeping room, and we now know that any light can deter sleep. A discussion ensues between a doctor and the maid of Lady Macbeth in Act 5, Scene 1.

Maid: Lo you, here she comes! This is her very guise; and, upon my life, fast asleep. Observe she; stand close.

Doctor: How came she by that light?

Maid: Why, it stood by her: she has light by her continually; 'tis her command.

Doctor: You see, her eyes are open.

Maid: Ay, but their sense is shut.

Doctor: What is it she does? Look, how she rubs her hands.

Maid: It is an accustomed action with her, to see thus washing her hand: I have known her to continue in this a quarter of an hour.

Lady Macbeth: Yet here's a spot.

Doctor: Hark! She speaks: I will set down what comes from her to satisfy my remembrance the more strongly.

Lady Macbeth: Out, damned spot! Out, I say! One, two .... Here's the smell of the blood still. All the perfumes of Arabia will not sweeten this little hand. Oh, oh, oh!

Doctor: What a sigh is there! The heart is sorely charged...This disease is beyond my practice: yet I have known those which have walked in their sleep, who have died in their beds.

Lady Macbeth: Wash your hands, put on your nightgown; look not so pale. I tell you yet again, Banquo's buried; he cannot come out [his] own grave.

Doctor: Even so?

Lady Macbeth: To bed, to bed! There's knocking at the gate: Come, come, come, come, give me your hand. What's done cannot be undone. To bed, to bed, to bed!

Doctor: Will she go now to bed?

Maid: Directly.

That wondrous scene can help us all understand sleepwalking a little better. There are similarities between sleep terrors and sleepwalking. In both conditions, (1) children are less responsive to parents while they are in the episode; (2) they are confused about what happened when they wake up; (3) sleep deprivation, noise, fever, stress, and certain medications can increase episodes; and (4) about one-third of the children who had night terrors also had sleepwalking later on in life.

How to Handle Sleepwalking and Sleep Terrors

Preventing these conditions is better than having to treat them. Remember to keep a child's room as dark as possible so that melatonin, the sleep hormone, can be created in the brain. Also keep sound off, or keep it very, very low so the child is not disturbed or kept awake. A regular evening routine helps a child associate their bed with sleep. Avoid a television set or radio in their room. Aim for a bedtime of 8 p.m. rather than 9 p.m. until teenage years.

What can parents do during these events? During a sleep terror, parents should remain calm. The episode is usually more frightening for the parent than for the child. Do not try to wake your child. Make sure your child cannot hurt herself or himself and try to keep your child in bed and safe. Be sure to tell other caretakers, such as family or babysitters, how to handle the sleep terrors if you are not there.

If your child is sleepwalking, do not try to wake him or her. Gently guide your child back to bed. If you are concerned about your child's sleep, try keeping a sleep diary. Record where your child sleeps, how much sleep he or she gets at night, how often sleep is disturbed, and the length of daytime naps. then share this information with your pediatrician.

Sleep researchers who have studied sleepwalking and sleep terrors learned these surprising facts. One third of children who had early sleep terrors later developed sleepwalking. Nearly half of those had one parent who was a sleepwalker as a child. If both parents were sleepwalkers, about two-thirds of their children were sleepwalkers. Researchers concluded that these conditions run in families.

This brings up the realization that some sleep problems may be inherited. Only a few have been proven to be inherited but others are suspected. Those inheritable diseases are Fatal Familial Insomnia, Familial Advanced Sleep-phase Syndrome, Chronic Primary Insomnia, and Narcolepsy with Cataplexy. Others suspected of a genetic basis are Nocturnal Bedwetting past the age of five, Restless Leg Syndrome, Sleep Paralysis (when awake), Bruxism (teeth grinding or clenching), Sleep Walking, Sleep Talking, and Night Terrors. More research will eventually clarify what can and cannot be done to prevent these sleep disorders.

We now have some idea about when sleep problems begin, and how they should be handled. For children, let us hope they get past their problems through the care of their parents. We can use our knowledge, some of which comes from dreams, to help us understand our problems and our lives. We can be detectives and use sleep and dreams as allies in finding the answers to life's problems. Let us examine dreams that helped some famous people.

Chapter Four
"I HAVE A DREAM!"

America is a country of change agents. That trait distinguishes us from other more tradition-bound nations. Change comes from ideas and many ideas come from dreams. Great people do not ask what are your ideas or plans but why are you planning these things? They listen to your beliefs, your feelings and your dreams.

When I was in psychoanalysis and lay on the couch talking about my favorite subject—myself—I would sometimes remember a dream. I would describe the dream and my psychoanalyst would ask me whether I thought it meant anything in particular. I would carry on and speculate, usually connecting it to something that had happened the previous day. He would ask me questions to help me connect the dream with various things in my life. Often, I dreamt about a struggle in a relationship or a work challenge. Several times over the course of years, I felt that dreams helped me understand things I worried about and was trying to work on. I won't tell you all those secrets, but it was worth keeping a pen by my bed to jot down a dream.

Feelings and dreams were created in human brains long before language. We share that with many animals who also dream. But we can go further than animals by understanding why we dream and what we dream about.

Martin Luther King, Jr. said on August 28, 1963: "I have a dream that my four little children will one day live in a nation where they will not be judged by the color of their skin but by the content of their character." He was not referring to an actual dream but to his goal. He was telling us why he planned what he did, what his beliefs were, and how he was going to change things. He was a true change agent and a good example of how we can break traditions to develop something new and better. America listened to his dream and many Americans became change agents to further his dream.

What Do We Dream About?

Let us skip the ancients and their dreams where they expected to foresee the future. Let us move up to the modern world to learn about dreams. Scientists can now solve the question that plagued Sigmund Freud: "Why do we dream?" He always thought that question would be answered by the field of biology. They did answer it. Further questions of what we dream about were answered through his studies and those of other researchers.

From Freud and psychoanalysts, we have learned that we work on the problems we face in life and we seek satisfaction for our wishes. From biological science, we have learned that dreams help us consolidate what we've learned through the day by practicing and figuring things out in sometimes symbolic forms.

Freud (1856-1939) studied dreams of patients, his own dreams, and the study of ancient people who believed dreams were valuable. He put his ideas into *The Interpretation of Dreams*. He knew people from many walks of life including scientist Albert Einstein, composer Gustav Mahler, artist Salvador Dali, and writers Thomas Mann and Virginia Woolf.

Freud explained that we try to work out our problems in dreams but the symbols can befuddle us. Also, he believed the real detectives were patients who offered possible interpretations, since they knew themselves better than anyone else. He explained to patients that their interpretations would trump his because he wasn't in their shoes. They knew better what things they were trying to figure out in real life so they could better interpret their own dreams than any outsider.

He wrote about a few meanings of things in dreams in his practice patients sometimes told the same kind of dream symbols. But sometimes, patients were lazy and wanted Freud to tell them the meaning of every little thing in their dreams. Being a cigar smoker, he said, "Sometimes a cigar is just a cigar."

Freud had most patients lie down upon his famous couch, which can still be seen in his Vienna office. He sat behind them and they gazed at his office while saying whatever came to mind, usually relevant to the issues they came to solve. Freud didn't distract them by his facial or physical reactions so they shared their "confessions" much as an unseen priest in the confessional booth.

It was a non-judgmental form of therapy in which patients were accepted without criticism. Many say that acceptance was the key to improvement. Unlike rituals to absolve guilt as a priest might do, Freud asked questions and emphasized what the patient seemed to be saying. If the patient discussed self-destructive or harmful urges, they were invited to discover where those arose and what they would accomplish if carried out. Nobody ever fell asleep because they were talking about themselves—the most interesting subject in the world! Occasionally, a therapist might fall asleep but hopefully the patient would not know that.

Freud would certainly celebrate new research about dreams. My Hungarian relative who took a class in Vienna taught by Freud told me of the professor's keen interest in dream research. These days, Freud would have learned that the stories we invent while sleeping are much more practical than he imagined. They don't always reflect unfulfilled sexual desires. Instead, we dream about the problems of personal and business life.

Freud had a sweet tooth and undoubtedly enjoyed this famous old recipe with all the right ingredients for an evening sleep inducer.

Austrian Walnut Balls

1 cup butter
6 tablespoons sugar

½ teaspoon vanilla
2 cups all-purpose flour
¼ teaspoon salt
16 ounces of walnuts
1¼ cups confectioners' sugar

Preheat the oven to 325 degrees. In a large bowl, with mixer at medium speed, beat butter, sugar and vanilla until creamy. Reduce speed to low and gradually beat in flour and salt just until blended, occasionally scraping the bowl. Stir in walnuts. Shape dough by rounded spoonfuls into 1-inch balls. Place balls, 1 inch apart, on ungreased large cookie sheet.

Bake 13 to 15 minutes or until bottoms are lightly brown. Place confectioners' sugar in a pie plate. While cookies are hot, transfer 4 or 5 cookies at a time to the pie plate and turn them with a fork to generously coat with sugar. Transfer them to a wire rack to cool. Repeat until all are done and enjoy. This recipe should yield 6 dozen walnut balls. Austrian balls can be frozen for as long as three months.

Sigmund Freud apparently never paid that much attention to eyelids of people when they were asleep. He might have noticed that his beloved dog, a chow he named Jofi who sat in his office when he saw patients, had quivering eyelids from time to time. However, nothing was ever written about eye movement and dreaming until the mid-1950s. Then work began on that subject and scientists eventually tied eyelid movements to dreaming.

Rapid Eye Movement (REM) and Dreams

Our brain creates the "movies" in our mind during rapid eye movement (REM) sleep. Dreaming is so important that animals deprived of REM sleep die after a few days. People deprived of REM sleep (by medicine, insomnia, torture, or other means) are unable to fully rest and cannot remember things they learned recently. Freud couldn't know in his day that chemicals flow into the brain during dreams to paralyze the body so we don't act out our dreams.

The peculiar chemistry in our brain during dreams is the reason that mammals have progressed so very far in the seemingly short period of 66 million years. What's so special about mammals that made them dream? The word "mammal" comes from the Latin word for breast. Animals called mammals have mammary glands, a neocortex region of the brain, hair, middle ear bones, temperature regulation through circulation, and a four-chambered heart. Each of those changes played a part but the neocortex, the new (neo) addition to the animal brain (cortex) made the biggest difference.

Why Do We Dream?

Why did higher animals begin to dream? An eye-opening 2001 sleep study described how scientists compared the brain patterns of rats running through a maze mapping with their brain patterns during REM sleep right after their activity. Scientists found that the brain patterns were so similar that they could tell what part of the maze the rates were "dreaming" about. The study fits with the idea that physical spaces, like the maze, are "encoded into long-term memory during REM sleep."

Earlier, researchers altered cat brains to disable the paralysis mechanism that inhibits movement during REM sleep. The sleeping cats raised their heads, suggesting they were watching objects; arched their backs; and appeared to stalk prey and get in fights. Cats likely see images during sleep, though they may not be dreams quite as we know them.

Most people who have dogs see their pet's eyes move when asleep, sometimes accompanied by small leg movements as if running. Pet owners may well be in the dreams of their animal. They may be running to us for food or running away from perceived threats from other animals or people.

Human dreams help us connect new events with old ones and adapt to change. They get us ready for challenges so we can cope better when we're awake. They help us get through emotional difficulties such as a terrible situation or losses. Death of a loved one or monetary worries or a job challenge may put us in mind of past losses. They help us learn from the day's events how we can apply techniques from our past or new ones we can practice in the safety of our own dreams.

Sleep is considered restful and peaceful in many songs and books. Our daily struggles go away for a while when we relax and sleep. We can even dream up scenarios where we get help for our loneliness or wishes for love and acceptance. The song *Mister Sandman* written by Pat Ballard was a big hit in 1954. The singer dreamed of a cute guy that she hoped to meet. Listeners were thrilled with words like these:

> Mister Sandman, bring me a dream
> Make him the cutest that I've ever seen.

Dreams, Creativity and Memory

Scientists have learned how indispensable REM sleep is for creativity. When German students were given a tedious task to transform a long list of numbers into a new set of number strings, there was a shortcut that could be uncovered if the subjects saw the subtle links between the different number sets. When students were allowed to sleep between trials, they suddenly became smarter and 59% were able to find the shortcut. When they were prevented from sleeping between trials, less than 25% of the students found the shortcut. Researchers postulated that dreaming allows us to mentally represent old ideas in new ways. We are like a rat in a maze looking for shortcuts to our cheese thinking "Who moved my cheese?" The cheese we seek is the answer to whatever problems we are dealing with in life.

An American neuroscientist gave subjects a variety of puzzles. Then they were instructed to take a nap. The subjects who went into REM during their nap solved 40% more puzzles than they did before their brief sleep. The amusing tests included sentences like "Chips are to salty as candy is to?" The answer is "sweet." The dramatic improvement in creativity was due to the fact that REM sleep allows us to integrate new information into our problem-solving approaches.

Writer John Steinbeck (1902-1968) said, "It is a common experience that a problem difficult at night is resolved in the morning after the committee of sleep has worked on it." Sleep eluded many of the characters in Steinbeck's stories and he undoubtedly found solutions to some of his dilemmas after a good night's sleep. He was most famous for *Of Mice and Men, East of Eden, Cannery Row* and *The Grapes of Wrath*.

We will see in the next section how sleep helped important people solve a variety of problems. Albert Einstein liked to sleep ten hours a night, unless he was working very hard on an idea and then it was eleven hours. He claimed that his "dreams" helped him to invent. He felt that naps refreshed the mind and helped him to be more creative.

Helpful Dreams of Famous People

The father of quantum mechanics, Niels Bohr (1885-1982), spoke of an inspirational dream that led to his discovery of the structure of the hydrogen atom. Bohr got his doctorate in 1911 and gained notoriety for deciphering complex problems in the world of physics. He wanted to understand the structure of the atom but none of his guesses would fit. Then one night he began dreaming about atoms. He pictured the nucleus of the hydrogen atom, with electrons spinning around it, much as planets spin around a sun. When he awoke, he returned to his lab and searched for evidence to support his theory. His vision of atomic structure turned out to be one of the greatest breakthroughs of his day. He was awarded a Nobel Prize for Physics.

Golfing legend Jack Nicklaus had a downward slope in his golfing career in 1964. He was hitting poorly and then suddenly his game improved. He attributed the change to a dream that he had about how to hit differently.

Teenager Mary Wollstonecraft (1797-1851) wrote *Frankenstein* in 1816 during a trip with her lover, poet Percy Bysshe Shelley (1792-1822). They were guests of writer and poet George Gordon, Lord Byron (1788-1824) in Geneva, Switzerland, who also invited his lover, Clair Clairmont. Mary explained in the introduction to her famous book that the idea for *Frankenstein* came to her in a dream.

However, it was not as simple as that. Mary's father, William Godwin, was involved with Italian physiologist Luigi Galvani, Alessandro Volta, and a nephew who applied electricity to the corpse of a recently executed criminal in London and reported the "jaw began to quiver, the adjoining muscles were horribly contorted, and the left eye actually opened." The word "volt" came from Alessandro Volta, and "galvanism" or electricity derived from a chemical battery came from Luigi Galvani. Mary made much out of those discoveries which must have been in the back of her mind.

Mary and Percy Shelley fashioned the final manuscript. Here are some of her words from the introduction of *Frankenstein: The Modern Prometheus*, printed in 1831:

Some volumes of ghost stories, translated from the German into French, fell into our hands. "We will each write a ghost story," said Lord Byron...There were four of us. I busied myself to think of a story--a story to rival those which had excited us to this task..." Have you thought of a story?" I was asked each morning, and each morning I was forced to reply with a mortifying negative...

When I placed my head on my pillow, I did not sleep...I saw with shut eyes but acute mental vision, I saw the pale student of unhallowed arts kneeling beside the thing he had put together. I saw the hideous phantasm of a man stretched out, and then, on the working of some powerful engine, show signs of life, and stir with an uneasy, half vital motion. Frightful must it be, for supremely frightful would be the effect of any human endeavor to mock the stupendous mechanism of the Creator of the world...He sleeps; but he is awakened; he opens his eyes; behold the horrid thing stands at his bedside, opening his curtains, and looking on him with yellow, watery, but speculative eyes. I opened mine in terror. The idea so possessed my mind, that a thrill of fear ran through me!

Some people did not see Frankenstein as a terrible creature. Mel Brooks, who produced the classic 1974 movie, *Young Frankenstein*, presented the monster as a sort of hero. In one scene, he directed actress Madeline Kahn as she "slept" with the monster to sing "Ah, sweet mystery of life!"

Opium and Dreams

Opium user Robert Louis Stevenson came from England to marry an American lady friend. In his 1892 book *Across the Plains,* he included "A Chapter on Dreams." It is rare for a writer to admire dreams, but the inventive Stevenson did just that. He shrewdly created the name Hyde for the split personality of the scientist who must hide his basic instincts in *The Strange Case of Dr. Jekyll and Mr. Hyde.* Stevenson gave credit to the "little people" in the theater of his mind and how they helped him construct plots such as that story.

The past...is witnessed in that small theatre of the brain which we keep brightly lighted all night long...I am awake now, and I know this trade; and yet I cannot better it....Who are the Little People?...That part which is done while I am sleeping is the Brownies' part beyond contention...I dress the whole in the best words and sentences that I can find....For two days I went about racking my brains for a plot of any sort; and on the second night I dreamed the scene at the window, and a scene afterward split in two, in which Hyde, pursued for some crime, took the powder and underwent the change in the presence of his pursuers. All the rest was made awake, and consciously, although I think I can trace much of it in the manner of my Brownies.

Stevenson was one of many drug users who used dreams from drugs to create literature. Another was Samuel Taylor Coleridge (1722-1834), author of *The Rime of the Ancient Mariner*. He used laudanum, a form of opium popular at the time. Few will forget his lines:

"Water, water everywhere
And all the boards did shrink;
Water, water everywhere
Nor any drop to drink."

Coleridge's second most important work was *Kubla Khan* or *A Vision in a Dream*. It was created after he awoke from a dream of the stately pleasure domes of a Chinese emperor. The opening lines from his dream were:

In Xanadu did Kubla Khan
A stately pleasure-dome decree:
Where Alph, the sacred river, ran
Through caverns measureless to man
Down to a sunless sea....

And all should cry, Beware! Beware!
His flashing eyes, his floating hair!
Weave a circle round him thrice
And close your eyes with holy dread
For he on honey-dew hath fed.
And drunk the milk of Paradise.

Coleridge drank too much "milk of Paradise" and died later from his addictions. Other writers who used drugs received some fame but often suffered from drug-related symptoms.

More recently, opium was obtained in Chinese establishments where people would use it and sleep around on the floor. Songs like *Kickin' the Gong Around* meant using opium. Cab Calloway used to sing that song in the 1930s. In such songs "junk" meant cocaine.

He was broke, and all his junk ran out;
"Tell me where is Minnie?
Oh, I want my little Minnie!
Has she been here,
Kickin' the gong around?"

Lewis Carroll (1832-1898) was in real life a mathematician, logician, deacon, and photographer named Charles Lutwidge Dodgson. He had a stammer and a seizure disorder. He invented a nyctograph, which was an instrument for note-taking in the dark. This suggests that he wanted to make notes about his dreams and ideas during the night. He was also fond of taking photographs and painting young girls in the nude. He appeared to be in love with an 11-year old girl named Alice. He gave up an opportunity for priesthood in later life for unknown reasons, about which we could speculate.

His gloriously interesting book is about a little girl's dream. Some phrases from his *Alice in Wonderland* suggest that he might have used opium. Those phrases come mostly from the caterpillar using a hookah in chapter five, partaking of a mushroom (similar to opiates), that created visual hallucinations:

This time Alice waited patiently until it chose to speak again. In a minute or two the Caterpillar took the hookah out of its mouth and yawned once or twice, and shook itself. Then it got down off the mushroom and crawled away in the grass, merely remarking as it went, 'One side will make you grow taller, and the other side will make you grow shorter.'

'One side of what? The other side of what? Thought Alice to herself.

'Of the mushroom,' said the Caterpillar, just as if she had asked it aloud; and in another moment, it was out of sight.

Alice remained looking at the mushroom for a minute...there was hardly room to open her mouth; but she did it at last, and managed to swallow a morsel of the left hand bit.
'Come, my head's free at last!' said Alice in a tone of delight, which changed into alarm in another moment, when...all she could see, when she looked down, was an immense length of neck...

Hookahs are water pipes that people use to smoke a specially made tobacco. Often the tobacco used in hookahs is flavored, which makes it more enjoyable. A hookah uses coal to burn tobacco. This creates either smoke or a vapor that is inhaled through a tube. People usually smoke a hookah as a group, passing the mouthpieces from one person to another. Group smoking spreads germs as well as herpes and other diseases.

According to recent studies, nearly one-fifth of high school seniors have smoked a hookah. The smoke inhaled contains both coal and tobacco. The smoke also has nicotine that makes people addicted to tobacco. That tobacco smoke contains more than 7,000 chemicals, including hundreds that are toxic and many that can cause cancer. The fact that it's a group activity is appealing because it's important for teens to feel like part of a group. Hookah groups have several sites on the Internet and many discuss sleeping problems due to smoking hookah with its nicotine high.

One study showed that for every cigarette smoked, sleep time decreases by 1.2 minutes. They found that nicotine may halt the normal sleep-wake cycle because of its stimulant effects. Physicians and researchers recommend that people should kick the habit, explore smoking cessation aids (like patches) or get their head in the game with meditation training.

Studies also showed that smoking increases the risk of developing sleep apnea. Inhaling smoke irritates the tissues in the nose and throat causing swelling that restricts air flow. Smokers struggle with restless sleep compared to non-smokers. People who have never smoked at all are the soundest sleepers. Furthermore, scientists have linked smoking cigarettes to serious cancers, heart disease, routine infections, anxiety, and depression, all of which cause sleep problems.

Englishman Thomas De Quincey (1785-1859) wrote of his addiction to opium and became instantly famous in 1821. He described taking 80 teaspoons a day mixed with alcohol and cinnamon. *Confessions of an English Opium Eater* was published in 1821. Charles Baudelaire (1821-1867), published a French translation of De Quincey's book called *The Artificial Paradise*. Baudelaire compared opium with wine: "Wine exalts the will, hashish destroys it and makes idlers of all those who use it." Baudelaire died of opium addiction seven years after that book was published.

Baudelaire was a member of the Club de Hachichins (Hashish Club) that met in Paris between 1844 and 1849. Members were portraitist Eugene Delacroix; authors Victor Hugo, Honore de Balzac, Theophile Gautier, and Alexandre Dumas; and Dr. Jacque Joseph Moreau. The latter was a physician interested in studying drug users since their symptoms resembled those of insane persons. He wrote *Hashish and Mental Illness* in 1845.

Victor Hugo used opium and claimed that opium dreams contributed to *The Hunchback of Notre Dame* and *Les Miserables*. Alexandre Dumas never wrote that any of his famous stories came from Hashish but his works include comments about it. He wrote *The Three Musketeers* and *The Count of Monte Cristo* in the year that the Hashish Club originated. Some 200+ movies have been made from the works of Dumas. Few object to his references about hashish. In *The Count of Monte Cristo*, the Count poses as Sinbad the Sailor who sailed the Seven Seas and offered hashish to a guest saying:

> Judge for yourself, Signor Aladdin...judge, but do not confine yourself to one trial. Like everything else we must habituate the senses to a fresh impression, gentle or violent, sad or joyous. There is a struggle in nature against this divine substance...Nature subdued must yield in the contest. The dream must succeed to reality and the dream reigns supreme, then the dream becomes life, and life becomes the dream... Taste the hashish, guest of mine.

Dumas (1802-1870), a half black son of a Haitian slave, went on to write a dictionary about cooking called *Le Grand Dictionnaire de Cuisine* in 1873. This was his recipe for Strawberry Omelette and it contains ingredients for a good night's sleep.

Alexandre Dumas Strawberry Omelette

Choose 10 big strawberries and cut them into quarters. Put them in a bowl with sugar, a little orange zest and two soup spoons of rum. Put 10 more strawberries through a fine sieve. Make enough puree to fill a (6 ounce) glass, sweeten it sufficiently, add a little orange flavored sugar and spread it on a plate and place briefly in a refrigerator.

Break ten eggs into a bowl. Mix into them a teaspoon of sugar and two teaspoons of cream. Beat together for a few seconds. Then melt some butter in a frying pan. When hot, add the eggs and let the omelet thicken while stirring. When about set, put the cut strawberries in the middle of the omelet. Fold the omelet over the berries to give it a pretty shape. Sprinkle lightly with sugar (flavored with vanilla). Retrieve the puree and pour into the middle of a plate. Place the omelet in the middle of the strawberry puree like an island in the middle of a red sea. Makes four servings.

We see the increase of drug users in today's world and wonder whether drugs and their dreams help or hurt creative people? What determines whether we meet the challenges in our life? According to *The Lessons of History* by American historians Will and Ariel Durant, we meet life's challenges by initiative, clarity of mind, energy of will, and effective responses to new situations. We don't meet challenges by saying what Rhett Butler said to Scarlett O'Hara in *Gone with the Wind*. "Frankly, my dear, I don't give a damn!"

Some Famous Dreamers

Charles Dickens (1812-1870), author of *Great Expectations* and other books, said "Dreams are the bright creatures of poem and legend, who sport on earth in the night seasons, and melt away in the first beam of the sun, which lights grim care and stern reality on their daily pilgrimage through the world." In 1852, Dickens wrote the essay "Lying Awake" where he said:

My uncle lay with his eyes half closed, and his nightcap drawn almost down to his nose. His fancy was already wandering, and began to mingle up the present scene with the crater of Vesuvius, the French Opera, the Coliseum at Rome, Dolly's Chop-house in London, and all the farrago of noted places with which the brain of a traveler is crammed; in a word, he was just falling asleep....I devote this paper to my train of thoughts as I lay awake: Most people lying awake sometimes, and having some interest in the subject—put me in mind of Benjamin Franklin's paper on the art of procuring pleasant dreams...

Before describing Ben Franklin's paper, here is an old English recipe from the time of Charles Dickens mentioned in Chapter V of *David Copperfield* where the following conversation takes place.

"How about pie? He said, rousing himself.

"It's pudding," I made answer.

"Pudding!" he exclaimed. "Why, bless me, so it is! What!" looking at it nearer. "You don't mean to say it's a batter-pudding?"

"Yes, it is indeed."

"Why, a batter-pudding," he said, taking up a tablespoon, "is my favorite pudding! Ain't that lucky! Come on, little 'un, and let's see who'll get most."

Baked Cherry Batter Pudding

Preheat the oven to 400 degrees. Prepare your own white cake batter, perhaps from a mix. Put half of it in a buttered baking dish. Then boil up a 4-6 ounces of cherries with a tablespoon of sugar and drain, saving the sauce. Put the drained cherries on the batter in the dish, and pour the rest of the batter over them. Bake at 400 degrees for 30 minutes until set and brown. Serve with the hot cherry sauce on top.

American Founders on Sleep and Dreams

Charles Dickens' ruminations about Benjamin Franklin's 1786 advice for sleep set us searching for Franklin's suggestions:

> As a great part of our life is spent in sleep, during which we have sometimes pleasant and sometimes painful dreams it becomes of some consequence to obtain the one kind and avoid the other...Restless nights follow hearty suppers after full dinners... Nothing is more common in the newspapers than instances of people who, after eating a hearty supper, are found dead abed in the morning. Another means of preserving health...is having a constant supply of fresh air in your bed chamber....

> By eating moderately, less perspirable matter is produced in a given time; hence the bedclothes receive it longer before they are saturated...When you are awakened by this uneasiness and find you cannot easily sleep again, get out of bed, beat up and turn your pillow, shake the bedclothes well with at least twenty shakes, then throw the bed open and leave it to cool; in the meanwhile continuing undressed, walk about your chamber till your skin has had time to discharge its load...

Ben Franklin's list of daily activities included only four hours for sleep. He wrote, "There will be sleeping enough in the grave," which matched Thomas Edison's view of sleep being a waste of time. Franklin (1706-1790) combined a "can do" attitude with inventively making every day count. He said: "Early to bed and early to rise makes a man health wealthy and wise." Of course, others have humorously countered that advice, like writer James Thurber, who said: "Early to rise and early to bed makes a man healthy and wealthy and dead."

Franklin's good friend, Thomas Jefferson (1743-1826), arose from sleep as soon as he could read the hands of the clock kept directly opposite his bed. Jefferson was rare for his day. He often bathed whereas Franklin opted to stand nude in the wind to take an "air bath." Jefferson claimed that he never went to bed without some time reading something moral to consider in the intervals of sleep when he was awake. Did he dream about his young black slave mistress, Sally Hemmings? Jefferson was unusually moderate in his consumption of meat and it was said (by his granddaughter) that he lived principally on vegetables.

Jefferson was a scientist. He invented the dumb waiter, copying machines, automatic doors, telescopes, and other instruments at the cutting edge of technology. He compared plants and animals, tasking Meriwether Lewis and William Clark to collect specimens, execute drawings, and send to him Native Americans so that he might construct a correct picture of life in the United States. He was the first archaeologist of America as he excavated Indian burials on his land, describing his finding layer by layer as he observed the remains of earlier man.

Jefferson lived life with a casual elegance. His lifestyle showed even in his cookbooks. *Thomas Jefferson's Cookbook* includes recipes from Jefferson's own notes, those of his wife, his friends and those who traveled with him to France. Follow a light meal with something sweet or include his Sweet Potato Pudding with your evening meal.

Thomas Jefferson Sweet Potato Pudding

1 lb. sweet potatoes
5 eggs
1 ½ cups sugar
1 cup butter

5 ounces of brandy
Zest of one lemon (thin outer peeling)
½ teaspoon nutmeg
Pie pastry
More zest of lemon or orange for topping

Peel and boil the potatoes until tender. Rub them through a sieve. Beat the eggs and add them, the sugar, butter, lemon zest, nutmeg and mix all together. Pour into a baking dish with pastry. Sprinkle with sugar and more citrus zest and bake in a slow oven (200 to 300 degrees) until set (testing with a knife to see when it is no longer wet).

Dreams Can Solve Problems

In 1845, American Elias Howe (1819-1867) introduced refinements to the sewing machine based on a dream about a needle. He dreamed that he was building a sewing machine for a savage king in a strange country. He was given 24 hours to complete the machine. If not finished in that time, death was to be the punishment. Howe worked and worked, and finally gave it up. In his dream, as he was taken out to be executed, he noticed that the warriors carried spears that were pierced near the head of the spear. While the inventor was begging for his life, he awoke and ran to his workshop where he built a needle with an eye at the point. He reinvented the eye of the sewing machine needle as if his life depended on it.

Albert Einstein (1879-1955) was curious about time and space. It took the fear of death to stimulate his sleeping brain to develop that theory. Oh, what a joy ride he must have had! In 1905, 26-year old Albert Einstein dreamed he was sledding down a steep mountainside, going so fast that he approached the speed of light. At that moment, the stars in his dream changed their appearance in relation to him. He awoke and meditated on this idea and formulated the kernel of his relativity theory.

Otto Loewi (1873-1961) was an innovative German pharmacologist who earned the Nobel Prize in 1936 for discovering acetylcholine, a neurotransmitter that sends substances between nerves that promote dreaming. Early in his studies, Loewi was bored with medical lectures but when he learned about scores of deaths from tuberculosis and pneumonia, he searched for cures.

In 1921, he believed that transmission of nerve impulses was chemical—not electrical. He could not figure how to test and prove his theory. It preyed upon his mind. He awoke one night after dreaming of an experiment to prove his theory. He jotted it down before returning to sleep. The next morning, he arose but couldn't read his midnight writings. The next evening, he dreamt about it in more detail. Upon awakening, he went to his lab to perform the experiment that successfully proved that nervous impulses are transmitted chemically.

His experiment to prove that nerves communicate chemically through substances was tested when he isolated the beating hearts of two frogs. Once a frog dies, the heart continues to beat for a short while just like a chicken running around with its head cut off. Loewi stimulated the vagus nerve of one frog with saline and it slowed the heart. He put that saline into the second frog's beating heart and it automatically slowed the heart rate. That nerve substance was identified by Henry Dale as acetylcholine and they shared the Nobel prize.

August Kekule (1829-1896) was also German and worked as a chemist. Most molecules have linear structures but benzene did not. He believed that benzene (an important organic compound found in crude oil and gasoline) had some different structure but couldn't pin it down. There are many eureka moments about mental images and Kekule had one. He slept on the problem and dreamed that the structure of the benzene ring was circular. Kekule recorded this 1865 dream of his realization of the ring structure:

I was sitting writing at my textbook but the work did not progress; my thoughts were elsewhere. I turned my chair to the fire and dozed. Again the atoms were gamboling before my eyes. This time the smaller groups kept modestly in the background. My mental eye, rendered more acute by the repeated visions of the kind could now distinguish larger structures of manifold confirmation: long rows, sometimes more closely fitted together all twining and twisting in snake-like motion. But look! What was that? One of the snakes had seized hold of its own tail and the form whirled mockingly before my eyes. As if by a flash of lightning I awoke; and this time also I spent the rest of the night in working out the rest of the hypothesis.

Musicians Dream of Lyrics and Melodies

We are all familiar with Hungarian composter Franz Liszt's (1811-1886) beautiful *Liebestraume Number 3—Dreams of Love*. We also know that German composer Robert Schumann composed *Traumerei--Day Dreams* which is one of the most popular piano solos. But some composers had dreams which helped their compositions.

When Wolfgang Amadeus Mozart (1756-1791) was only fifteen years old, he wrote *Il Sogno de Scipione* in 1772. That was a one-act opera about the Dream of Scipio, who was a governor during the collapse of the Roman Empire. The famous dream of Scipio was that people would serve the governor and their just and compassionate empire would somehow bring coordination among the planets around the sun and heavenly music would be heard by those on earth.

Italian violinist Giuseppe Tartini (1692-1770) wrote a book called *Lalande's Voyage d'un Francois en Italie* about 1765. In that book he described a dream which led to his composition "Devil's Trill Sonata." This three-part 15-minute complex luscious composition draws violinists to play well enough to tackle this trill—especially the third part called Grave. He described his dream:

One night, in the year 1713 I dreamed I had made a pact with the devil for my soul...My new servant anticipated my every desire...I gave him my violin to see if he could play. How great was my astonishment on hearing a sonata so wonderful and so beautiful, played with such great art and intelligence...I awoke. I immediately grasped my violin in order to retain, in part at least, the impression of my dream. In vain! The music which I at this time composed is indeed the best that I ever wrote, and I still call it the "Devil's Trill."

Robert Schumann (1810-1856) mentioned above composed the beautiful *Violin Concerto*. It had a particular theme which came to him in a dream and he later composed the dream theme in a piece called *Ghost Variations*. It was published after Schumann's death by young protégé Johannes Brahms (1833-1897). Schumann dreamt that he was hearing angelic music. Then he thought he heard angels dictating a "spirit theme" which came from his *Concerto* and he expanded it in the *Ghost Variations*.

Anton Stepanovich Arensky (1861-1906) wrote an opera called *Son no Volge* (A Dream on the Volga River) in 1888. Arensky was influenced strongly by Rimsky-Korsakov and Tchaikovsky. The opera was about a governor who loved two women and imprisoned them when they would not come to him freely. They dreamed of freedom and that was eventually granted to them. Igor Stravinsky attended the opera and found it dull.

Russian-born composer Igor Stravinksy (1822-1871), who was greatly influenced by American jazz in his later life, was known for *The Rite of Spring* in the United States. That composition is a wild riot of sounds depicting how life begins anew each spring. He was working on another composition in 1918 called *L'Histoire du Soldat* or *The Tale of a Soldier*. One night, he dreamt that a young gypsy woman appeared at the side of a road with a child in her lap. The woman was playing the violin to entertain the child. The child was very enthusiastic and applauded wildly with his little hands. Igor told others that he incorporated this dream into the composition.

Leo Tolsoy's Dreams and his Literature

One of the characteristics of sleep deprivation is that one begins to speak almost as if one is drunk. Russian Count Leo Tolstoy (1828-1910) wrote a comical scene in his 1877 book *Anna Karenina* about Anna's brother, Stepan Arkadyevich who was trying to help Anna. However, he blurted out things in his sleepy state that ruined her reputation. He became conscious of a peculiar heaviness in his head and began to mix up dreams and reality:

> The most incongruous ideas were running through his mind...How good a smoke would be now!...To be saved, one need only believe, and the monks don't know how the thing's to be done, but Countess Lydia Ivanovana does know...And why is my head so heavy? Is it the cognac, or all this being so strange? Anyway, I think I've done nothing objectionable so far. But, even so, it won't do to ask her now. They say they make one say one's prayers. I only hope they won't make me! That'll be too absurd. And what nonsense she's reading! But she has a good accent...

Shakespeare's Works and Dreams

This sort of foolishness in a sleepy person is contrasted with the dramatic seriousness of Hamlet and his fear of dreams. In 1603, William Shakespeare wrote *Hamlet* in which the Dane described the possibility of bad dreams. He learned that his uncle killed his father, the late king, and married his mother so he pondered suicide or murder. Hamlet's original soliloquy began:

To be or not to be, aye, there's the point. To die, to sleep, is that all? Aye, all: No, to sleep, to dream, Aye there it goes, for in that dream of death when we awake, and borne before an everlasting judge from whence no passenger ever returned, the undiscovered country, at whose sight the happy smile, and the accursed damn'd...

By 1605 he improved it to be worded as we know it. Hamlet's moral and mental anguish is at its height in this emotional centerpiece of the play:

To be, or not to be, that is the question, Whether 'tis nobler in the mind to suffer the slings and arrows of outrageous fortune, or to take arms against a sea of troubles, and by opposing, end them--to die, to sleep no more, and by a sleep to say we end the heartache and the thousand natural shocks that flesh is heir to; 'tis a consummation devoutly to be wished. To die, to sleep, to sleep perchance to dream, aye, there's the rub, for in that sleep of death what dreams may come when we have shuffled off this mortal coil must give us pause.

Fyodor Dostoyevsky's Dreams and Writings

Dreams are powerful. Dmitri's dream in Fyodor Dostoyevsky's 1880 *The Brothers Karamazov* made him admit to something he didn't do. In Book 9, chapter 8, Dmitri had been grilled by people who thought he killed someone. He was exhausted and gradually fell asleep. After they permitted him to sleep a few minutes, he awoke from a dream where he observed strange sights. When his captors gave him a form and a pen, he signed saying that he had killed someone even though he had not. It was a false confession from feelings of guilt for the plight of others that he dreamed about.

His eyes were closing with fatigue... Then he had a strange dream. A peasant was driving him in a cart with a pair of horses, somewhere in the Steppes, through snow and sleet. He was cold... Not far off was a village—he could see the black huts... there was a little baby crying... "Why are they crying?" he asked.

"Why, they're poor people, burnt out. They've no bread..."

"Why are they poor?... Why don't they feed the babe?"... And he felt that a passion of pity, such as he'd never known before, was rising in his heart, that he wanted to cry, that he wanted to do something for them all, so that the babe would weep no more... He exclaimed opening his eyes and sitting up... He was suddenly struck by the fact that there was a pillow under his head, which hadn't been there when he'd fallen asleep... "Who put that pillow under my head? Who was so kind?" he cried, with a sort of ecstatic gratitude, with tears in his voice, as though some great kindness had been shown him.

This false confession is the very reason that sleep deprivation has turned out to be a bad method of handling prisoners in real life. Dostoyevsky (1821-1881) was a prisoner along with a group of Utopian socialist group members. They were taken to Siberia after being sentenced to a firing squad. He was in the second row of men to be shot when a note arrived commuting the sentence. He was held in Siberia in such close quarters people could not lie down to sleep and filth was a foot deep. He suffered from epilepsy and had many seizures before, during, and after his five years in prison. He was allowed only to read *The Bible* and finally became a Christian.

Thomas Mann's Dreams of His Heroic Characters

German novelist and social critic, Thomas Mann (1875-1955) wrote about the snow blizzard dream of a young man in *The Magic Mountain* in 1927. His protagonist, Hans Castorp, visited a friend with tuberculosis in a sanitarium on a beautiful mountain. While there, he contracted the disease and stayed for many months. He and patients discussed everything from international politics to art, food and love. As he healed one day he went out to ski and ran into a blizzard. In the cold, he got mixed up, went farther from the sanitarium. He dreamt of death but it turned out to be a dream of no longer being alone that left him unafraid to die. He died soon after he left the sanitarium because he was conscripted as a soldier. Here is the description of his dreamy condition in the life-threatening blizzard:

Hans Castorp decided to stop for the present... "suppose I take a sip of port—it might strengthen me... Quiet, quiet...if the head be heavy, let it droop."

Youths were at work with horses, running hand on halters alongside their whinnying head-tossing charges...A lovely boy, with full hair drawn sideways across his brow, sat directly beneath him... This lad looked up, turned his gaze upward and looked at him... An icy coldness held him. He would have covered his eyes and fled, but could not... He tried desperately to escape—and found himself lying by his hut in the snow, leaning against one arm...

Dostoyevsky's Dream About Conscience

Fyodor Dostoyevsky composed a novella called *The Dream of a Ridiculous Man*. It presented an interesting point of view about the role of guilt and truth to a dreamer. He wrote this about one's conscience:

For instance, a strange reflection suddenly occurred
to me, that if I had lived before on the moon or on
Mars and there had committed the most disgraceful
and dishonorable action and had been put to such
shame and ignominy as one can only conceive and
realize in dreams, in nightmares, and if, finding
myself afterwards on earth, I were able to retain the
memory of what I had done on the other planet and
at the same time knew that I should never, under any
circumstances, return there, then looking from the
earth to the moon—should I care or not? Should I
feel shame for that action or not?...

But does it matter whether it was a dream or reality,
if the dream made known to me the truth? If once
one has recognized the truth and seen it, you know
that it is the truth and that there is no other and there
cannot be, whether you are asleep or awake."

Great writers show us how they value dreams. Through their
descriptions, we see compassion for others, consequences of actions,
and the impact that dreams can have upon our waking life.

Adolf Hitler's Dream

One infamous person, Adolf Hitler, had a dream which he wrote
about. This Austrian artist wanted to serve in World War I but the
Austrian Army ruled him unfit for service. He had been an art student,
attended operas, and was mostly vegetarian. He liked good food
but had little income from his art and ate poorly. He left Austria for
Bavaria where he was accepted and served in the German Army as
a message runner with the rank of corporal. He was wounded in his
thigh in 1914. Then he was hurt again, badly in 1918 near Ypres.

During that battle, Hitler was temporarily blinded and covered
in sores from mustard gas--a combination of chlorine and sulfur

which emits a mustard-like scent. He was treated for "shell shock" as well as the physical effects of the chemicals in the gas. Treatment consisted of strong bleaches to the skin, eye masks, and pain killers. Later, he wrote *Mein Kampf (My Struggle)* while imprisoned for an unsuccessful coup with his German Workers Party. He described his war wounds and described feeling that his eyes were like hot coals. He concluded: "That I would ever be able to draw or design once again was naturally out of the question."

In Hitler's somnolent condition at the hospital, he experienced a "vision" from "another world" which he described in Volume 1, Chapter 7 of *Mein Kampf*:

> As I lay there, the realization came to me that I would liberate Germany, that I would make it great. I knew immediately that it would be realized.

During World War II, Hitler ordered the collection of art from museums across the countries of German occupation to be saved. They were placed in a castle featured in the movie *The Monuments Men* with George Clooney. Hitler painted a lovely picture of this castle, Neuschswanstein, in his early life. It was a fairy tale castle built on the "Romantic Road" in the Bavarian Alps. His picture sold to a buyer from China in 2016 for just over $93,000. The castle was ordered by King Ludwig II who died before it was completed in 1886. Walt Disney was so impressed by this castle that he used it as the model for his "Magic Kingdom."

In addition, Hitler mentioned in *Mein Kampf* that automotive magnate Henry Ford blamed the Jews for instigating World War I saying, "I know who caused the war: German-Jewish bankers." Henry Ford was very anti-Semitic and in 1915 stated in his company newspaper that the Jews had started World War I. Ford was the only American mentioned in Hitler's book, probably because Ford's statement justified Hitler's plan to eliminate Jews.

How do you portray a dream? We generally have about five dreams a night and remember only the last, if that. Patients tell psychoanalysts about the little bits of a dream they can recall. The psychoanalyst then questions them since only the patient knows what the dream might be about. The psychoanalyst or patient might have an idea but dream symbols are not universal and do not mean the same thing to everyone.

A Dream Portrayed in a Movie--*Spellbound*

How does Hollywood portray a dream? The director usually figures out what they want the viewer to know. Then they inject it into some crazy half-symbolic art work. The 1945 movie, *Spellbound,* had a psychoanalyst as a consultant on the picture. David O. Selznick had problems in his relationship with Jennifer Jones (who later became his wife) and consulted analyst Dr. May E. Romm, who was born in Russia and trained in the U.S. He hired her as his movie consultant for $1,500. She and Director Alfred Hitchcock did not see eye to eye so the movie symbolism lacks some credibility. Even so, Selznick valued her advice.

One of the most notable dream scenes was in the movie with Gregory Peck. He was a patient of psychoanalyst Ingrid Bergman. The dream sequence was designed by surrealistic artist Salvador Dali. Director Alfred Hitchcock said he wanted the dream to have clarity and vividness while remaining absurd. Dali's work is like a dream with its eerie perspective and weird images. The dream also suggested clues about the actual murderer by a confrontation with a masked man in a tuxedo. Ski lines on a mountain of white snow in the final scene transport the viewer toward the movie's resolution.

David O. Selznick produced the movie and had his own ideas of what Dali and Hitchcock should do, so some of their ideas were sacrificed. Hitchcock, a great mystery director, thought that the length of a film should be directly related to the endurance of the human bladder.

Hitchcock's favorite food was a soufflé. Being an Englishman, he undoubtedly sampled many of these traditional English desserts.

He knew that soufflés work best if all your ingredients are at room temperature before beginning.

English Lemon Soufflé Pudding Cake

1 cup sugar, divided
3 tablespoons butter at room temperature
3 eggs separated
1 teaspoon vanilla extract
2 tablespoons lemon zest (2 lemons needed)
1/3 cup flour
¼ teaspoon salt
1/3 cup fresh lemon juice
1 cup whole milk
1/8 teaspoon cream of tartar

Preheat oven to 325 degrees. Place the rack in the center of the oven. Butter and dust with sugar a six-cup dish. Set aside 2 tablespoons of the sugar to use when whipping the egg whites. Place the remaining sugar in a bowl. Add the lemon zest and use a beater on low speed to mix them together. Add the softened butter and add the three egg yolks, one at a time, beating until all are incorporated. Beat in the vanilla. Add the flour and salt and beat until combined but do not over mix. With beater on low, gradually pour in the lemon juice and milk.

Set this aside while you beat the egg whites in a separate bowl until frothy. Add the cream of tartar and gradually add the remaining 2 tablespoons of sugar until stiff peaks form. Gently fold the egg whites into the batter, in three additions, mixing just barely until incorporated. Carefully pour the batter into the prepared dish. Place that dish in a larger baking pan and boil up some water to place in the pan for a water bath. Put enough water to go halfway up the sides of the dish and carefully slide it into the oven. Bake about 40-45 minutes or until the sponge cakes are golden brown and a toothpick inserted comes out clean. Remove the dish from the water bath and cool slightly before serving at room temperature. Dust the top with confectioners' sugar, fresh berries, or lemon slices.

How might creatures on other planets sleep and dream? How do they live and learn? Are we the only ones who lost our nights and our sleep? How do their days and nights differ from ours?

Chapter Five

IS THE UNIVERSE ON CIRCADIAN RHYTHM?

One of the monumental discoveries of the 20th and early 21st centuries is that science is neutral. It has no conscience or agenda. It can kill as readily as it can heal. The science of dreams and sleep at night only comes about because of the way our particular planet operates.

Our day and night and moon and stars become involved in the way we think, live, love, measure time, and spend our hours. As children, my family used to lie outside on blankets upon the grass watching stars and the occasional meteors or "shooting stars" as we called them. It was a nice time for relaxing and telling stories and planning for the next day. It was the only time our family came together because my father's work took him away so very much. Little did I know that creatures on other planets we saw did not have experiences anything like ours.

Night viewers throughout the ages and scientists have created a method of learning about our solar system and all of life. The scientific method tests guesses about things and throws out wrong guesses until it finds the right guesses. Science teaches us about the deepest issues of our species, our planets, and the Universe. It teaches us about where, when, and who we are in creation. The scientific method is a way to call the bluff of those who pretend to tell us something is correct.

How Day and Night Changed on Our Planet

Thomas Edison (1847-1931), the great inventor, changed our day and night. His 1883 electric lamp finally liberated people from ending their days at sunset. He was already admired because he brought moving pictures into being. We loved the nickelodeons where we could watch a few minutes of motion as photographs with tiny changes were advanced and whirred in front of our eyes. We spent a nickel for that!

Edison's new incandescent electric lamp lit up our night. After many guesses and discards of wrong guesses, his bulb was accomplished by heating a filament high enough to emit radiation in the visible range to produce a white glow. Argon gas prevented the tungsten filament from burning up. The clear glass light bulb was a harsh light but illuminated a room brightly. The search for a softer light went on until 1925 when Marvin Pipkin invented the frosted incandescent light bulb.

The invention of light at night kept everybody from sleeping as much. Edison proudly claimed he worked so intently on his inventions that he needed little sleep. His attitude about wasting time on sleep was clear in his words: "I have got so much to do and life is so short, I am going to hustle."

Edison was said to have only three months of schooling, but he was a great reader. His imagination, optimism and self-confidence enabled him to spend long hours inventing things that would make life better for all. His was the first voice to be recorded when he read the poem *Mary Had a Little Lamb* in 1878. It can be heard on Internet.

Thomas Edison and the Vagabonds

Between 1915 and 1924, Thomas Edison, Henry Ford (1863-1947--auto manufacturer), Harvey Firestone (1868-1938--tire manufacturer), and naturalist John Burroughs (1837-1921), calling themselves the Four Vagabonds, embarked on a series of summer camping trips. These geniuses set out to meet nature in magnificent cars, elaborate camps with large staffs, and invited famous guests to join them. These four men changed how we spend our lives now. They changed how we move about our habitat. They changed our livelihoods and everything that we do.

It all began when Ford, Edison and Firestone were in California for the Panama-Pacific Exposition of 1915. They decided to visit horticulturalist Luther Burbank (1849-1926) and then drove from Riverside to San Diego. They enjoyed it so much that they planned a trip the next year.

In 1916, Burroughs, Edison, Ford, and Firestone journeyed through the New England mountains. World War I soon changed everyone's preoccupation so trips were not made from 1917 to 1920. In the late fall of 1920, the four friends proceeded to Woodchuck Lodge. That was Burroughs' home in Roxbury, New York.

One of the vagabonds, Henry Ford, was a health guru in addition to creating and producing automobiles. He saw the possibilities of soybeans in food, milk, paint, plastics, and many other things before 1930. In his fast-growing automobile industry, the soybean played a big part in manufacturing commercial products. His friend, George Washington Carver (1864-1943) the black botanical chemist at Tuskegee Institute in Alabama, had researched the peanut and found three hundred commercial uses for it. Ford had his chef, Jan Willemse, research soy with Carver's scientists.

Willemse developed several soy recipes and one was dubbed Model T Crackers. This was Mr. Ford's favorite because the crackers were emblazoned with the design from the hubcap saying "Ford Made in U.S.A." Ford gave his chef an actual hubcap to use as the cookie cutter. This recipe was served on August 17, 1934, at the Ford Building of Chicago's Century of Progress Exposition. You can use your own cracker recipe but with soybean flour, margarine and milk or this old Civil War cracker recipe where I've inserted his ingredients. An excellent snack in late evening is a cracker like this with a bit of cheese. This recipe can be rolled out and cut up to look like Ford's hubcap.

Henry Ford Model-T Crackers

1 cup soybean flour
1 cup whole wheat flour
½ teaspoon salt
¾ cup sour cream

Preheat oven to 350 degrees. Mix flours and salt. Add enough sour cream to make a soft manageable dough. Roll it out. Cut it in squares. Bake a few minutes until brown. If desired, you can add a bit of dried rosemary and ½ cup of parmesan.

Edison, like Ford, was a driven man. He wanted to illuminate the night, and his discovery of the electric light bulb changed our circadian rhythm from the end of the 19th century forever. Circadian rhythms are the biological processes in all animals and plants driven by our 24-hour day/night cycle. Our world now operates 24 hours a day due to electricity and light. Edison was our first sleep thief! But we didn't blame him. We thanked him.

According to research, the usual amount of sleep per night has been declining among American adults over the last twenty years. The median sleep time for adults aged forty to seventy-nine years was eight hours per night in 1959. Adult median sleep time has decreased to seven hours per night, with more than one third of adults sleeping fewer than seven hours.

The Circadian Rhythm of Life on Other Planets

Much of our world of industry and communication functions on a 24-hour day so sleep patterns are affected. How did our body adapt to this change? We said, "Why should I do this?" Most people saw more possibilities in staying awake after dark. We just started changing our sleep-wake patterns, we got used to "jet lag" when flying west to east when one's body is out of phase and won't go to sleep at a new time. Most of us adapted within a few days to a time change when traveling, but some required more time.

The circadian rhythm of life on Earth evolved over some 4.6 billion years after planet Earth was created. This rhythm is connected with the Earth's rotation, the movement of the moon, and the seasonal variation, thanks to Earth's tilt. It regulates our body chemistry so we are alert during the day and asleep at night during a 24-hour cycle.

What would life be like somewhere else? As they said in the movie *Contact:* "Do you think there's life on other planets?" The answer was: "I don't know, but I guess I'd say that if it is just us— seems like an awful waste of space."

If we went to another planet in our solar system or a planet in a different solar system, their orbits would not match ours. If another planet's axis is tilted, it might have seasons but they would probably not correspond to ours in length. We would have adjustment problems on a planet where day plus night doesn't add up to 24 hours. However, our time frames are not in our bones. It is in our hormones and habits that can be adapted without much difference just as we finally adapt to jet lag.

What Is the Length of Night and Day on Other Planets?

The closest solar system to ours is the Alpha Centauri star group. There are three stars—Alpha A, Alpha B, and Proximus Centauri in that Alpha Centauri star group. The latter is a red dwarf star a little older (4.85 billion years) than our Sun 4.6 billion years. A planet slightly larger than Earth (1.3 times the size) is rotating around that star every 11 days. It is in the habitable zone with a daily temperature of 86 to 104 degrees if it has an atmosphere like we do, but if it doesn't, an estimated -22 to -40 degrees would be extremely cold. Half of the planet receives its somewhat dim full sunlight but the back of the planet may be very cold if it is locked into axial tilt and having no seasons.

A group of philanthropists and international scientists have formed a company called Breaththrough Starshot. They are planning to send a number of small rockets to this star system to beam back pictures of possible planets to see if there might be life forms on any of them. Famous English theoretical physicist, cosmologist, and author Steven Hawking has said "With light beams and light aircraft we can launch a mission to Alpha Centauri within a generation... We commit to this next great loop into the cosmos because we are human and our nature is to fly."

Some more possibly habitable planets are only 14 light years away. Some such planets were discovered on December 17, 2015. Their solar system has three planets orbiting around a red dwarf star called Wolf 1061. Wolf has 79% of the luminosity of our sun and is a darkish color of reddish-brown. One planet is 1.4 the mass of the Earth and it orbits Wolf every five days. The next one, 4.5 times larger than Earth rotates every 18 days. The largest, 5.5 times the size of the Earth, rotates every 67 days. The middle one may be rocky and may have water but only one side faces its sun so there will be extreme temperature changes from one side of the planet to the other. That would be like our moon where only one side is visible to us on Earth and the invisible back side is extremely cold.

Every few days, discoveries of more earthlike planets are emerging. Planets that resemble the earth kind of follow the Goldilocks theory. Some are too hot, some are too cold, and some are just right! If such planets were to be colonized, pioneers might want to transport plants and perhaps creatures to supply food if they can grow in the conditions on another planet. But those life forms would need to survive the long (several years or generations of humans) time necessary to reach the planet.

What Do Astronauts Eat and Drink?

In 2016, scientists predicted that the United States could develop the capability to land humans on Mars and return them to Earth some twenty to forty years from now at a cost of half a trillion dollars. However, the risks are that prolonged exposure of astronauts to the space environment has demonstrated debilitating effects caused by their microgravity environment. There is too little gravity for Earth people in space vehicles and on certain planets.

On Earth, the birds and bees pollinate our plants and the sea contains chemicals and a variety of life that nourishes our edible foods. Could we live on the plants and creatures of other planets? Would there be bacteria that could kill us?

What do we already know about food from years of astronaut travel into outer space?

Originally, astronauts ate toothpaste-type tubes of condensed meat, drank Tang, a fruit-flavored drink developed for space flight, and ate low residue food to reduce the chance of defecation in flight. Gradually, items such as shrimp cocktail, chicken and vegetables, toast squares, butterscotch pudding, and apple juice were added for American astronauts in space. Spoon bowls were added to allow more normal eating practices. Recently, Lobster Newburg was added along with ice cream. Then, perhaps responding to Paul Masson's motto "We will sell no wine before it's time," astronauts requested alcohol and Paul Masson Cream Sherry was permitted for one flight. However, the sherry triggered the gag reflex and it was abandoned.

Some Russian cosmonauts enjoyed "space vodka" and tubes of borscht, canned beef tongue, bread, and caviar. Recently, their diet included curds, nuts, mashed potatoes, jellied pike fish, perch, goulash with buckwheat, black currant juice, broccoli and cheese, peaches, and grape juice.

Rehydratable flavored Japanese ramen with pork, chicken, rice, sushi, and miso soup was offered Chinese and Japanese astronauts. Koreans partook of kimchi, a fermented cabbage dish. Italians enjoyed hot drinks such as tea, hot chocolate, broth and espresso. A Swedish astronaut wanted reindeer jerky but had to go with moose instead.

These days, astronauts have a greater variety of foods such as fruit salad, spaghetti, nuts, cookies, granola bars, etc. Carbonated drinks were tried in space but caused belching because of so little gravity producing "wet burps" or vomiting. Coffee, tortillas, and beef steak have been added as well as foods that have a longer "shelf life."

Barley harvested from crops grown for several generations in space has also been brought back to Earth to produce beer. While not a space food, the study did demonstrate that ingredients grown in space on very long flights are safe for production and consumption. Long flights to Mars might require growing food in the space vehicle to feed astronauts because it would be impossible to carry enough food for the lengthy trips.

Some Astronaut Food Induces Sleep

On November 6, 1979, NASA at the Johnson Space Center in Houston issued a public news bulletin: "New Food for Third Skylab Mission." It stated that a new high energy food bar was added to the menu for Skylab astronauts who spend as many as 85 days circling the Earth. The crew could eat these bars every third day along with the regular Skylab food such as sausage, pork, chicken, spaghetti, potatoes, grapefruit drink, and dried apricots. Each bar has about 300 calories. Here are examples of those bars that contain high tryptophan and fiber ingredients should you care to try them.

NASA Fruit/Veggie Space Food Sticks

1 cup peanut butter
½ cup honey
2 cups dry powdered milk
½ cup raisins
½ cup finely grated carrots
1 cup uncooked oatmeal
¼ cup wheat germ
¼ cup coconut (optional)
Little water

Mix all of the ingredients except coconut thoroughly. Shape into sticks the size of fingers. Roll in coconut if desired.

NASA Sunflower Seed Space Food Sticks

1 cup peanut butter
1 cup honey
2 cups milk powder
½ cup raisins
½ cup hulled sunflower seeds

Knead together and roll into small logs. Wrap in waxed paper for individual snacks.

More recently, NASA chefs and trainers recommended a breakfast that doesn't really require a recipe. It would be good as an evening snacks to help produce melatonin.

Astronaut Breakfast Cereal

Place 1 cup of your favorite crunchy cold cereal, 1/3 cup of powdered milk, and 1 teaspoon of sugar in a sealable plastic sandwich bag. When ready to eat, add ½ cup cold water and reseal the bag. Shake to dissolve milk and sugar. Open the bag and eat with a spoon.

How Do Astronauts Change Their Circadian Rhythm?

Since circadian rhythms on other planets would be quite different from ours; we have explored trying to adapt to the rhythm on another planet. A trip to Mars might present more problems because daylight is yellowish-brown and on earth it's blue green. Melatonin production is suppressed more by some wavelengths of light than others plus the Martian day is 24 hours and 29 minutes. That may not sound like much but researchers studying Mars have reported problems.

The Mars Explorer team that ran the Sojourner and Intrepid instruments on Mars had to adapt their lives to Mars' rotational cycle of more than 24 hours. Within days, many on the team started to complain about symptoms similar to jet lag. Yet they had to continue the longer day for the extent of the mission, which lasted many months.

Whole families were affected and those who had to interface with our 24-hour day suffered the most. The two periods that began in sync, slipped further and further out of phase until the crew who worked days found themselves on the night shift in about two weeks and then back again to days just two weeks later. Most people can adapt to a sudden change, as long as their circadian rhythm is not stressed for prolonged times.

Furthermore, NASA studied sleep loss and concluded in 2016 that more research is needed to evaluate whether observed sex differences in physiology lead to altered performance in spaceflight and on the ground. Of course, we could have told them that men and women are different and as the French say: "Viva la difference!"

Possible future trips to Mars have been studied in much depth recently. Mars doesn't have a major moon but it has two asteroids—Phobos and Demos—that can be seen daily. Sunlight is weaker on Mars than on Earth so agriculture would consist of shade-loving plants. Colder temperatures would require protective environmental suits when venturing outside of a man-made facility or space ship. Confinement in such facilities would be difficult emotionally. The longer days would take several generations for people to adapt.

What Happens to the Human Body in Space?

Humans have evolved in a certain gravity field on Earth. Our bodies react, according to studies of astronauts, by losing bone, muscle, and heart mass when there is no gravity. We would have to develop exercises to duplicate Earth's gravity or our bodies would deteriorate rapidly. Furthermore, astronauts sleep poorly in space. Up to 50% of the crew take sleeping pills and still average about two hours less sleep each night in space than they get on Earth. Why? Excitement and the circling of the Earth every night where the sun rises and sets for them every 1½ hours make it hard to sleep. It is never completely dark in their space capsule so melatonin is hard to produce by the brain.

Fatigue is a big problem because it affects performance, decreases concentration, increases irritability, and slows reaction time. Scientists must measure fatigue by having astronauts wear a wrist Actiwatch that tracks sleep patterns and light exposure. This helps researchers learn what affects sleep the most during space flights—light, temperature, noise, or other things.

NASA is interested in whether hypnotic drugs used thus far by astronauts are helpful or harmful. About three quarters of the International Space Station crews took sleeping pills and anti-anxiety medicine, as well as caffeine and a Dexedrine-like stimulant to stay alert. Because of FDA warnings about abnormal thinking and amnesia associated with these drugs, they want to know whether an astronaut's performance could be impaired if suddenly awakened in the middle of the night for some emergency.

There were also problems in space with wetting themselves. When my mother heard that people were going to the moon, she asked "How can they go to the bathroom in those space suits?" Here's the answer.

Astronauts wear maximum absorbency garments—nappies—while they sleep. There were problems with orthostatic hypotension (dizziness) and weakening of bones but they have turned to osteoporosis drugs and treadmill running. They also receive more radiation in space than on earth but try to limit those effects. Scientists concluded that sleep deficiency in astronauts was prevalent during space shuttle and Space Station missions as well as preflight training. Use of sleep-promoting drugs was pervasive because chronic sleep loss leads to performance decrements and the search continues for the development of effective countermeasures to promote sleep.

The latest health report in November, 2016, showed that among the twenty-four astronauts to the moon and the space station, seven have died and three of those died of cardiovascular disease. Those who studied the effects of spaceflight on the cardiovascular system for more than two decades wondered if radiation was impacting the cardiovascular system in astronauts as it impacted mice, who were tested in extra radiation. The deaths are much higher than that found in astronauts who did not go to the moon or the international space station.

Despite all these problems, NASA is preparing for a manned space flight to Mars. You might not want to go but many astronauts would.

Sleep Problems in Stressful Climates and Conditions

Scientists have also tested those who live in polar twilight in the two polar circles on Earth where they have no true daylight. In the Norwegian territory of Svalbard and in Dikson, Russia, there is only a faint glow of light visible at midday for more than a month. There is just enough night for normal outdoor activities and street lamps remain on for 24 hours. Some people suffer from a kind of depression that occurs because they have little light. Those who have that disorder must seek therapy with artificial light. They have the greatest depression during the season with the least light. A study of Norwegians and Russians in those areas have noted that those people have a sense of unreality that anything exists other than what little can be seen and done.

Little attention has been paid to sleep and fatigue differences in particular latitudes and longitudes. A study of people by states has demonstrated that there are sleep and fatigue differences across the United States. Scientists found that the people in Western states reported the fewest complaints and the Southern states reported the most sleep complaints.

A psychological movie entitled *Insomnia* was made in 1998 and set in Norway. It was remade in 2002 in Alaska with the same name and starred Al Pacino, Hilary Swank and Robin Williams. Pacino played a police investigator sent to Alaska with another policeman to investigate a murder. In this land with a midnight sun and no dark, there is nowhere to hide. There is only the constant "unblinking eye of God." Pacino's role features a weary older man who becomes increasingly rattled and guilt-ridden, fearing that he will be blamed for the accidental murder of his colleague. The movie presents the ravages of sleep deprivation on Pacino's character. Day and night, sunlight and cloudiness/darkness are clearly linked with our mental and physical health, a realization that has been clear to mankind for centuries.

Sleep Deprivation as a Torture Technique

Sleep deprivation (called "Operation Sandman" by the military psychiatrists who created it) is one of the torture techniques used on enemies, and was used on Guantanamo prisoners. It would proceed with 15 hours of interrogation, five hours of sleep in a cell, then transfer to a new cell every 30 minutes for the rest of the 24-hour period. A nickname for that procedure was "frequent flyer program" because of the frequent moves.

These sleep deprivation procedures make a person more suggestible, reduce psychological resistance, reduce the body's capacity to resist pain, impair memory and thinking processes, decrease short term memory, impair speech, yield false confessions, foster hallucinations and psychosis, lower immunity to disease, increase blood pressure and cardiovascular disease, stress, anxiety and depression. Sleep deprivation strategies were to keep subjects standing for up to 180 hours. Do people undergoing these strategies tell the truth or do they say anything to stop the torture and get some sleep?

For many of us, how we sleep is connected with the person or persons or animals we sleep with. This is an area that has not been examined in enough detail by sleep specialists. It is likely to become much more important for people who are undergoing treatment for sleep problems. They will have to work out changes in their routines and adaptations to new devices with sleep partners if their therapy is to be effective. Therefore, we will spend quite some time examining sleep mates.

Chapter Six
PEOPLE SLEEPING TOGETHER

How Men and Women Coupled in Days of Yore

In ancient times, men and women did not have bedrooms. They slept together anywhere they could for three million or more years. They moved from place to place in search of prey and plant food. Hunter gatherers had a rather egalitarian life style in bands of twenty to fifty people. They had few individual possessions, and depended upon each other for safety. They chose sleeping partners using various obvious methods. Some of those methods have been observed by anthropologists studying recently discovered primitive hunter-gatherer groups in Africa, Asia and South America during the last 125 years.

I have only rarely slept outside. Camping trips yield that experience where some nights go better than others because of climate and creatures. However, there is something awesome about camping out in a natural setting. We recreate the wonder, fears, pleasures, discomforts, and intimacies that early men and women endured for eons before us.

For some five million years since the time of primates, life and sleep has been spent in the natural environment. In Japan, an interesting research study used 420 people wandering through 35 forests to walk, bathe, sleep, and sit around together. The researchers found that the subjects had lower blood pressures, lower heart rates, and increased parasympathetic nervous system activation providing greater relaxation. The wood touches, wood smells, and bathing in natural water were found to be especially relaxing. We can draw our own conclusions about how we might relax ourselves outdoors. Luckily, we do not have to worry about most of the predators that challenged our ancestors.

Researchers have studied how hunter gatherers maintained their egalitarian ways. These people were observed to use consensual decision-making in their small groups. They also were seen to ridicule those who boasted or put on airs. They had very permissive child-rearing practices and playfulness was part of their daily life. In fact, adults could be silly together in delightful ways. Couples would develop years of memories and enjoyed sexual intercourse and pair-bonding.

Women chose men as mates when they offered better protection, displayed more survival skills, gathered more provisions and food, and participated in caring for children. Females offered those men a high degree of fidelity and sexual responsiveness, including orgasm.

It became traditional among people to mate with outsiders to presumably strengthen a tribe. Many of these unions occurred because of the need for peace with nearby tribes and they may have been on the order of arranged marriages. This undoubtedly reduced the incidence of incestuous genetic problems from inbreeding.

What Happened to Couples Ten Thousand Years Ago?

Things changed about ten thousand years ago with the advent of agriculture in many parts of the world. Groups no longer had to keep moving regularly since they could farm vegetables and fruits and domesticate certain animals. This led to the development of villages, mutual protection, and the building projects of kivas and temples. Coordinated control of natural resources developed so that people would not overuse what must be shared.

Land ownership brought inheritance of property. Some property was more valuable because of its natural resources. Chiefdoms gradually replaced elders. Some women were undoubtedly chosen by chiefs and the egalitarian earlier lifestyle may have been abandoned. Women were used in bartering for peace with nearby threatening groups. Exchange of goods, wars, games to the death, and other strategies promoted survival of tribes in villages. Some women became sexual slaves and their sleep quarters and patterns were changed abruptly in new areas where they were taken.

By historic times, marriages usually consisted of a man and woman and their children. Sometimes there were more wives. According to the American Standard Version of the Bible, 1929, Abraham had two wives and one concubine. Jacob had four wives. These husbands and wives produced the twelve patriarchs—the twelve tribes of Israel. Solomon had 700 wives and 300 concubines say some records. Apparently, they wanted to have many male heirs.

After the time of Jesus, Paul of Tarsus generated a number of Christian colonies whom he advised in epistles and letters to their leaders. When asked about sexual problems that arose in Christian sects, he wrote "It is good for a man *not* to touch a woman. Nevertheless, to avoid fornication, let every man have his own wife, and let every woman have her own husband."

Arranged marriages became more commonplace but marriage for romantic love existed on a small scale. As time passed, peace between groups was maintained through marriages to outsiders and trades of goods, animals, crops, dowries, and promises. Individual choices for a mate became rare. There is no doubt that sleeping with an enemy occurred and did not contribute to a good night's rest. Marrying for romantic love was usually suppressed in favor of arranged marriages which avoided short-lived infatuations.

Romantic Love and Sleep

Around 500 A.D., "courtly love" developed popularity. The Knights of King Arthur who held court in a place called Camelot in either

Wales or England captivated the imagination. Knights continued to venture about Europe to win the admiration of women as they slew bad people. These avengers pledged their troth to women and promised to lay down their lives for them.

Romantic love was prominent in Middle Ages literature. Alighieri Dante's famous book, *The Divine Comedy*, portrayed the love of his life, Beatrice, as a guide through Paradise. Written in 1300, Beatrice was based on a girl he met when he was nine years old. He fell for her but she married another as he later did. She died at 24 but he had encountered her at parties shortly before her death. His was a platonic affair based on his love for this young woman and it set heads spinning to see how much love of a girl could influence a man for the rest of his life.

One story of a knight was *Don Quixote de la Mancha*, the amusing tale by Miguel Cervantes. He, tongue-in-cheek, described knight-errant heroic deeds on behalf of the idyllic Dulcinea. Herein lies one of the problems of romantic love. He idolized his female, exaggerated the evils he had to overcome to obtain her love, and unlike his realistic riding companion, Sancho Panza, was never able to just fool around with his beloved. There was not a lot of time in bed with the opposite sex in many such chivalrous tales.

Who Could Afford a Bed?

From the 1600s, personal privacy grew as the upper classes separated from the lower classes. Private sleeping quarters developed and monarchs began to sleep on wooden frames with lattices of palm reeds and leather thongs in the center—the first beds. Decorated headboards and floor boards gradually developed. By the 1800s, these beds included brass and iron. Mattresses contained feathers, straw and cotton. Box springs did not appear until the 1900s. The Japanese slept on futons--supple pads of cotton, wool or softer materials that people rolled out at bed time.

By the Industrial Age around 1820, the United States was so prosperous that most people had homes and beds—in fact, a double bed. How a family slept had much to do with their wealth. Before that time, poverty kept most people together in one bedroom or in one large room in a small dwelling. The prosperous few had more rooms and more beds. The importance of beds cannot be exaggerated because they were where people slept, made love, recovered from illness, told stories, bore children, and died.

The Muslim religion permits as many as four wives at one time and husbands must pledge to support their wives and children in a reasonable style. Osama bin Laden's father had many wives according to Muslim traditions since he married and divorced keeping a current roster of only four at one time. Osama was one of 54 children. He had four wives, each usually living in different locations.

There is little talk of research in religion. It is a set of faiths made up by fallible humans. It becomes a way of life to believe without testing ideas given to congregations. For those scientifically minded, there is a constant fear—"You might be mistaken, you've been wrong before!" Which leaders of faith acknowledge that their beliefs might be incomplete or erroneous?

Scientists test ideas and let the chips fall where they may. As Benjamin Franklin said, "How many pretty systems do we build, which we soon find ourselves obliged to destroy?" Such untested ideas in religious believers have led to horrendous results such as in the following sect.

Mormons Sleeping Together

Some Americans were in favor of several wives. Joseph Smith, founder of the Mormon religion (Church of Latter Day Saints), said he received the beliefs of the church from the angel Moroni. Included in those beliefs was polygamy. He established the pattern of arranged marriages in which parents were offered special salvation and incentives to allow him to take their daughter as a wife. He was married to over 50 women, the youngest being 14 years old.

Brigham Young, who led the Mormons after Smith's death, had at least 55 marriages and the youngest was 14. He cited the rules of

Mormon life which said "The only men who become Gods, even the Sons of Gods, are those who enter into polygamy," according to the *Journal of Discourses,* 1877, VII.

Both men have been called pedophiles since they included young teenagers among their wives. Unlike the Muslim or Islamic religions which limited a man to four wives at a time, Mormon husbands could have as many wives as they liked. Smith had a large house with a separate living quarters for each wife—giving each a parlor, a bedroom, and a key for their door.

When Brigham Young died in 1877, Joseph Ferdinand Keppler painted a picture called: "In Memoriam Brigham Young." Below the title is this phrase: "And the place which knew him shall know him no more." The picture depicts thirteen weeping women in a large bed, with Young's boots at the foot of the bed and his hat and neck scarf at the head of the bed.

Mormon men usually did not sleep with more than one woman at a time, despite how this picture shows Young's bed with thirteen mourning women in it. Each wife usually had her own dwelling area to offer privacy and eliminate jealous feelings among each other.

One of Brigham's children recalled the immense meals at her father's table in Utah. He particularly loved codfish, doughnuts, wine, and hard cider. Here was his recipe for doughnuts and one might serve this as an evening sweet. This was passed down through Mary Van Cott, former wife of Brigham Young and relative of this book's proof-reader, Edgar Van Cott.

Brigham Young Doughnuts

2 cups buttermilk
1 cup sugar
2 eggs
1 teaspoons nutmeg
2 teaspoon baking soda
1 teaspoon baking powder
1 teaspoon salt

5 cups flour

¼ cup melted butter or shortening

Combine buttermilk, sugar, eggs, and blend well. Blend in sifted dry ingredients, then stir in melted butter. Roll or pat dough on floured board about 1/4" thick and cut with 2 ½ inch doughnut cutter. Fry in hot fat until golden brown on both sides. Drain and sprinkle with sugar, if desired. Makes 2 dozen doughnuts.

In 2011, Warren Jeffs was sentenced to life in prison for having sex with young children. He was the leader of the Fundamentalist Latter Day Saints (Morman religion) with 70 wives, the youngest being 12 years old. At his trial, tapes were played of his instructions to girls about how they were to dress and please their husbands, whose property they were.

Sleeping Together in Arranged Marriages

The benefits of arranged marriages are many. The United States culture tells us that "love conquers all," but being in love is not a good reason to get married. Marriage is about the long haul. Arranged marriage is based on the concept that love is a fleeting emotional response, and is hardly important enough to be the basis for a lifetime marriage. In an arranged marriage, you love your wife because she is your wife, and because she is the mother of your children.

The main benefits of the two types of marriage may be summarized. Benefits of an Arranged Marriage are (1) Reduction of incompatibilities (same religion, dietary preference, linguistic group, socioeconomic background, etc.) (2) Love can be just infatuation. (3) Lower divorce rates. (4) Lower expectations—neither spouse knows what to expect so they are pleasantly surprised by how good their marriage is. Benefits of Love Marriage are (1) Autonomy—it's your life, so you should choose who to spend it with. (2) Informed decision—you know your partner well so you know what to expect. (3) Love will conquer all. (4) Individual interest—you can choose a partner who is best for you—not what is best for the family.

Low divorce rates in countries with arranged marriages point to their success. High divorce rates in countries with marriages based on romantic love indicate that perhaps this form of marriage does not work as well. But in India, where arranged marriages are the "norm," love marriages are becoming increasing popular.

Mohandas Gandhi's Strange Sex Life

Mohandas K. Gandhi (1869-1948) was known in India as "Mahatma," which means "Great Soul." He wrote about his own marriage in *The Story of My Experiments with Truth/Part I/Playing the Husband.* Here are some words about his arranged marriage to Kasturbai.

> I must say I was passionately fond of her. Even at school I used to think of her, and the thought of nightfall and our subsequent meeting was ever haunting me. Separation was unbearable. I used to keep her awake till late in the night with my idle talk...I was very anxious to teach her [to read] but lustful love left me no time...My efforts to instruct Kasturbai in our youth were unsuccessful. And when I awoke from the sleep of lust, I had already launched forth into public life...Had my love for her been absolutely untainted with lust, she would be a learned lady today...

After Gandhi began public life and saw less of his wife, he vowed never to be sexually involved with other women. To accomplish this, he had the strange habit of asking young 17 or 18-year-old relatives to spend the night with him in his bed, massaging him and sleeping nude with him so that he would learn to resist temptation. This continued until the night he was assassinated while sleeping next to them.

Gandhi experimented with food also. He wrote *Diet and Diet Reform* published the year after his death in 1949. He concluded that the best food he could eat was a plantain with ground nuts upon it—a banana with peanut butter spread on it. This is an excellent sweet with protein for the last snack of the evening.

Tevye and Golde in *Fiddler on the Roof*

Perhaps these two types of marriages can be illustrated in songs. Tevye, a Russian Jew in the *Fiddler on the Roof*, the 1971 musical by Jerry Bock and Sheldon Harnick, sings this song to his wife Golde.

Tevye asks Golde "Do You Love Me?"

Golde: Do I love you? For twenty-five years, I've washed your clothes, cooked your meals, cleaned your house, given you children, milked your cow about twenty-five years. Why talk about love right now?...

Tevye: I know...but do you love me?

Golde: Do I love him? For twenty-five years I've lived with him, fought with him, starved with him. Twenty-five years my bed is his. If that's not love, what is.

Tevye: Then you love me?...

Golde: I suppose I do.

Both: It doesn't change a thing but even so, after twenty-five years it's nice to know.

Perle Mesta in *Call Me Madam*

Irving Berlin wrote a song about romantic love for the 1953 musical *Call Me Madam*. Madam, played by Ethel Merman, is a take-off on Perle Mesta, a real-life "hostess with the mostest". She financed the Democratic campaign during Truman's candidacy. In the musical, she was invited to become the ambassador to the tiny nation of Lichtenstein where she expected to do a financial deal benefitting America. A journalist played by Donald O'Connor accompanied her. He fell for a princess played by Vera Ellen so Merman and O'Connor sang "You're Not Sick, You're Just in Love."

> I keep tossing in my sleep at night
> And what's more I've lost my appetite
> Stars that used to twinkle in the skies
> Are twinkling in my eyes, I wonder why.
>
> You don't need analyzing
> It is not so surprising
> That you feel very strange but nice
> Your heart goes pitter patter
> I know just what's the matter
> Because I've been there once or twice.

Obviously, Irving Berlin understood a lot about romance. His first marriage ended after six months when his wife died of typhoid fever which she contracted on their honeymoon in Havana. It took him years to fall in love again. His second wife was a Catholic and he was a Russian Jew. Her father sent her to Europe hoping she would forget him, but Berlin was unforgettable. Romantic love prevailed over the parents' wish to choose whom their daughter married. Berlin introduced the first American music (ragtime) to the world and continued his musical career to the age of 100.

To write lyrics about physical symptoms of love, Berlin knew from experience that there are changes in the body when one is in love.

Sleep, Sex and Hormones

Primitive areas of the brain are involved in romantic love, say scientists. These areas light up on brain scans when we talk about a loved one. These areas can stay lit up for a long time for some couples.

As we fall in love, chemicals associated with the reward circuit flood our brain. They produce racing hearts, sweaty palms, flushed cheeks, and feelings of passion and anxiety. Cortisol, the stress hormone, increases to get our bodies ready to cope with a crisis. Low levels of serotonin send intrusive, maddeningly preoccupying thoughts, hopes, and terrors into our brains which resemble obsessive-compulsive behaviors. Your song might be "Can't Get You Out of My Mind."

Romantic love also releases high levels of dopamine, a chemical that gets the reward system going. Dopamine brings on feelings of euphoria like the use of cocaine or alcohol. Oxytocin and vasopressin, hormones that have roles in pregnancy, nursing, and mother-infant attachment, are present in romance. Released during sex and heightened by skin-to-skin contact, oxytocin deepens feelings of attachment and makes couples feel closer to one another after having sex. Oxytocin, the love hormone, creates feelings of contentment, calmness, and security, which are associated with mate bonding. Vasopressin accompanies behavior that produces long-term, monogamous relationships. Those two hormones may explain why passionate love fades as attachment grows.

We Americans like to mate with someone we love, not someone chosen for us. When we are feeling romantic, critical assessments of other people shut down. Love is blind, as they say. The roller coaster of emotions calms down within one or two years, say psychiatrists who have studied this. The passion is there but the stress is gone because cortisol and serotonin levels return to normal. Compassionate love grows out of passionate love.

Long-term marriages move from passionate infatuation to compassionate attachment. At that point, people make choices, usually at about four years into a marriage. For those who are hooked on the highs, the hormones that make us walk on air, may move on or look for something like that in another partner. The rest stay and enjoy the attachment, but often magnify excitement using their own inventive romantic notions.

Why would Americans feel the need to end a stable, but less exotic marriage for a passionate one? Is romantic love an addiction that needs to be addressed? If love is an addiction, this may account for why the most cited cause for divorce is infidelity. If a couple manage to stay together following infidelity, the relationship is certainly traumatized. Psychoanalyst and social philosopher Erich Fromm wrote *The Art of Loving* and described the confusion and failure when romance ceases to exist.

Fromm said that Americans spend more time trying to become acceptable rather than learning to love oneself and each other. He argued that we exert ourselves for business, career, power, and money. In fact, our lives may be hectic as we rush about to attain those things. Love is left as a passive, rather than an active, part of our lives. He emphasized that love requires us to care, respect, learn about and have concern for a loved one. Continued love takes discipline, concentration, patience, commitment, and will power. Marriage needs humor, stimulating lifestyle, and excitement. We no longer need extended family support systems. Finally, he thought we must see and accept our beloved as they are, rather than believe in a Hollywood romance based on fantasy.

One scientist, Helen Fisher who has studied the subject for years, gave romantic infatuation two years in her book. The joy of discovery is part of infatuation and passion. Insights propel you to the next stage where you love a mate more for who she or he really is. That becomes attachment. Things that destroy attachment are dissimilar interests and goals, sexual dysfunction, antipathy for each other's friends and family, fear of loss of personal freedom, inability to argue productively, and boredom or lack of novelty. You have to continually have adventures and do new things together. If you can keep introducing fresh experiences into the relations, you can lengthen the duration of romantic love or have a burst of that old feeling with the attachment stage.

One can try prolonging infatuation by making improvements in your physical appearance. By that we mean perhaps losing ten pounds, diminishing gray hair, dressing more attractively, and smelling clean and good. Getting back the euphoric feelings of romance with massages and sexual adventures can help a lot.

Sometimes, people fail to keep enough romance going and seek infatuation elsewhere. For those who strayed, there were dangers if they talked in their sleep. *If You Talk in Your Sleep Don't Mention My Name* was a cute little 1911 ditty by Nat Ayer and Seymour Brown sung by many, including Elvis Presley.

> Love is so much sweeter when it's borrowed
> I'll feel a little easier tomorrow
> Don't give our secret away, be careful what you say
> If you talk in your sleep don't mention my name
> If you walk in your sleep forget where you came.

Elvis had a recipe with sleep-inducing ingredients which we can all enjoy. It has been printed in many newspapers and nobody knows the exact amounts in the recipe. Elvis told a club owner what he wanted to eat so he could get some sleep before he performed one night.

Elvis Presley Peanut Butter and Banana Sandwich

Elvis didn't give the owner a recipe but these are the ingredients he requested. Banana, whole wheat bread, peanut butter and bacon-- are all good sources of tryptophan. If you go easy on the butter used to fry it, this sandwich will be healthier. Mix and mash the bananas and peanut butter if you wish.

There is another recipe that could possibly contribute to sleep even more—or so it would seem. Gertrude Stein was an American writer who went to Paris in the 1920s. She was famous less for her writings or phrases ("A rose is a rose is a rose" and "Sugar is not a vegetable") than for mentoring writers and artists in Paris.

A recipe from *The Alice B. Toklas Cook Book* of 1954 became rather famous. The book was written by Gertrude's lover, Alice Babette Toklas. This recipe was served to their friends including Ernest Hemingway, F. Scott Fitzgerald, Pablo Picasso, Thornton Wilder, Josephine Baker, Sherwood Anderson, and others. Those who have tried it say there is no particular effect from the hashish and it is very heavy on the stomach. The details of the recipe can be found in that book but here are the general features.

Alice B. Toklas Hashish Fudge

The ingredients include black peppercorns, nutmeg, cinnamon, coriander and they should be pulverized in a mortar. The next step is to chop dates, almonds and peanuts and add them. A bunch of *cannabis sativa* (hashish made from a hemp plant slightly more psychoactive than a marijuana plant) is then pulverized and kneaded together with the other ingredients. Sugar and butter are then mixed in. The stuff is rolled into a cake and cut in pieces or made into balls about the size of a walnut. It should be eaten with care. The recipe did not call for baking it. The recipe was given to Toklas and Stein by their itinerant friend, Brion Gysin. He was shocked to find it in their book as he gave it to them in jest.

In those early days, there was marijuana use in America as well as France and many other countries. In fact, when singing actress Judy Garland was thirteen, she joined her two older sisters, when they sang *La Cucaracha* as the Gumm Sisters in 1936. They were in a 19-minute comedy called *La Fiesta de Santa Fe*. They sang the words in Spanish, never realizing what they were really saying:

La cucaracha, la cucaracha, ya no puede caminar
Porque no tiene, porque le falta, marijuana que fumar.

The cockroach, the cockroach, can't walk anymore,
Because it doesn't have, because it's lacking marijuana
to smoke.

The song came from the Mexican Revolution around 1910 to 1920 when Pancho Villa got his men (smoking cockroaches—the name given to a cigarette held in a paper clip to smoke more of it) to march and fight for him by supplying them with marijuana. Isn't it curious that Judy Garland died of a drug overdose years later?

The song was nominated for the Academy Award. Perhaps some people knew what it was really about including Gilbert Roland and Leo Carillo who were in the movie. Other stars in that little production were Warner Baxter, Ida Lupino, Robert Taylor, Harpo Marx, Andy Devine, and Gary Cooper.

Sleeping Together in Literature and Movies

In the 1930s, people were traveling about by foot, car, bus, train and ship. Writers were beginning to cover events in other countries along with reporters. Movies were showing more foreigners (Greta Garbo, Theda Bara, Hedy Lamarr, and Marlene Dietrich) and villains were often from other countries. Imbibing alcohol appeared cosmopolitan. One famous detective couple drank their way through many mystery movies. They were Nick and Nora Charles in the *Thin Man* movies. In *The Thin Man* by Dashiell Hammett on page 599 (*Dashiell Hammett Five Complete Novels,*) Nora told Nick she was unable to sleep despite reading a dull book and smoking a cigarette. This was the dialogue in the book:

"Don't you think maybe a drink would help you to sleep?"
"No thanks."

"Maybe it would if I took one."

Nora sighed. "I wish you were sober enough to talk to." She leaned over to take of sip of my drink.

Staying asleep can be a problem when drinking alcohol because when that sugar travels through the blood stream, it may waken people with a glucose hit in the wee hours of the night. What happens is called a "GABA-glutamine neurotransmitter rebound". Advice is being given to people to keep an evening drink small and have it early—a night cap. When we fall asleep after drinking alcohol, slow waves increase and we sleep well until midnight. Then we go into a lighter sleep as an excitatory neurotransmitter (glutamate) fills our blood vessels.

Virginia Woolf wrote: "One cannot think well, love well, sleep well, if one has not dined well." Dashiell Hammett lived with writer Lillian Hellman and they both drank a great deal and dined well. Her last book was *Eating Together: Recollections and Recipes.* This recipe following an evening meal could add the sweets necessary to help tryptophan in a meaty meal enter the brain and turn on the sleep hormone. One wine glass of this dessert before bedtime won't keep you awake in the middle of the night.

Lillian Hellmann Strawberries with Grand Marnier

This really wasn't a recipe because Lillian just mixed sliced strawberries with some Grand Marnier about an hour before serving them in wine glasses.

The *Thin Man* movies with William Powell and Myrna Loy and their dog, Asta, were quite a hit. The movie series always had a sophisticated mystery with comic touches. It was not a film noir movie.

The Big Sleep is a 1946 film noir movie taken from Raymond Chandler's 1939 novel of the same name. Film noir "dark" movies used low level lighting and were dreamlike and sometimes brutal.

Humphrey Bogart played private detective Philip Marlowe in *The Big Sleep*. Lauren Bacall co-starred in this hard-boiled story about a criminal investigation. Death was called "the big sleep" by gangsters of that era. Bogart and Bacall became very mushy in that movie. They had just married and seemed to be having a lot of fun.

Bedroom Eyes

Sometimes movie stars in film noir movies had bedroom eyes. Certainly, Lauren Bacall swept Bogart (and her movie audiences) off his feet with her sultry eyes and sexual seductiveness. These are eyes that look half-closed, in a sweet drowsy state, or in a sidelong glance.

Such male actors were Charles Boyer, Paul Newman, Brad Pitt and Jack Nicholson. Actresses with "bedroom eyes" might include Lauren Bacall, Greta Garbo, and Marlene Dietrich. There is something that draws us to people with "bedroom eyes. It appears to indicate a desire to lie down and do things done in bed. Is sleepiness seductive?

Humphrey was a fount of wisdom for his young wife and could create a healthy dish or two. He could also put her to sleep with his dessert which you can reproduce easily.

Humphrey Bogart Coconut Spanish Cream

You can duplicate his dessert by making a nice vanilla pudding, and then add a cup of shredded coconut and orange extract to the pudding. When set, serve it with orange sections.

Did Humphrey ever tell his wife the line he told Ingrid Bergman so many times in *Casablanca?* "Here's looking at you, kid!" Humphrey Bogart was in another film noir movie by Dashiell Hammett called *The Maltese Falcon*. This 1941 film included lines about the significance of the falcon statuette. Bogart said it contained "the stuff that dreams are made of." That line comes from Shakespeare's *The Tempest*, Act

4, Scene 1, where Prospero said "We are such stuff as dreams are made on: and our little life is rounded (finished) with a sleep."

Humphrey Bogart understood something about touch. He realized by his own life and observing others that people who are anxious try to calm themselves using touch. In movie after movie he touched his face, or his nose, or fingered a wine glass or a cigarette or his neck in movements that promoted self-relaxation. The movie where this was most notable was *The Caine Mutiny* made in 1954 where he played Captain Queeg. In one scene as he underwent interrogation, he fingered some Baoding iron balls in his hand, a Chinese stress reducer. The scene proved his undoing and he was relieved of command. These Baoding balls have even been used for eons to help people become sleepy.

Sleep and dreams don't come easy to some lovers. William James, who was an assistant professor of the new science of psychology at Harvard in 1876, was in love. He lay awake thinking about his future wife, Alice Gibbens. After seven weeks of insomnia, he decided to propose to her. Later, he suffered from insomnia again when his ground-breaking book about the *Principles of Psychology* met with instant success. His insomnia was so bad that he used chloroform to fall asleep.

One movie lothario was John Wayne. Despite three Mexican wives, he was said to have "slept" around quite a bit with lovers such as Marlene Dietrich and Maureen O'Hara.

German actress Marlene wrote *ABC: Wit, Wisdom & Recipes* in 1984. The book is in alphabetic order. Next to "Sleeping Potion" she advised the reader to stop by a delicatessen and get a sardine-onion sandwich on rye. That is certainly a questionable sleep remedy.

Sleeping Apart

Many men and women sleep together throughout most of their entire marriages. How do they sleep? Forty percent of spouses sleep on their side with the knees slightly bent upward toward the chest. This permits a couple to cuddle together as they fall asleep. Sleeping on the back or the stomach may be preferred by a person but does not lend itself to as much physical closeness to their mate.

Sleeping next to each other was celebrated in the 1908 song "Cuddle Up a Little Closer, Lovey Mine, Cuddle Up and Be My Little Clinging Vine". Composers Karl Hoschna and Otto Harbach must have had good marriages.

Some couples have trouble sleeping together. Circumstances involving health, schedule differences, and sleeping problems may interrupt sleeping together. News stories have come out about Queen Elizabeth II and her husband Prince Philip of Wales. They are said to have slept together until at least 2007. It was later reported that they had moved to separate bedrooms. The Queen's cousin, Lady Pamela Hicks, explained the sleeping by saying they had the choice to avoid the flying leg syndrome.

We do not know whether the Queen or Prince Philip snore. Of course, the cure for snoring is to never sleep, but that won't do! Unfortunately, the snorer usually goes to bed first. "Laugh and the world laughs with you. Snore and you sleep alone." For those who choose not to sleep separately like this royal couple, inserting ear plugs or white noise might help obscure snoring noises. Let us hope that the snorer has been evaluated to be sure there is no sleep apnea or other problem requiring treatment.

Queen Elizabeth enjoyed a version of scones which is like American pancakes. She ordered them when President Dwight Eisenhower visited Balmoral Castle in 1959. The chef sent Eisenhower this recipe which was finally made available to the public on the *National Archives* on June 10, 2011. This is a nice final evening treat to send one off to dreamland.

Queen Elizabeth Drop Scones

3 cups all-purpose flour
2 teaspoons baking soda
3 teaspoons cream of tartar

(If you have no tartar, use 5 teaspoons of baking powder and skip the soda)
¼ teaspoon salt
2 eggs
¼ cup sugar plus 1 teaspoon more
1 ½ cup whole milk
2 tablespoons butter, melted

Whisk together the flour, baking soda, cream of tartar and salt in a bowl. In a separate bowl, whisk together the eggs and sugar. Then whisk in most of the milk. Make a well in the middle of the flour and pour in the milk-egg mixture. Whisk until smooth, adding more milk until you get the right consistency—thin enough to spread on the pan but not so thin as to run. Fold in the melted butter.

Heat a griddle or frying pan to medium low. Coat the pan with a little butter, spreading it with a folded paper tower. Drop large spoonfuls of batter on the griddle to form pancakes. When bubbles start to appear on the surface (2-3 minutes), use a spatula to flip the pancakes over. Cook another minute until lightly browned. Remove to a plate and cover with a clean tea towel to keep warm while you cook the rest of the drop scones. Serve with butter, jam, or syrup. Makes about 16 American-sized pancakes.

A 2005 survey found that one in four couples sleep in separate beds in America. What? Why? A 2006 study at the University of Vienna in Austria showed that sharing a bed with a partner reduces brain power in men because they performed cognitive tests worse than when they slept alone. Is this why coaches tell athletes not to have sex the night before big games? Did Viennese women share beds with men to help smarten them up? No, people say they like the feeling of having their partner next to them when they are asleep. But you have to be awake to feel that.

To lie in bed and touch your partner at night is something you don't ever do with anyone else. It is not always a pleasant experience to share a bed with someone, but it is rather unique and shows the married condition. Disconnection decreases intimacy. Sleeping alone means physical distance, which can lead to emotional distance.

Some long-married couples are embracing the realities of aging with two master bedrooms. Snoring, medical issues, conflicting schedules and other obstacles to a good night's sleep have caused more dual-bedrooms to be built. Design Basics of Omaha offers several floor plans with dual master bedroom suites for couples.

The National Association of Home Builders predicted in 2007 that 60 percent of custom homes would offer dual bedrooms by 2015. That has not proved to be true, but there is much more interest in plans with dual master suites in recent years. People are living longer, which means they're married longer, and it may get harder to sleep as we age.

Sometimes a separate space makes it too easy to avoid relationship troubles. One way to manage the anger in a long-term commitment is two master suites. That doesn't resolve the problem but it lowers the heat, which may allow the couple to find workable strategies for healing rifts.

Interviews of couples have revealed that some who slept in two bedrooms to avoid duels were well-rested and happier at the breakfast table. Some couples do this experimentally at first but discover that they don't like sleeping apart much. They miss the warmth of having someone next to them. Some even confessed they were only alive because their spouse was sleeping next to them when they experienced a heart attack or went into a diabetic coma.

Psychologists and psychiatrists warn people to reconsider sleeping separately. They say one of the greatest gifts you can give to a loved one is to be close and loving with each other. Independence is not a bad thing, but it isn't really what being in a relationship is about. If you want to have a closer relationship, sleep closer to your mate.

Marriage and family therapists surmise that when at least one of the parties is pulling away from the other, they'll spend less and less time together, sex will come to a halt and one member of the relationship will feel ignored. The marriage suffers as a result.

Those therapists recommend that couples make cuddling and sex a top priority. Be willing to compromise. Make the bed neat, tidy and attractive. Remove clutter from the bedroom. Create an emotional oasis. Keep Fido on the floor. You're in bed to snuggle with your honey, not your schnauzer. Minimize technology. Be sensitive to a loved one's desire to talk or cuddle. A note for men: Women may love having their backs rubbed firmly, but gently.

Some of the biggest news about President Donald Trump in 2017 was that he and his wife, Slovenian model Melania, do not sleep together. The differences in age, responsibilities, locations, and preferences may play a part. Perhaps more information will surface regarding their relationship as time goes by.

Sleep Positions

The Better Sleep Council prepared a flyer on healthy sleep positions. The Healthy Living Section of www.medicaldaily.com invited an orthopedist, psychologist, and an internist to evaluate those sleep positions. There are basically three positions—side, back and stomach. In a survey of the most used positions, 41% slept in a fetal position with knees slightly bent slightly upwards toward the chest. For those with a bad back, they may place a pillow between the legs to alleviate pressure on the hips and lower back. This position is the easiest for cuddling with your bed mate as the two of you are shaped in a sort of curved arrangement next to each other.

Some 7% sleep on their stomach with the head turned to one side. This position is the least healthy and should be done without a pillow so the neck is not in an awkward position. This position is associated with considerable tossing and turning. While it should be avoided for those with neck or back pain, it may be beneficial for snorers as it helps keep the upper airways open.

About 15% of people sleep on their side with arms and legs in a straight line like a log. Pregnant women should sleep on their left side for optimal blood flow and to reduce acid reflux. However, it can strain the liver, lungs, and stomach. Sleeping on the right side can worsen heartburn. About 13% sleep on their side with legs straight but arms out in front of the body.

Sleeping on the back is done by 5% of the population but some sleep specialists consider it the best. It is certainly the best for infants to avoid sudden death syndrome. In adults, it may create lower back pain and even episodes of sleep apnea. A soft pillow or rolled up towel under the knees facilitates the natural curve of the spine. It prevents facial wrinkles and skin breakouts, and is best done with the head of the bed elevated slightly. This will allow digested food substances to move downward and therefore prevents acid reflux. Some who sleep on their back have their hands and arms up near the pillow and some do not, but those with arms up add pressure to the shoulder nerves which leads to pain.

Those who teach about relationship lifestyle describe some sleep solutions. If your partner kicks in his sleep and wakes you up, buy a larger mattress such as a queen-size. If your partner likes it hot and you like it cool, set the temperature at 60-65 degrees Fahrenheit and invest in a dual-control electric blanket for a warmer blanket half.

If your partner snores keeping you awake, use earplugs or buy anti-snore pillows. It is possible that sprays or nasal strips could help a snorer breath more easily. If your partner tosses and turns, check the mattress for comfort and support. If your partner loves to cuddle but you like space to sleep, compromise and spend some time snuggling and then agree to sleep slightly apart.

If your sleep schedules don't match, find a bedtime that works for both of you and use a personal book light until you're sleepy rather than keeping overhead lights on. If your bedroom feels more like an office than a place to sleep, keep work laptops, PDAs and television out of the bedroom. Use the bedroom only for sleep and sex.

There is more to be said about temperature. Men are usually larger and warmer than women. In fact, many women like to snuggle closer to a man for the warmth of his body whereas men may need to sleep farther from a woman to stay cooler. Sometimes one party will use extra blankets or switch on their half of an electric blanket. This may impact their partner who prefers less heat. A dear petite friend of mine said her marriage (to a larger man) has lasted 60 years thanks to dual control electric blankets. The important thing is to talk about temperature preferences and come up with a plan that works for both sleep mates.

Sleeping Nude Together

How did we all start sleeping together back in days of yore? Nobody had pajamas. Nobody had beds. People started messing around with each other and just threw animal skins over themselves to keep warm.

People who create nightwear would love for you to buy something to cover yourself in bed but what are the results? Do you want to snuggle up to somebody who wears pajamas? Do you want to fondle somebody in a nightgown? Take it off. Take it all off if you want be close to your mate, say family and marriage counselors. Ask any woman who wears a bra what she thinks when she rips it off at night. She'll probably say—"Free at last, free at last!"

The Cotton USA experts quizzed 1004 Britons about their sleep habits and whether or not they felt happy in their relationships. Some 57% of nude couples claimed to be happy compared with 48% in pajamas, and others who wore something in bed. They suggested that nudity encouraged openness and intimacy, and therefore led to greater happiness.

Five things learned from couples sleeping naked included the following:

(1) Sleeping less than one inch apart. Those who touched each other were happier than those who had no contact.

(2) Having no children. Childless men and women out of 5,000 in Great Britain were more satisfied and felt more valued by their partner.

(3) Egalitarian relations brought more stability and sexual satisfaction than authoritarian control with one person on top and the other below.

(4) Gratitude, thank you's, and compliments preserved bonds.

(5) Honest arguments without insults brought more closeness.

A final note from those Cotton experts was: "Ageism be damned. It's the over-55 crowd who are most likely to sleep naked. It shows: I want to be close to you!"

Bedding Materials Affect Sleep Quality

The garments worn, if any, for sleeping and the bedding materials can affect the quality of your sleep. Korean females were studied sleeping three consecutive nights on five different sets of clothing and bedding. They were measured from softest/ to hardest/ roughest. One-fifth of the sample reported that they slept better in softer T-shirts and pants and on softer bedding on mattress cover, pillowcase and covering blanket. Some subjects called the texture they liked fluffy, cozy, cuddly, smooth, warm, relaxing, and comforting. The other fabrics were called scratchy, rough, itchy, coarse, bumpy, or cold. There was less body movement during the sleeping periods with the softer textures. Overnight secretions of adrenaline and noradrenaline in their urine were significantly less with the soft type than the hard type.

Researchers concluded that softer texture materials might be more comfortable due to less tactile stimulation of the skin. Apparently, soft textures result in neurophysiological relaxation which provides better sleep quality. One study showed that people's perception of what is soft or hard is influenced by how moist their fingertips were. This would make some difference for towels when getting out of the shower or bath.

Studies with similar results were done in an 1895 article in the *American Journal of Psychiatry* and a 1937 study suggested that people find smooth and soft fabrics "relaxing." Recent studies have found that many people mentioned wool when they were described fabrics that were itchy or cold. The favored beddings over time have been silk, satin, fleece and cotton. Cotton absorbs body moisture but silk does not. Fleece from the llama is often considered the choice for a wheelchair as tender skin of an impaired person needs protection.

The Cotton USA company was proud to claim that cotton conveyed a sense of cleanliness to relationships. But companies who make satin sheets and pillowcases swear by their more expensive, cooler, and slicker products. Beware that you don't slide right off the bed on a satin sheet during sex play but to preserve a hairdo, ladies might prefer a satin pillow case.

Flower Aromas Affect Sleep Length and Quality

Today, aromatherapy is being considered as an alternative medical approach to sleep and other problems. In principle, the sense of smell plays an important role in overall health as well as physical and mental relaxation as the brain responds emotionally to aroma. Studies have shown some actual physical changes in sleep by flower aromas inhaled in the bedroom.

While little research has been done on physical changes due to aromas, some small sample studies show the following results:

Jasmine reduces anxiety levels. Lavender helps women and babies go to sleep quicker and sleep deeper. Gardenias relieve anxiety and promote sleep. Damask Roses or rose oil calm and relax people, are antibacterial, antispasmodic (like Chamomile), and may benefit people with dementia because of their central nervous system effect. Their petals are used in many Middle East dishes and desserts. Valerian will help you fall asleep and have a better quality of sleep. Lemon will not help you sleep and will perhaps keep you awake. Lavender oil used to bathe babies relaxes the baby and the mother who is applying the oil at bedtime. It also relaxes both parties and reduces crying in a baby when the mother and child look at each other smiling while the bathing and rubbing is done.

The names of such studies are interesting. "The Sleep Enhancing Effect of Valerian Inhalation and Sleep Shortening Effects of Lemon Inhaled." "Lavender Bath Oil Reduces Stress and Crying and Enhances Sleep in Very Young Infants." "Wheeling Jesuit University Professor and Students Find Jasmine Odor Leads to More Restful Sleep, Decreased Anxiety and Greater Mental Performance." "Rosa Damascena as Holy Ancient Herb with Novel Applications."

Many of these aromatic flowers have been used by putting four drops of their oil on a cotton ball, inhaling it about 10 sniffs, and setting it next to the sleeper on a side table (hopefully within 1 ½ feet). Some people like to rub a drop of lavender or rose or other oils on the forehead before reclining.

The Damask Rose from Damascus, Syria, is popular in the Middle East and Europe. It can be bought in the U.S. and blooms mainly in July and August. It has nicknames such as Rose of the Prophet Muhammad, and the Rose of Castile (in Spain). Some people like to put rose petals on their bed for sleeping. Rose petals, usually dried, can be made into a tea but lose some of their hypnotic effect in the boiling. The petals are also eaten in ice cream or yogurt or other foods such as marzipan or chicken with roses.

Flowers are less powerful than their oil but have some relaxing aromatic effects on the sleepers in the room. It should be noted, however, that unfortunately it is very hard to keep gardenias by the bedside because they need much sunlight during the day. They might be cut and brought into the bedroom at night from some other place where they are growing.

The field of aromatherapy may have more to offer later in medical practice, pleasurable uses, and aesthetic decorations. A common Valentine gift is roses. Restaurants sometimes offer a rose for females upon arrival. But their use and other flowers for sleeping still requires more study to determine whether they can replace other things now used.

Teas with hypnotic properties are quite commonly recommended for sleep. Studies of flowers for those results often take place with human subjects but emotions can play some part in reactions. Some flower studies for sleep involve animals like rats. They may not care whether something looks pretty but will fall asleep for periods of time if the right flower is inhaled. Scientists will count how quickly they fall asleep, how long they sleep, body movements, and wakefulness. But this is an area we can all study for ourselves.

Sleep Needs May Differ

Of course, those who study sleep recommend using earplugs for snoring, headphones for the partner not yet ready for bed, keeping handy medicines like decongestants to reduce snoring, finding a better pillow or mattress, getting a mattress pad for your side of the bed to dampen any movements of your partner, making a plan for who will sleep while the other tends to a child who wakes you at night, using eye covers for total darkness, using a soothing lavender scent on covers, and restricting fluids to reduce bathroom trips.

The main thing is to communicate about sleep problems and make a plan concentrating on teamwork and compromise. Changes don't occur overnight. There will be some trial and error to see what works. And it goes without saying, brush your teeth just before bedtime no matter what.

A chief problem in sleeping together is different preferences for the time to go to bed. Researchers were looking closely at morning people and night people, often referred to as "larks" or "owls." That terminology was used by Sir William Osler, the physician who set his sights on better development of medical students. He wrote about those students thusly:

There are also the two great types, the student-lark who loves to see the sun rise, who comes to breakfast with a cheerful morning face, never so "fit" as at 6 a.m. We all know the type. What a contrast to the student-owl with his saturnine (gloomy) morning face, thoroughly unhappy, cheated by the wretched breakfast bell of the two best hours of the day for sleep.

However, the good news is that you and I can adjust our internal clocks. Camping out can help us reset our natural sleep time to be more in harmony with nature.

Heather Gunn is a sleep researcher at the University of Pittsburgh. She's learned that couples don't need to sleep at the same time to have a healthy relationship. She advised couples who sleep at different times to make sure they find other times to connect such as the morning or evening or weekend. She believed, however, that most people feel the need for closeness and security whether they go to bed at the same time or not.

Why do couples sleep together? The perception is you're having sex and people are afraid to admit to sleeping apart. Studies have shown that they sleep more soundly when they sleep alone, but the findings show that despite that fact they prefer to sleep with their partner. We sleep together because we are affectionate beings. We need camaraderie and intimacy and whispering. It's enjoyable to talk about the day laying side by side. We cuddle, we laugh. At the end of each day we remove our public face and lie next to our best friends to know we're not in it alone.

Medical Discoveries about Sex and Sleep

Divorced people have more sleep problems than married or single people according to studies. Studies of marital quality and the marital bed noted that a bed partner is an important source of data in the sleep evaluation of their mate. Sleep problems and medical illness occur together which affects exercise, and adherence to medical treatment. Most couples engage in health behavior together.

Life events and sleep disturbances can cause declines in marital quality. Sleep deprivation affects mood regulation, frustration tolerance, and cognitive functioning, which lead to more negative marital interactions. In many cases, improving a snoring problem has a positive impact on a couple's happiness within the marriage.

Women in studies reported that they prefer co-sleeping because they feel more "secure" with a partner, whereas men preferred co-sleeping out of habit. Sleep occurs most often when one feels secure enough to lower vigilance and alertness. Going to bed with a trusted and secure partner provided a couple with a chance to unwind and decrease the stresses of the day before falling asleep. A supportive confidante reduces the intrusive thoughts that disturb sleep.

Although light is the most important disrupter of sleep-wake cycles, meal time, pre-bedtime routines, exercise, and conflict affect couples and their sleep greatly. Hostile behavior during couple discussions raise blood pressure and stress hormones. Such behavior increases vigilance and avoidance. Not only that, hostile behavior and disrupted sleep also increased physical inflammation and led to bacterial and viral infections because of reduced resistance.

Researchers also found that the oxytocin hormone may link social relationships to health and sleep. It has widespread central nervous system effects and is present in both males and females. It is most associated with maternal contractions during childbirth and lactation. But it plays a role in pair-bonding and sexual behavior. Oxytocin has recently been found to relax cardiovascular stress responses in both rats and humans. This suggests that emotional closeness and physical intimacy during the daytime and prior to bedtime may promote sleep.

Researchers did not ignore financial resources, noise and overcrowding, difficult work conditions, parenthood, shift work, and illness. However, they pointed out that a supportive spouse could be a "powerful stress buffer" leading to less sleep disturbance. In contrast, unhealthy relationships may lead to greater sleep disturbances by increasing vigilance, increasing risk for physical and psychiatric disorders, and creating unhealthy sleep-related behaviors and sleep disorders.

Researchers Must Study Sleep Partners
to Understand Sleep Problems

Studying sleep as a dyadic, rather than an individual phenomenon, is clearly in its infancy. Recognizing the social context of sleep and incorporating such knowledge into both clinical practice and research in sleep medicine may elucidate key mechanisms in the etiology and maintenance of both sleep disorders and relationship problems and may ultimately inform novel treatments.

Julia Roberts from Texas starred in many movies, one of the most important of which was *Sleeping with the Enemy*. This psychological thriller featured her unable to sleep with a husband who had anger management problems to say the least. She certainly would not have said: "Keep your friends close and your enemies closer." One evening she stole away and found a new life until her husband caught up with her. This movie explored the dangers of sleeping with someone who cannot be trusted because she feared he would take her life. Trust takes considerable time to develop. Only slowly does a woman, who is physically less powerful than a man, feel able to totally relax and be herself in bed with a man.

Sleep deprivation increases negative emotions and decreases friendliness, elation, positive mood, and empathy. Sleep-deprived individuals tend to blame others when frustrated, which leads to marital dissolution. Considering sleep and relationships as a mutually interacting system may not only provide a more ecologically valid model but may also help to uncover the role of relationships with effects on health and function both day and night.

Psychiatric disorders are associated with sleep disturbances and one of those is Alzheimer's Disease. Alzheimer plaques disrupt sleep and, conversely, a lack of sleep promotes Alzheimer plaques. In one study, patients whose sleep efficiency was below 75% were five times more likely to have pre-clinical Alzheimer disease than good sleepers. It appeared that amyloid deposits in the brain from Alzheimer disease caused people to have worse quality sleeping but there was no change in the amount of sleeping time. Most of the Alzheimer patients tested for two weeks tended to nap three or more days per week.

Now here's a subject that might interest us! Does sleep have an impact on female sexual response behavior? One study found that more sleep was related to greater next day sexual desire. A 1-hour increase in sleep length corresponded to a 14% increase in the odds of engaging in partnered sexual activity. Scientists concluded that obtaining sufficient sleep was important to the promotion of healthy sexual desire and response, as well as the likelihood of engaging in partnered sexual activity. So a good night's sleep results in a female being much more interested in sexual activity the following day or evening.

Sleep problems might better be treated at a couple-level phenomenon than an individual one. Middle-aged couples were sampled during the annual medical exams in one study. Husbands' anxiety and depression had a stronger effect on wives than the other way around. If a husband has anxiety or depression, a shorter sleep duration is predicted for his wife.

The medical articles about sleep and dyadic relationships in this chapter illustrate that evaluating sleep problems requires taking a full history from the couple who live together. The problems and the solutions will involve both members of the couple. This will require longer evaluations and more costly testing, but may result in better understanding of problems and better treatment compliance.

What if there are sleep problems at the top of our society—at the presidential level? What are we to do if our leaders are impaired and sleep-deprived when making decisions regarding world matters? How have world leaders been handling sleep problems as they fly internationally across many time zones to negotiate peace and war?

Chapter Seven
SLEEP AND WORLD LEADERS. ARE WE SAFE?

After World War II, travel got a lot faster. No longer were horses, coaches, cars, and buses taking people about the country. Railroad trains provided a faster trip at fairly low costs. Rail revolutionized travel and daily life. Each community in the United States defined its own time by the location of the sun at noon. That caused lots of problems because train travelers had to keep re-adjusting their watches in every city according to the local time. So the railroad companies adopted time zones.

The United States have four time zones—Pacific, Mountain, Central, and Eastern—plus several more for Alaska, the Aleuts, Hawaii and Canadian provinces. These zones began operation at noon on November 18, 1883. Other countries have their own time zones.

In the beginning, train travel was extremely uncomfortable and one could get little sleep on the benches people had to share. There was usually no food available. Trains did not have sleeping areas. That is why Fred Harvey finally established a chain of railroad hotels and restaurants on railroad lines. Gradually, trains began to serve meals and arrange tables for people to play cards, or relax, and enjoy a variety of beverages from a bar.

As a child, I used to love to travel by train. The motion and vibrations were hypnotic, so I often fell asleep even when I was enjoying the countryside from the window. The long trips to see relatives made me look forward to things yet to come. Travel was so slow by train, that I never had to accommodate myself to time changes. Travel by ship was the same way, pleasant conversations with people from all over the world, interesting activities, and no time pressure to adapt quickly. That all changed when I began to fly to and from exciting places in my teen age years.

The Horrors of Early Train Travel in America

Englishman Robert Louis Stevenson wrote about his train trip in the United States when he came to visit the woman he would later marry. The year was 1879 and he wrote of the trip from Council Bluffs, Iowa, heading for California.

> I suppose the reader has some notion of an American railroad-car, that long, narrow wooden box, like a flat-roofed Noah's ark, with a stove and a convenience... The benches are too short for anything but a young child. Where there is scarce elbow-room for two to sit, there will not be space enough for one to lie. Hence the Company... have conceived a plan for the better accommodation of travelers. They prevail on every two to chum together. To each of the chums they sell a board and three square cushions stuffed with straw, and covered with thin cotton. On the approach of night, the boards are laid from bench to bench, making a couch wide enough for two.

It is no wonder that things gradually improved on trains by the agreement between Fred Harvey and the Santa Fe Railway to offer meals across the country. In fact, my father used to travel that route for business and brought home the old recipe book from Santa Fe. I still have that Super Chief recipe book for meals served from 1941 to 1947. Here is a typical example of one dish. This might be a recipe for a good night's sleep if one had a better accommodation than Stevenson described.

Santa Fe Railroad Hot Strawberry Sundae

1 pint strawberries, cut in half
4 tablespoons Jamaican rum
4 tablespoons lemon juice
Rind of 1 orange, cut in strips
¼ cup honey

Marinate strawberries in rum for one hour. Bring honey, lemon juice, and orange peel to a boil; removed orange rind and combine flavored honey with strawberries. Serve over ice cream immediately. Serves two.

Returning to the relationship between the United States and England, our citizens became interested when Edward VIII, King of England, abdicated the throne in in 1936 to marry an American divorcee, Wallis Simpson. Before he became the Prime Minister, his title had been Prince of Wales and after his abdication, a new title was created for him—the Duke of Windsor.

The first Prince of Wales was Queen Victoria's oldest son by Prince Albert, Edward who was called "Bertie". While waiting for his mother to die before he could reign, he became popular as a rake. Despite his marriage to Princess Alexandra of Denmark, he had affairs with English actress Lillie Langtry and French actress Sarah Bernhardt. His crazy hours and lack of sleep plus his reputation was well known to English and American women who loved to make a Prince of Wales Cake.

When Victoria died in 1901, he reigned until his death in 1910. With his humor and his many liaisons in Europe, he was fondly remembered and nicknamed "Uncle of Europe." My family enjoyed this cake from the Daughters of the American Revolution recipe passed down the family line. A little might go a long way toward making you sleep better than Bertie did.

Prince of Wales Cake

1 cup sugar
½ cup shortening (oleo or butter are substitutes)
1 egg
½ c. maple (or pancake) syrup
2 cups flour
1 teaspoon baking soda
1 teaspoon vanilla
½ teaspoon each cinnamon, nutmeg and ground cloves
1 cup sour milk (1 tablespoon of lemon or vinegar to sour)
Optional: raisins and/or nuts

Cream the sugar, shortening, and egg. Add syrup. Sift the dry ingredients and add with sour milk and vanilla. Add raisins and nuts if desired. Bake in a greased 13x9 inch pan at 350 degrees for 30 minutes or until done. Dust with confectioner's sugar if desired.

Sleep in England During World War II

Before World War II, there was still little air travel by the general public so jet lag was not even in the lexicon. The world had yet to discover how airplanes would change things after their use in World War II. That awareness began when British Prime Minister Neville Chamberlain announced the following on September 30, 1938.

I have returned from Germany with peace for our time. This morning I had another talk with the German Chancellor, Herr Hitler, and here is the paper which bears his name upon it as well as mine. Go home and get a nice quiet sleep.

Within two years, young John Kennedy was very upset with this British attitude. He wrote his thesis at Harvard in 1940 entitled *Why England Slept*. His father, who was the American ambassador to England at that time, made sure the thesis was published. In fact, his father bought out most copies so that it became a so-called best seller. This was done even though he did not agree with his son's dire predictions about eminent war with Germany.

England was attacked and it took British Prime Minister Winston Churchill some time before he could persuade President Franklin D. Roosevelt to declare war on Germany. Churchill was a man who claimed to sleep only six hours a night during World War II. Yet his age, weight, smoking and drinking habits suggested that he should become sleepy from time to time. He napped for 1½ to 2 hours many days. He once said, "You must sleep sometime between lunch and dinner and no halfway measures. Take off your clothes and get into bed. That's what I always do...When the war started, I had to sleep during the day because that was the only way I could cope with my responsibilities."

What did the English people drink at the end of the evening before bedtime? The Syllabub is a frothy English evening drink popular from the 1500s until about 1940 when it was replaced by ice cream. The milk and fruits contain tryptophan and melatonin. The wine curdles the milk. Look up Syllabub pictures on the Internet for creative serving ideas.

English Syllabub

This English drink is served looking like a sundae. A Syllabub is made with 1 cup white wine added to 1/8 cup sugar, 1/4 teaspoon nutmeg, and 2 cups cold milk mixed in a blender. If desired, top with whipped cream, perhaps mixed with cinnamon. Vary the ingredients by including blueberries, raspberries, or top it with lemon or orange zest, or even a stick of rosemary to dress it up. Serves 2 to 4.

Sleep and Travel

Thirty years after the widespread growth of railroads, aircraft began to show their capabilities at air shows. Although airplanes were used in World War I, they were not affordable as a method of transportation until World War II. Soon they became the most common form of transportation across long distances. In days gone by, people could sleep on long flights but movies, lights, tighter seating, and commotion have made sleep more and more difficult, which adds to jet lag problems.

Hundreds of songs about sleep during World War II emerged during the early 1940s. Dinah Shore sang on radio and in movies as well as later having her own television show. One of her big hits was *I'm Getting Tired So I Can Sleep* composed by Irving Berlin in 1942. During World War II, men and women both used sleep and dreams to feel less lonely. Here are some of the lyrics from that song:

> I'm getting tired so I can sleep
> I want to sleep so I can dream
> I want to dream so I can be with you.

The Jet Lag Was Created

As travel got faster, people had to adjust their body to move two or three thousand miles in a few hours. The "jet lag" was born. Perhaps those impacted most were world leaders and corporate heads who must get off their plane and negotiate business without any sleep. Sleep problems were notorious during World War II and continued during the Cold War. Constant air travel for peace negotiators ensued, creating jet lag in all who travel across time zones within a few hours.

Jet lag can start wars! In 1956, United States Secretary of State John Foster Dulles arrived back in Washington after a long flight to learn that the Egyptians had just bought a substantial amount of Russian arms. Dulles immediately canceled an agreement he had made with Egypt's Colonel Nasser to bankroll the Aswan Dam project. That opened the door for Nasser to work with the Soviet Union to fund the project and improve their position in the Middle East. Years later Dulles admitted that he had made a mistake in acting so hastily. He blamed it on the effects of jet lag.

When U-2 American pilot Gary Powers was shot down over Russia in 1960, he did not commit suicide as instructed and was captured. Nikita Sergeyevich Khrushchev was jumping with joy when he cabled President Dwight D. Eisenhower to say they had an American plane. Eisenhower claimed it was a weather plane. Nikita then revealed that they had the pilot who was "alive and kicking." The picture of the crashed U-2 and Powers were broadcast on television across the Soviet Union when Lee Harvey Oswald lived there, as I learned in researching my book *The Mind of Oswald*. (Oswald was the man who tried to shoot Major General Edwin Walker on April 10, 1963, but missed, and six months later assassinated President John F. Kennedy on November 22, 1963.)

Gary Powers was imprisoned for 21 months and subjected to sleep deprivation, bright spot lights, and death threats. That spy plane incident ruined Eisenhower's hope to tame the Cold War by the end of his term. A 2015 movie, *Bridge of Spies* with Tom Hanks, depicted the exchange of Gary Powers for Soviet spy Rudolph Abel.

During the Cold War, Anastas Mikoyan represented the Soviet Union in negotiations with the United States and Cuba. In 1936, he was the Commissar of the Food Industry and was sent to the U.S. by Joseph Stalin to get ideas on American cooking. Stalin wanted to improve food and prove that things were better in Russia than before he took over. Mikoyan brought back recipes for ketchup and ice cream and in 1939 produced a book of recipes for homemakers across Russia. *Book of Tasty and Healthy Food* by Mikoyan is now available in English. Besides ice cream, his most popular contribution was cornflakes and the Kotleti or cutlet, which copied the American hamburger without the bun. This recipe followed by a bit of ice cream produces a meal with ingredients that encourage melatonin production.

Anastas Mikoyan Cutlets (Russian Hamburger Patties)

1 ½ pounds ground beef (could use pork, chicken or fish)
2 slices stale bread (soak in water 5 minutes and squeeze)
1 small onion, chopped
2 garlic cloves, crushed
2 tablespoons chopped dill or parsley
2 ½ tablespoons mayonnaise
1 teaspoon Kosher or Mediterranean salt
½ teaspoon ground black pepper
2-3 cups fine dried bread crumbs for coating
2 tablespoons oil and pat of butter for frying

Mix all ingredients down to pepper in a large ball covered with plastic wrap. Keep in the refrigerator 30 minutes. Then shape into oval patties 3 ½ inches long. Coat with crumbs pressing for crumbs to adhere. Heat the skillet and bring oil and butter to a sizzle. Fry cutlets at medium heat until golden brown—about 4 minutes on each side. Then cover pan and heat on low flame 2-3 more minutes. Drain on paper towels and serve. Russians serve them with fried potatoes.

World Leaders and Their Sleep Problems

On June 18, 1973, Soviet Party Secretary Leonid Brezhnev told President Richard Nixon's translator that he was so happy to meet Nixon at Camp David. He did most of the talking at the private meeting with the translator, which is available on the Internet.

Brezhnev, who replaced Khrushchev, suffered from insomnia, took sleeping pills, consumed large amounts of alcohol and suffered from emphysema due to lifelong smoking. He commented in the first few minutes that he had a cigarette box with a mechanism that he couldn't open for one hour. Nixon laughed and reassured him for having a good way to discipline himself about smoking.

This was just after John Dean had released the taped conversations in the White House, staffers John Ehrlichman and H. R. (Bob) Haldeman had resigned, and Elliott Richardson had been appointed the new Attorney General. Brezhnev knew of all these problems and comforted Nixon by telling him that Nixon's staff members had spoken highly of him. Brezhnev talked by far the most, which made some people worry about his sobriety for carrying on.

Brezhnev went on to discuss the similarities between the U.S. and U.S.S.R. and how he wanted to begin a lasting relationship to obtain peace. He added that he would use the lunch break to have a little nap because he was still a little weak due to time differences. Nixon said he would arrange it.

Leonid Brezhnev was surprised by a special treat of an upscale car contributed by the Ford Automotive Association. He could not contain his excitement about the car and drove President Nixon about to try it out, scaring poor Nixon to death with his speed and sudden stops. Some speculated that his erratic driving may have been the effects of jet lag.

Political pundits have mentioned Henry Kissinger's jet lag when he traveled as President Nixon's National Security Advisor and as Secretary of State. He recalled his negotiations with North Vietnamese diplomat Le Duc Tho saying he was on the verge of losing his temper at the North Vietnamese insolence. From then on he never began a negotiation immediately after a long flight.

Kissinger applied this rule in dealing with his Soviet interlocutors. He told the Soviet Ambassador that he never negotiated immediately after a long flight across many time zones and would not be prepared to begin talks until Sunday morning Moscow time, more than 36 hours away.

How World Leaders Handled Jet Lag

Kissinger prepared for international trips by changing his waking/ sleeping schedule over the period of a week before a trip so the schedule matched the place he landed. According to authors Lynne W. Scanlon and Charles F. Ehret, he began to follow directions in their book *Overcoming Jet Lag* published in 1983.

Their directions were to eat normally four days before you fly but skip alcohol and caffeine and have only carbohydrates for suppers that make you sleepy. Three days before leaving, have a light protein breakfast and lunch and just have fruit for supper. Two days before leaving, have a high protein breakfast and lunch but high carbohydrate supper. The day of flight eat a high protein breakfast and lunch and high carbohydrate supper. Between 7 p.m. and 11 p.m. relax, avoid alcohol, and try to sleep. The arrival morning, eat a high protein breakfast, wash your face, brush your teeth and stay awake for the day. Some of these instructions seem strange to us because we rarely fly that far or skip alcohol that long!

President Ronald Reagan followed the Scanlon Ehret recommendations before going to Japan, China and Viet Nam's Demilitarized Zone in late 1983. This was his third year in office and he stated that what caused him to lose sleep was the thought of soldiers going into Beirut and being slaughtered. He did, however, have problems staying awake.

President Ronald Reagan and Sleep

The older Reagan got, the more sleep problems he had. At one 1991 meeting with the press, famed UPI reporter Helen Thomas asked him about his sleep.

Thomas: "How come you can't sleep these nights?" President: "What?" Thomas: "Jet lag?" President: "Doing fine. Please don't worry about that." Thomas: "I'm really worried." President: "You wake up at night. I'll tell you, it's crazy." Thomas: "We're all worried." President: "All right, here we go."

President Reagan then left the room, while offering rides to reporters. Some accompanied him as he drove them around the area to show that he had no sleep problem right then.

Other times President Ronald Reagan recognized his sleep problem and said with his delightful self-denigrating humor: "No matter what time it is, wake me up, even if it's in the middle of a cabinet meeting." It is well known that he slept through Pope John Paul II's speech after flying to meet him in 1982. Reagan also fell asleep when Paraguayan President Stroessner was welcoming him to that country. His wife, Nancy, had to keep poking and waking him.

As a personal aside, let me explain that Nancy Reagan's Just Say No program for children to fight drugs was untested. Because I was the "Drug Czar" of Dallas, she expected me to spread a program to fight drugs with a simple slogan like that. The slogan was something that a child from five to ten could memorize and say by rote if somebody offered a drug, but that didn't happen much in Dallas. It was the older children from age ten up that tried drugs and we had to find other methods to fight drugs.

Thanks to the nation's drug czar, William Bennett, we came up with more valid strategies. However, drugs have overwhelmed our world and our country so that solutions become harder as seemingly intelligent people approve more and more mind-bending drugs. Ronald Reagan's best after dinner sweet was the jelly bean and a handful of those will help one drift off to sleep.

John Kerry, who ran for the Presidency and was defeated, served as Secretary of State for President Barack Obama. He traveled to many countries and humorously described his method of dealing with jet lag. He stated that he simply listens to one of his own speech on his iPod, takes an Ambien, and he's out in seconds.

President George H. W. Bush and Sleep

In 1992, President George H. W. Bush was in Japan on the 10th of a 12-day 26,000-mile tour of four Asian countries. At a state dinner in his honor, the president suddenly felt ill and vomited on himself and his host, Japanese Prime Minister Miyazawa. This attack of gastroenteritis could have been brought on by jet lag, said presidential spokesperson Marlin Fitzwater. During that year, Bush was also advised not to use controversial sleeping pills like Halcion because it might cause depression, amnesia, paranoia and hallucinations. Great Britain had banned that drug the year before.

Fortunately, the elder George Bush could laugh at himself and his problems. One illustration of his humor was a letter to President Bill Clinton on January 23, 2008. The letter was published in his 2013 book *All the Best, George Bush*. He described how he saw Bill trying to keep his eyes open during a Martin Luther King Day sermon. He explained that he had been there and how difficult it is to fly about and then fall asleep at the worst times. Bush went on to describe the problems many leaders such as Dick Cheney had with sleep, and there was even an in-group award bestowed upon the person who had fallen asleep but covered it up the best.

When President Bush's son, George W. Bush, was elected president, several reporters discussed the elder Bush "syntax" or malapropisms during his presidential terms. They indicated that these might be the result of some kind of medical problem, medicines, travel or insomnia. His malapropisms were first noted in 2000: "They misunderestimated me." 2002 speaking in Tennessee: "There's an old saying in Tennessee, I know it's in Texas, probably in Tennessee— that says 'Fool me once, shame on—shame on you. Fool me—you can't get fooled again.'" 2003: "Free nations don't attack each other. Free nations don't develop weapons of mass destruction." 2004: "Too many good docs are getting out of the business. Too many OB-GYNs aren't able to practice their love with women all across this country." 2008: "This is still a dangerous world of madmen and uncertainty and potential mental losses." He was supposed to say "missile launchers" so his concern about mental loss accidentally surfaced here. I call it a "Freudian slip!"

These may sound like critical comments of people appointed to high offices and the presidency. Rather, this information is intended to demonstrate that medicines, jet lag, and physical illnesses might put our country at risk. The best medical help must be available to world leaders accompanied by advice regarding conditioning for trips and rest.

British Prime Minister Margaret Thatcher and Sleep

British Prime Minister Margaret Thatcher said while preparing for a trip to Japan, she described how jet lag is an awful nuisance when you're going straight into talks and negotiations, but promised she would cope. Tony Blair, a more recent British Prime Minister from 1997-2007, was married to Cherie Blair. She wrote a book called *Speaking for Myself: My Life from Liverpool to Downing Street* in 2008. She explained that after two days of campaigning followed by a 12-hour flight, she and Tony were shattered and jet-lagged.

The English have a sense of humor, don't they? They even have funny names for their food such as "Spotted Dick". Dick stands for pudding and spotted refers to raisins. A nice evening treat to aid your sleep comes from this old English recipe. You can be sure that British prime ministers and most Englishmen have eaten this dish.

Old English Spotted Dick

1 cup raisins
2/3 cups mincemeat
3 tablespoons brandy
1 cup self-rising flour
2 tablespoons baking powder
¼ teaspoon salt
¼ cup dark brown sugar
1 egg
1 tablespoon butter
Zest of 2 lemons
¼ cup cream

Warm the brandy, mincemeat and raisins in a pan and set aside. Whisk the flour, baking powder, salt, brown sugar, and then add egg to the flour mixture. Then add butter, lemon zest, and cream to the flour mixture. Mix and then roll out on a floured surface into a rectangle. Spread the raisin-mincemeat across the top. Roll up. Place it in greased parchment paper and tie the ends with string. Put into a bowl which will fit inside a crock pot. Place enough water in the crock pot to come half way up the bowl containing the spotted dick. Cook for four hours to steam the pudding. Slice and serve warm or at room temperature with whipped cream or drizzle some warm syrup over if desired.

In 2005, the younger Bush, President George W. Bush, was to meet the new Chinese President. As the Chinese minister was being introduced, the announcer mistakenly said "Republic of China" instead of "People's Republic of China". A protestor took offense and was finally ejected from the meeting. Meanwhile, despite all this commotion, President Bush fell asleep. He was questioned later by reporters. "In your statement this morning with President Hu, you seemed a little off your game... Was something bothering you?" President Bush responded: "Have you ever heard of jet lag?"

The National Sleep Foundation has found that individuals over 50 years of age are more susceptible to jet lag and its effects may last for more than one day.

Secretary of State Hillary Clinton and Sleep

During Hillary Clinton's four years as Secretary of State under President Obama, she visited 112 of the world's 200 countries spending some 87 full days on a plane as well as being on the road 401 days. State Department officials worried about her grueling schedule and had her cut back on it. On one of those trips, in

December 2012, she suffered from gastroenteritis that may have been a result of jet lag.

President Barack Obama claimed to sleep about six hours a night during his presidency. But he described his fatigue in the 2007 campaign as overwhelming. He blamed jet lag for an error where he said the death toll from tornadoes in Kansas was "ten thousand" when it was only twelve.

Do we sleep less than people in other countries? Are there different sleep patterns and needs according to age or gender or ethnic group? Why don't people all sleep the same on Earth?

Chapter Eight
SLEEP IN VARIOUS CULTURES: WHO SLEEPS WITH WHOM?

Who sleeps by whom is not merely a personal or private activity. Instead, it is a social practice like eating meals with your family, or honoring the practice of a monogamous marriage, which is invested with moral and social meaning for a person's reputation and good standing in the community.

In my travels to some 48 countries, some observed sleeping patterns were quite different from Americans. I shall never forget sleeping in London where the custom was to sleep with windows open on cold nights. As a travel agent, my lodging was one room of an old church across the street from Selfridge's Department Store on Oxford Street. The only way to sleep was to drop a six-pence into a little stove which ran for thirty minutes, and hope that you were asleep by the time it turned off. In Paris when I first married, we set a fire in the fireplace before bed so the room would warm up and laid coats and blankets upon us, windows again open. We awoke at sunrise and went out for croissants and café au lait, read, or watched passersby before going to work.

Only a few cultures are described here to suggest the variety of sleep practices across the world.

Where a Baby Sleeps Differs by Culture

Each country has their own lifestyle, which depends upon the kind of money and housing of each rung of society. Some sleeping practices should at least be examined so that we can select what works best for us and our loved ones.

Some researchers believe that people have overestimated the need for infants to sleep separately in order to assure "independence" from their parents. The American practice of separating infants from parents for sleep is at odds with the practices of most other cultures.

American children are trained to be self-reliant and to display their individuality by sleeping alone. Japanese children are taught to "harmonize with the group" and, hence, to "co-sleep" with their parents. In Japan, an infant is seen as separated from the beginning and needs to be drawn into relations with others. In America, an infant is seen as dependent and in order to develop properly, needs to be made independent of others.

The Japanese think the United States culture is merciless by pushing small children toward such independence at night. Japanese infants and children usually sleep adjacent to their mothers on futons and children sleep with someone (fathers or extended family members) through the age of fifteen. Touch is much used and skin-to-skin contact is deemed important.

Vietnamese mothers were told about sudden infant death syndrome. They felt that the custom of being with the baby would prevent this problem. They believed that if mothers are sleeping with the baby, they always sleep lightly. They notice if the baby's breathing changes. They felt that babies should not be left alone.

Mayan mothers from Guatemala believe that sleeping alone is so difficult for adult Guatemalans that in the absence of family members, adults seek out friends with whom they can share sleep. Upon hearing that American babies are made to sleep alone, Mayan women thought that practice was child neglect. No particular bedtime routines were observed in Mayan communities but sleeping alone was considered undesirable. Mayans considered it a pity if an infant was forced to sleep alone.

But some American physicians advise parents that sleeping with a baby or child is abnormal. Cultural psychologists at the University of Chicago studied the role of sleep in character development. They found that sleep recommendations are guided by: (1) protecting the separateness of children from the husband-wife relationship, (2) avoiding the appearance of incest, and (3) teaching the child self-reliance and independence.

What are the results when American children slept with their parents at an early age? In a survey of adult college subjects, males who co-slept with their parents up to five years of age had significantly higher self-esteem, less guilt and anxiety, and more sex. Women who co-slept with parents as children also had higher self-esteem than those who did not. This may have reflected an attitude of parental acceptance instead of rejection. Furthermore, a study of 1,400 subjects from five ethnic groups of Chicago and New York found more positive outcomes and satisfaction with life in those who co-slept with parents as a child.

A study of 36 American families with children aged one to three were compared to a Dutch sample of 66 families with children from six months to eight years of age. The Dutch babies slept two hours longer than the American infants. The three traditions of Dutch child-rearing were rest, regulation and cleanliness. They believe infants need much sleep and should not be over-stimulated day or night. Their babies are put down to sleep earlier because parents worry that too much stimulation will threaten their ability to sleep at night.

Thousands of American parents were buying books to solve the problems associated with solitary infant sleep. Dr. Benjamin Spock in *Baby and Child Care* had recommended that mothers minimize contact and feeding during the night.

In Japan and Korea where co-sleeping is normal, children usually don't suck their thumbs or use transitional objects (doll or blanket or shirt). In Turkey where children are left alone to fall asleep, 96% of infants were thumb suckers.

Some researchers have surveyed the sleeping practices of over a hundred cultures and found that mothers slept in the same bed with their infants in the majority. In one-fifth of these cases, the father slept in the same bed as well. In none of the cultures was the infant actually isolated at bedtime. The baby was always placed in close proximity of another person.

One survey of U.S. pediatricians in 1984 found that almost all disapproved of co-sleeping. But in 1992, Eastern Kentucky infant-parent co-sleeping was prevalent among white Americans who seemed uninterested in what doctors said about the issue. As one Eastern Kentucky woman phrased it: "How can you expect to hold on to them later in life if you begin their lives by pushing them away?"

In the early 1990s, psychological experiments began to produce more scientific data on children's sleep. The main theme of these reports was that children in the beginning of the 20th century did not get enough sleep. A German study concluded that German school children had insufficient sleep time and one author implied that inadequate sleep led to the development of criminal behavior.

Italian Children Are More Involved in All Family Life

In the 1990s, Italian preschool children two to four years old were reported to have a shorter nightly sleep duration than did children in other countries. They went to bed later and woke up earlier. Compared with American children, they had no clear bedtime schedules, no consistent bedtime rituals because they often participated in evening social activities with adults and fell asleep before they were put to bed.

Actress Sophia Loren from Italy is an example of this kind of upbringing. She wrote in her cookbook *Sophia Loren's Recipes and Memories*, "The kitchen is where the whole family is united." From morning to night the family gathered for meal preparations, meal eating, meal clearing, confessions, debates, advice, and resolution of mini-tragedies that cropped up in daily lives. She said that children were left out of nothing.

A splendid cook, Loren concocted her own Minestrone soups with ingredients growing wherever she lived at the time. She suggested that people should adapt their ingredients according to the season and what they find in their own market. Her Minestrone contains vegetables, and if followed by a sweet, may bring a good night's sleep.

Sophia Loren Minestrone

Pick and chop your own fresh vegetables of the season, she advised. Hers included onion, carrots, potatoes, zucchinis, spinach, celery, cauliflower, a can of cannellini or Great Northern beans, and tomatoes. She cooked up some bacon. Then she added the fresh vegetables to cook in the bacon grease around ten minutes until lightly browned. Then she covered the vegetables in water and let everything except the beans simmer 20 minutes. Then she added the beans and Italian seasonings and heated the soup until it was warm. She served Minestrone in bowls with a ribbon of olive oil on each serving for those who desired it.

Some Cultures Believe Sleeping Alone May Bring Loss of the Soul

In Bali, infants are held continuously, day and night, by a variety of adults or older children. Being alone for even brief periods during sleep is considered undesirable. Bali religion preaches that sleeping alone leaves one vulnerable to spiritual risks and loss of the soul. The Balinese people have regular periods of sleep avoidance of one or two days per week. Because children are included in all adult social activities, they sleep and wake according to their own innate impulses just as the adults do.

Soul loss is also a Latin American phenomenon called *susto,*

This includes the common notion that human souls wander from the body during sleep. Awakening a sleeper too abruptly or at the wrong time may result in the soul's inability to return to the body properly.

Sleep in Young and Older Children

American pre-sleep rituals for children include an after-dinner bath, dressing in a particular night clothing, telling stories and singing lullabies, good-night kisses, then leaving the child alone in his or her room. Frequently, children insist on sleeping with a light on or taking a treasured object to bed with them such as a doll or toy or blanket or pacifier. They repeatedly call their parents after being put to bed, asking for another drink or another story.

The newest guidelines on sleep for children come from the American Academy of Sleep Medicine and were released at their annual meeting in Denver, Colorado in June 2016. The Academy recommended that children aged three to five sleep 10 to 13 hours per day, children six to twelve should sleep 9 to 12 hours per day, and teenagers thirteen to eighteen should sleep 8 to 10 hours. Their guidelines added that all screens such as televisions and computers be turned off half an hour before bedtime. They further recommended that parents not allow children to have screens or anything with blue lights or other lights in their bedrooms while sleeping.

A study of nearly 1,400 public school children aged five to seven with sleep apnea found that even mild problems such as snoring had a negative effect on children's thinking abilities. Researchers recommended that simple brain function tests should be used by pediatricians to evaluate children with habitual snoring to detect and treat sleep apnea.

Some 2.5 million people in the United States have sleep apnea. Sleep apnea and narcolepsy used to be called the Pickwickian Syndrome. Obesity and narcolepsy are closely related. One of Charles Dickens' characters in the *Pickwick Papers* was a fat red-faced boy called Joe who was always falling asleep. Here is one conversation about Joe from Dickens' book:

"Sleep!" said the old gentleman, "he's always asleep. Goes on errands fast asleep, and snores as he waits at table."

"How very odd!" said Mr. Pickwick.

"Ah! Odd indeed," returned the old gentleman. "I'm proud of that boy—wouldn't part with him on any account—he's a natural curiosity."

Most parents don't want their child to be a "natural curiosity". They try to keep their children on a regular sleeping pattern at home with rituals like reading stories, flipping on nightlights, and getting stuffed animals for them to sleep with. If these things don't work, they talk with physicians and some are sent for sleep studies and further evaluations. While these may seem like complex solutions for a simple problem, the sleep problems of children in earlier times were often very severe.

By the age of 15, many American adolescents have regular part-time employment. This occurred also in England in the early 1900s. In American as well as the British Isles and European countries, boys by the age of twelve worked for payment before and after school delivering milk, bedding horses, selling newspapers, and various other jobs. Girls were busy with the numerous household chores and caring for other siblings. Only in the last twenty years have part-time jobs for teenagers diminished in the United States.

In the past, children worked extremely long hours before child labor laws were enacted in most countries. A 13-year old girl who was overworked and sleepless was described in the 1888 short story, "Sleepy," by Russian author Anton Chekov, who was a physician.

Nursemaid Varka, aged thirteen, rocks the cradle where a baby lies and murmurs, almost inaudibly...

"Nurse will sing a song to you."....

The child cries. It has long been hoarse and weak from crying, but still it cries, and who can say when it will be comforted? And Varka wants to sleep. Her eyelids drop, her head hangs, her neck pains her. She can hardly move her eyelids or her lips...

Varka goes into the woods and cries, and suddenly someone slaps her with such force that her head bangs against a birch tree. She lifts her head, and sees her master, the boot maker.

"What are you doing, scabby?" he asks. "The child is crying and you are asleep."

He gives her a slap on the ear; and she shakes her head, rocks the cradle and murmurs her lullaby...

She wants to sleep, wants passionately to sleep. Varka lays her head on the edge of the cradle and rocks it with her whole body so as to drive away sleep; but her eyelids droop again, and her head is heavy.

"Varka, light the stove!"...

As she hears the cry of the baby, she finds the enemy who is crushing her heart. The enemy is the child...

Varka steals to the cradle and bends over it with outspread fingers which afterward close tightly. Then, laughing, with joy at the thought that now she can sleep, in a moment she sleeps as soundly as the dead child.

Russian tennis champ Maria Sharapova has won many titles in her career. She lived in Belarus until Chernobyl when her family moved to Siberia to escape the nuclear fallout and danger. When she was seven, her father brought her to Miami, Florida, to see if a tennis trainer thought she was worthy of coaching. She knew no English but lived with Americans who shunned her and kept her awake at night while they partied leaving her out. She gradually improved and developed a goal to win tournaments and to raise awareness of nuclear dangers. She described the lung cancer and other diseases which Russians in the path of Chernobyl fallout still suffer.

When she was banned from major tennis tournaments for a medicine that enhanced performance, she turned her attention to developing desserts. This is one of her tasty recipes for a good night's sleep. She said of sleep, "I love to sleep. It's my hobby." She has now returned to tennis but her recipe is online for readers. Here is the gist of her recommendation for a sweet.

Maria Sharapova Ginger Cookies

Use a recipe for your favorite ordinary vanilla cookies but instead of putting in chocolate chips or raisins, put in 1½ teaspoons of ground ginger. Throw in a little packed dark brown sugar and bake your cookies at 350 degrees until slightly brown.

Comparing Sleep Problems of Teens

These days, teenagers often do not have adult responsibilities but are juggling classes, after-school activities, and social lives which leave them chronically sleep deprived. A telephone poll surveying youngsters from eleven to seventeen years of age was conducted by The National Science Foundation. The scientists found that 56% slept less than needed, 15% slept more than needed. Some 54% of high school seniors went to bed at 11:00 p.m. or later on school nights and woke at 6:30 a.m., leaving many without the sleep growing children need.

One scary statistic was that 5% of those teenagers had nodded off while driving (twenty-one of them) and one quarter of those had been in traffic accidents. Traffic crashes are the leading cause of death in young people in the United States, taking the lives of at least 5,600 teens each year according to the National Highway Traffic Safety Administration.

A survey of college students identified sleep problems as the third biggest barrier to academic performance. They rated stress and anxiety higher. This sent researchers off to study college students in 2014. They found that 50% report daytime sleepiness and 70% attain insufficient sleep. The results are lowered grade point averages, academic failure, compromised learning, impaired mood, and increased motor vehicle accidents. Researchers concluded that if college students understood their sleep problems and learned methods to combat them, the consequences of sleepiness could be reduced.

A 2016 study of college students explored whether an on-line sleep education program would change their sleep behavior. The students who took the sleep course by computer did change. They stopped using electronics earlier in the evening, arose earlier on weekends, stuck to a regular sleep schedule, took fewer naps, lowered risky drinking, and reported less depression.

Research has revealed both racial/ethnic disparities in sleep and correlations between race-based stress and sleep. A 2010 study by the National Sleep Foundation revealed notable racial/ethnic differences in sleep duration between Black and White adults. Specifically, Blacks reported getting an average of 38 minutes less sleep on workdays or weekdays than Whites.

There are many probable causes for less sleep among Blacks. Researchers proposed these: (1) perceived discrimination, (2) lower economical sociographic levels, (3) early negative experiences embedded in memory, (4) the decreased likelihood of success on tests, and (5) less likelihood of getting hired. All of these may magnify sleep-disruptive stress. Awareness and anticipation of barriers may contribute to poor sleep and less ability to learn and remember new information. Interventions proposed by researchers were positive racial socialization messages, seeking a trusted person to talk through stressful feelings, and positive sleep hygiene practices such as a consistent bedtime.

Little was known about sleep patterns in China so a study of adolescents and parents was conducted in March and April of 2005. Participants included 625 boys and 441 girls from 7th through 10th grades. Their average morning waking time was 5:56 a.m. and sleep duration was 7.5 hours. Sleep insufficiency, insomnia, and daytime sleepiness was prevalent in these Chinese adolescents. Parental history of insomnia was associated with an elevated risk for insomnia in their offspring.

Insomnia in young people may be accompanied by other problems such as depression and suicidal thoughts. Suicide rates in university students are particularly high in South Korea. Insomnia has been found in those students with suicidal ideas. A sample of 552 South Korean young adults found that more insomnia symptoms were associated with feelings of loneliness. Suicidal ideas were possible solutions in the minds of some who felt terribly alone. Researchers urged physicians and university clinics to question those who report insomnia to see if depression and/or suicidal thoughts are present, so treatment may be recommended.

The study was called "Is Insomnia Lonely?" Among the reasons explored was the keen interest of Korean parents in their children's education and grades. Children may perceive this as pressure to achieve and Koreans are generally high achievers. This popular Korean drink might help these young people sleep better.

Korean Strawberry Drink:

Slice a cup of strawberries and mix with ½ cup of sugar. Boil up ¼ cup of sugar with 2 cups of water. Cool the sugar syrup. Pour over the strawberries. Sprinkle 1 ½ tablespoons pine nuts on top. Serves four in little cups with a spoon.

International Comparison of Adult Sleep Problems

An interesting study of 42,116 people fifty years or older compared sleep problems in nine countries. Poland had the most sleep problems with 17% of the sample, and China had the least sleep problems at 2.8%. The other rankings were: India 15%, Finland 9.6%, South Africa 9.6%, Russia 9%, Spain 8.1%, Ghana 7.1%, and Mexico 5.8%. Subjects were asked about other medical problems such as angina, arthritis, asthma, diabetes, depression, lung disease and stroke. The more medical problems a person had, the higher the risk for sleep problems. The study warned that insomnia increases with age and treatment is challenging due to the coexistence of other disorders and many medicines being taken.

Poland's insomniacs included Polish pianist Wladsziu Valentino Liberace (1919-1987) known as Liberace. He entertained into the late hours along with his violinist brother at public venues. He performed on television through the 1950s and 1960s. Stage settings featured glittering chandeliers. His home base in later years was Las Vegas where this child prodigy developed flamboyant flourishes for his piano solos.

He entertained his gay and straight friends by cooking up dishes that came from his mother and from his own rich imagination. He created a recipe called Liberace's Exceptional and Extraordinary Angel Bling Cake Pie. If you have, oh, so little a bit of it, after your evening meal, you may drift off to sleep from its contribution to melatonin production. We won't give away his recipe but we'll tell you how he got his "bling".

Liberace Angel Bling Cake

Make your favorite white cake and cover it with a fluffy white icing. Then to create the "bling," dot the topping with little colored fake jewels picked up from some arts and crafts store. Warn eaters that the jewels are not edible.

Sleepless in Japan and Suicide

Look at the current insomnia problem in Japan. "The Japanese are working themselves to death—literally" said a *USA Today* article in 2016. The article began with a 24-year-old girl who leaped to her death from her company window on Christmas Day. The Tokyo Labor Bureau investigators ruled her suicide *karoshi*—death by overwork. She had posted messages on social media accounts complaining of her crushing workload and indicating that she was considering suicide. Her parents reported that she was working 130 hours of overtime in a month.

Claims for compensation for *karoshi* rose to an all-time high in 2015, according to labor ministry data. However, the secretary general of the National Defense Counsel for Victims of *karoshi* said the real number was probably ten times higher, as the government is reluctant to recognize such incidents. Some 38% of the workforce are on non-standard contracts and are allowed to work 100+ hours overtime per month. This is a way for companies to keep labor costs down, but it is also a path that leads to death by overwork.

There are also cardiovascular deaths called *karoshi* if the employee worked 100 hours of overtime in the month beforehand, or 80 hours of overtime in two or more consecutive months in the previous six. Japan has no legal limits on working hours.

Yoko Ono was the Japanese wife of John Lennon who sang with the Beatles. The two of them were a notable pair until he was assassinated by Mark David Chapman on December 8, 1980. Ono was twelve when Hiroshima was destroyed by the atom bomb and she and Lennon tried to energize people to avoid war, and especially the Viet Nam War. She and Lennon did a Bed-in for Peace in 1969 inviting reporters to cover them sitting in their bed as they protested war and nuclear weapons. They were photographed on that bed for hours—but never sleeping.

She wrote this recipe in a curious and mystical way as if the salad represented something more special than just simple food. The answer lies in a play she wrote called *Hiroshima* where a little girl follows the Japanese tradition of making little paper cranes to fly into the sky but dies of radiation before she can complete her paper cranes picture. This dish is perfect for evening dining and sleep.

Yoko Ono Fruit Salad

Her salad contained spinach, green apple, edamame, dried cranberries and pecans. Her dressing contained grapefruit juice, sesame oil, chopped ginger, honey, brown mustard and soy sauce. Her instructions were: Make a salad. After you have eaten the salad, draw a picture of the sky. Send the picture to a friend.

American Sleep Habits Vary by State

A large sleep study of 1.1 million people found that the longest survival rates in the United States were among people who slept about 6 to 7 hours a night and didn't use sleeping pills. The study took place in San Diego from 1982 and was finally completed in 2002. The study, "Mortality Associated with Sleep Duration and Insomnia," was a surprise since it suggests that sleeping less than seven hours does not shorten life.

Another large national study of sleep covered approximately 700,000 Americans. This study appeared in *Sleep* in May 2016. Subjects were asked "On average, how many hours of sleep do you get in a 24-hour period?" Those who slept the least were employed males of many races who were divorced and depressed. They also found that people in the mid-Atlantic region slept less than the rest of country.

Those results matched another project from 2014 called "Prevalence of Healthy Sleep Duration among Adults—United States, 2014." The project analyzed data from 444,306 persons aged eighteen to sixty in all fifty states. Researchers concluded that more than one third of Americans reported sleeping less than seven hours per night. Those who slept the least were in Hawaii and those who slept longest were in South Dakota. Those living in the Great Plains states slept the longest. The shortest sleepers resided in the southeastern United States in states along the Appalachian Mountains where there is a greater degree of obesity and other chronic health conditions. Perhaps this gives a wake-up call for people to improve sleep by losing weight and taking good care of their health.

Who Sleeps Better—Men or Women?

People have wondered which sex has more insomnia. Insomnia is diagnosed when there is sleep difficulty at least three nights per week for a minimum of one month. In France, those conditions were found in more French women--12% with insomnia versus 6% of men with insomnia. That study of 12,778 French people was published in the *Journal of Sleep Research* in 2000.

Once upon a time, all a French person needed to sleep was l'amour, wine, and a nice meal. Alexandre Dumas understood this very well. He designed his stories about the *Three Musketeers* around those ingredients. He had this recipe to offer for a veal stew which may be accompanied by your favorite wine or small dessert for a carbohydrate. His wine would have been white wine with this recipe.

Alexandre Dumas Veal Stew

2 -3 tablespoons butter
2 tablespoons flour
1 lb. veal
2 cups water or beef stock
Salt and pepper to taste
1 bay leaf
1 tablespoon fresh or 1 teaspoon dried thyme
3 chopped onions
1 cup chopped mushrooms
½ cup chopped carrots

Melt butter in a pan. Add flour and mix to make a roux pasty mixture. Add veal and stir about in the roux paste. Heat water or beef stock and pour over the veal. Stir until it comes to a boil. Add the salt, pepper, bay leaf and thyme. Let it boil one hour. Add the vegetables and cook another 30 minutes.

Females usually have more insomnia than males regardless of the countries surveyed according to a 2011 study. In Asia, women had 1.29 times more insomnia cases than men. In Australia, women had 1.4 times more insomnia than men. In the United States and Europe, women have 1.5 times the insomnia cases than men. The greatest number of women suffering from insomnia was found to be the elderly African women who had 1.7 times the amount of insomnia of men.

A total of 19,500 Canadians over age fifteen were surveyed in 2005 with the conclusion that women reported more trouble falling or staying asleep than men. In the same year, a Swedish study of 645,429 elderly people (seventy-five to eighty-nine years) found that 27% of women and 18% of men were dispensed at least one hypnotic or sedative drug during the four-month study period.

Whoa! Wait a minute on this idea that women have more insomnia than men! A 2009 study published in the *Journal of Sleep Research* found something a little different in American females and males. The researchers of that study used 1,324 Pennsylvania residents and found that women, compared with men, had a higher percentage of sleep time, a lower percentage of stage 1 sleep, and a higher percentage of *slow wave sleep*. Even more interesting, was the finding that young, healthy women compared with men experienced less sleep disturbance when awakened for blood draws.

They concluded that the sleep of young women is more resistant to stressors. They even surmised that this better sleep by women might contribute to women's lower cardiovascular risks and greater longevity.

The First Night in a New Place Causes Sleep Problems

Most people recognize that when they travel to a new place, they have more trouble sleeping the first night. What is this about? It's about how our bodies are built to handle danger and change.

Researchers observed sleep waves in thirty-five college students, finding that the left side of the brain stays somewhat awake while the right brain sleeps during the first night when sleeping in a new place. This phenomenon has been recognized in animals for some fifty years. The left brain is alert for danger in the way that many animals sleep such as whales, seals, dolphins and ducks. Studies of sleeping ducks in a line have found that the two ducks on each end are staying half-awake to assess danger. The ducks in the middle are completely asleep.

This vigilance task goes away for most people after one night of sleeping in a new environment. Dolphins sleep with one brain hemisphere asleep and the other awake to recognize predators. Many animals do that and man is no exception.

Even highly developed societies maintain sleep wake vigilance such as the Japanese. Commuters on subway trains have short naps called *inemuri*, a word meaning "to be present" and "sleep." Those commuters are asleep but they awaken at the precise time the train reaches its stop, preserving just enough vigilance to wake when action is required. Many sleep standing up as they are packed in tightly by "pushers" that pack more riders in from the loading platforms. Apparently, *inemuri* has been practiced in Japan for perhaps hundreds of years.

This built-in waking vigilance protective mechanism served man well when nights were filled with more danger than they are in today's world. Business travelers might arrive at their destination one night earlier than an important presentation or negotiation. Thus, the poor first night of sleep in a new place is offset by a decent second night of sleep when less vigilance is needed.

What Ever Happened to Siestas?

Napping and siesta cultures of Italy, Mexico, China, Chile and Greece are fading during the last fifty years or so. Those countries are gradually avoiding their day-time sleeping in favor of sleeping all night and doing more business during the day.

In 2014, *The Wall Street Journal* reported on a study of the working hours of people across the world showing some connections with sleep deprivation. People in Singapore have the most sleep deprivation and work the longest hours—2,300 hours per year. People in the United States average 1,790 work hours per year, and people in Europe (France being the prime example) work 1,480 hours per year. When I lived in Paris, stores closed at noon and re-opened about 3:00 p.m. for siesta time. After lunch, sleepiness follows so a nap was in order. When they came back to work in the afternoon, they stayed open until 7:00 p.m. or so and that meant a later meal time for supper. In Spain, dinners were even later such at 10:00 p.m. because siesta closings were longer.

Dean Martin used to sing a song called *Siesta* by Barkan and Raleigh about 1964. The words are so very familiar that we can almost join in to sing them.

> I don't get much workin' done but I sure have a lot
> of fun
> Fiesta ends, it's almost dawnin'
> So how'm I gonna get up in the mornin'
> When I get up at noon each day, it's time for siesta
> And after siesta comes fiesta.

The Spanish word "siesta" comes from the Latin term for the sixth hour from sunrise. Siestas go way back in time and were common mostly in the Mediterranean area, India, Southeast Asia and South America where temperatures were high and residents were poor. This quotation from *Don Quixote de la Mancha* by Miguel de Cervantes was written in 1615. Sancho Panza, Quixote's traveling companion, had more common sense than his boss but travelled on a burro instead of a mighty steed.

The Duchess begged Sancho, if he wasn't feeling too excessive sleepy, to come and spend the afternoon with her and her maidens in a lovely cool room. Sancho replied that although he did usually sleep four or five hours on a summer afternoon he would, for her goodness' sake, try with all his might not to sleep for a single hour that particular afternoon, and would obey her command.

A study done in Jerusalem reported that siestas were usually found among mostly males and especially older males, and they were associated with higher mortality. Siesta studies in the Rancho-Bernardo cohort (diabetes and heart disease) from southern California have found siestas associated with increased all-cause mortality. In Germany, they were associated with atherosclerosis, which was also found in another study from Israel. In patients at high risk of coronary disease, especially those with diabetes, napping may lead to higher mortality.

A Greek study of siesta examined 23,681 Greeks aged twenty to eight-six for over six years. At enrollment, none had coronary heart disease, stroke or cancer. The men and women who did occasional napping had a 12% lower coronary mortality than those who did not nap. Those who napped systematically had an even lower coronary mortality of 37% against those who did not nap. The result was that siestas in healthy individuals had lower coronary mortality, which was particularly evident among working men. They concluded that among healthy adults, siesta, possibly on account of stress-releasing consequences, may reduce coronary mortality.

Although daytime napping has not been a British tradition, its prevalence is likely to increase with the rapidly aging population. So researchers studied 25,639 British men and women aged forty to seventy-nine from 1993 to 1997. They further followed 16,374 of them up to 2011. Daytime napping was associated with a more pronounced risk of death from respiratory diseases. They concluded that daytime napping might be a health risk due to respiratory problems, especially among those 65 years of age or older. So, take your pick about whether siestas in seniors hurt or help.

One senior actress, Bette Davis, understood a lot about aging. She said: "Old age ain't for sissies!" Seniors have more trouble with sleep than young people. One of the largest national studies of sleep in older adults (199,896 seniors aged sixty-five or older) showed that *unmarried* seniors with *lower* socioeconomic status were most likely to sleep less than six hours or have poor quality sleep. So if you are a senior, don't give up on the idea of getting married to improve your sleep and your socio-economic status. Seniors have long had these adages: "Marry a nurse with a purse" and "It's as easy to marry a rich man as a poor man but it may be harder to find a rich one."

Another study reported in November, 2016, put a dollar cost on sleeplessness around the world. "Why Sleep Matters: Quantifying the Economic Costs of Insufficient Sleep" costs Americans $411 billion per year. The costs stem from an estimated 1.23 million missed working days per year from the U.S. workforce (due to the increased risk for infections illness, fatigue, and depression).

Japan lost as much as $138 billion and 604,000 working days a year. The United Kingdom lost $50 billion and 207,000 working day a year. Germany lost $60 billion and 209,000 working days a year. Their research has shown that if Americans who sleep less than six hours a night increased their nightly sleep to between six and seven hours a night, this could add $226.4 billion to the U.S. economy.

Despite these findings, many executives and heads of state have said they get by on very little or no sleep. President Obama told *Vanity Fair* in 2012 that he didn't turn off the White House lights until 1 a.m. and arose before 6 a.m. President Donald Trump, wrote in his 2004 book *Think Like a Billionaire* that he sleeps only about four hours a night, and recommended "Don't sleep any more than you have to."

We haven't looked at where and when sleep deprivation is

dangerous not only to oneself but to others--many others. This is the scariest part of sleep deprivation. We may be responsible for others and could injure countless numbers through our own incapacities due to lack of sleep. If we can't control our sleep problems, others must step in to control us. Where is this happening? Where are others having to take over for us because we aren't making good choices to obtain adequate sleep?

Chapter Nine
DROWSY DRIVING

Most people think that drowsy driving is a new phenomenon. But it began in the early 1900s as people began to try out automobiles despite a lack of roads. Automobiles were such fun.

I shall never forget my first car. After my return from France, I went to work at Southwestern Medical School and Parkland Hospital every morning and needed transportation because of the poor bus service in Dallas. I made a first payment on a darling old yellow English convertible TR-3. By the third payment, I realized that I was speeding too much, my hair was messed if the top was down, and there were too many problems for the local gas station mechanic to fix. It was a wonderful three-month experience with that thrilling first car.

The Fun of Gas-Fueled Cars

In the early days, cars were just a play toy for the rich, and fellows loved to take a girl out for an exciting ride. Irving Berlin wrote *Keep Away from the Fellow Who Owns an Automobile* in 1912. A fellow took a girl out far from her home and they ran out of gas. The song warns of the dire straits she is in:

He'll take you far in his motorcar,
Too darn far from your Ma and Pa,
If his forty horsepower, goes sixty miles an hour,

> Say goodbye forever, goodbye forever,
> There's no chance to talk, squawk or balk,
> You must kiss him or get out and walk,
> Keep away from the fellow
> Who owns an automobile.

The National Old Trails Road was completed in 1915 and it was intended to draw drivers to the 1915 Panama-Pacific International Exposition to be held in San Francisco. The event would celebrate the opening of the Panama Canal and San Francisco's recovery from the earthquake and subsequent fires of 1906.

That exposition attracted the attention of a New York journalist named Emily Post. Before her books on etiquette, she drove west in 1915 with a cousin and her son Ned, a Harvard student. She intended to write a newspaper series about whether a woman could drive across the United States. However, she could not find a map. Along the way, they stayed at various Fred Harvey hotels because there were few decent places to stay and their drives were extremely long. They arose sleep-deprived in places where the beds, bugs, and noise made sleep difficult. Often, it was difficult to find a place to get gas so many long, long walks were encountered on their trip. She described the drive in her 1916 book *By Motor to the Golden Gate*.

> Of course, if we had had a breakdown, we would have been marooned out in a wilderness! No living being knew our whereabouts and we might quite easily have been dust before anyone would have passed our way.

Emily suffered chronic insomnia and her snoring could be heard by people walking along the street outside. She didn't warn people about her snoring but she gave good advice for the host to try out the guest bed first to be sure someone can sleep in it.

In 1916, writer Ernest Hemingway's mother had a 1916 Detroit electric car. They were easier for ladies to drive because they didn't have to be cranked to start. Thomas Edison developed a battery-powered car. In those days, there were few paved roads connecting cities so only horses or gas-propelled cars could drive longer distances.

Another automobile driver was Judge Harry Truman (later United States president). He lived in Kansas City where he was elected president of the National Old Trails Road Association in 1925, after selling an extraordinary number of memberships in the Kansas City Automobile Club. His campaign for county judge was conducted by driving around the state and talking face to face with people. The western half of the National Old Trails Road was designated as Route 66.

After Bess and Harry Truman left the White House upon Eisenhower's inauguration, they took a long driving trip through several states. Harry made a special point of not being a drowsy driver as described in a 2009 book by Matthew Algeo—*Harry Truman's Excellent Adventure: The True Story of the Great American Road Trip*. Bess rewarded Harry when they returned home from trips. He either got a martini or this pudding—a sweet for the evening after dinner, with all the right ingredients for a good night's sleep.

Harry Truman Ozark Pudding

1 egg
¾ cup sugar
2 tablespoons all-purpose flour
1 ¼ teaspoon baking powder
¼ teaspoon salt
½ cup chopped peeled apples
½ cup chopped nuts
1 teaspoon vanilla extract
Whipped cream with a touch of rum or vanilla ice cream

Preheat the oven to 350 degrees. Grease a 10-inch pie pan. Beat the egg and sugar together until smooth. Add the flour, baking powder and salt. Blend well. Fold in the apples, nuts and vanilla. Pour into the pie pan and bake for 30-35 minutes. Remove from the oven. The pudding will fall, but it's supposed to. Serve with whipped cream or ice cream if desired.

The Economy of Electric and Self-Driving Cars

The current research in self-driving cars is propelled by the fact that 94% of car wrecks are human errors. The recent introduction of UBER and LYFT have reduced accidents. People use their cell phone to call for a ride when they cannot drive for one reason or another—often because they are too sleepy. We have the capability for cars and trucks to detect drowsiness, but it is little used in private vehicles. However, since two-thirds of the cost of a trip is the driver, UBER and LYFT could save money and reduce accidents if cars could be programmed to drive safely.

Self-driving cars would reduce hot takeoffs, they would handle night vision better than human drivers, and they could detect traffic signs and lights. But can they understand a duck crossing sign or calculate rules of the road which change from place to place. Suppose a street was re-tarred covering lane markings. Could a self-driving car safely negotiate its route? What about directional cones and signs with arrows?

Do self-driving cars fill a pressing need? Are they economically viable? Are there unintended consequences? We've had self-driving vehicles for a long time. We've had elevators without drivers, Disney monorails without drivers, Amazon workforce robots that move merchandise rather than having human pickers and packers.

Self-driving cars are being built to match a human brain. But they need to know how to do updates and downloads at the right time and place. There are legal concerns. If a policeman directs traffic at an intersection, how must the car be programmed to be reliable and trusted?

In 1987, a famous race in Australia from Darwin to Adelaide (2000 miles) was held using solar powered cars. General Motors entered and won the SunRayce, as the driver whizzed by Ayers Rock, camels and kangaroos.

It will probably be 10 to 20 years before a 50-50 mix of humans and robots are driving cars. Meanwhile, sensors can be added to cars such as cruise control, GPS, drowsiness detectors, a foot vibrator for cars driving to the left or to the right of the designated lane, etc. Contraptions could be placed on the top or the sides of cars with these sensors. But how could we prevent hackers from taking over steering, horns, brakes, PIN numbers to start a car, a computer shutdown at 70 miles per hour, etc. For now, we must go with what we've got in technology.

Drowsy driving can be fatal to the driver, others in the car, and others who may be hit by an impaired driver. "Drowsy Driving and Automobile Crashes" is a 2016 publication put together by an expert panel on Driver Fatigue and Sleepiness sponsored by the National Center on Sleep Disorders Research and the National Highway Traffic Safety Administration. The document was designed to provide direction for an educational campaign to combat drowsy driving and is available on-line.

How and When Do Drowsy Driving Crashes Occur?

Sleepiness causes auto crashes because it impairs performance and can ultimately lead to the inability to resist falling asleep at the wheel. How do detectives know that a crash is related to sleepiness? Such a crash occurs during the late night/early morning or midafternoon. It is likely to be serious. The vehicle leaves the roadway. The crash occurs on a high-speed road. The driver doesn't attempt to avoid a crash by braking. The driver is usually alone in the vehicle. Those characteristics lead to the presumption of an accident caused by sleep deprivation.

The 2016 Drowsy Driving document above was aimed at young males ages sixteen to twenty-four. The goal was to reduce risks, promote rumble strips; and educate drivers about the dangers of drowsy driving. The National Sleep Foundation has set the second week of November as Drowsy Driving Prevention Week to educate the public about the hazards of driving while sleepy. This week was selected because it precedes two holidays where considerable long-distance driving occurs.

Most drowsy drivers have sleep loss, may have taken a sedating medication, have untreated sleep disorders, and may have consumed alcohol or other drugs. Males are five times more likely than females to be involved in drowsy-driving crashes. These may be due to their macho ideas about being tough despite fatigue.

Perhaps the most famous song about drowsy driving is *Show Me the Way to Go Home* written in 1925 by Jimmy Campbell and Reg Connelly.

> Show me the way to go home,
> I'm tired and I want to go to bed.
> Had a little drink about an hour ago
> And it went right to my head.
>
> Wherever I may roam
> O'er land or sea or foam,
> You always hear my singing this song
> Show me the way to go home.

Jaws, starring Richard Dreyfuss, Robert Shaw and Roy Scheider, featured that song. The three of them were getting tipsy singing the song on their boat just before a horrendous Great White Shark attacked them. That song has been sung on many a ride home where a group has been drinking or are wearied from activities.

Sleep researcher William Dement said: "We're beginning to realize that drowsiness or sleep deprivation fatigue is beginning to outstrip alcohol as a cause of accidents in transportation, particularly on the highway."

The National Highway Traffic Safety Administration (NHTSA) reported an increased number of people who died in vehicles during 2015. The deaths in 2014 were 32,675. In 2015 they were 9.3% higher at 35,200. This was the first increase since 2008 (37,423 deaths from driving). NHTSA believed the recent increase is due to low fuel costs and distractions by mobile devices. In 2008, the increase had less to do with mobile devices and more to do with such a bad economy that people gave up foreign trips in favor of driving to vacation spots in America.

Who Has Tried to Prevent Drowsy Driving Accidents?

President Dwight D. Eisenhower took office in 1953 and came to office with a goal in mind. In his book *At Ease,* he wrote about German roads and autobahn 4-lane highways as the model of how traffic accidents could be reduced. This led to the interstate highway system in the United States.

The main highway countermeasures to keep auto drivers awake are the rumble strips that create a noise and vibration that wake up drowsy drivers. In 1997, it was estimated that rumble strips reduced drive-off the road crashes by 30 to 50%, according to the National Sleep Foundation. Drivers should react to the rumble by pulling over somewhere to get some sleep and/or quickly get about two cups of coffee.

Various state Departments of Transportation have designed alerts for drivers with attention-getting comments. In 2016, the Arizona Department of Transportation used the "Star Wars" theme on lighted announcements to drivers. Examples are: "Trust the Force but always buckle up!" "Aggressive driving is the path to the dark side!" "Toast away this New Year. Just don't get behind the wheel toasted." "We've got a fever and the only cure is sober drivers." Other departments use announcements like "Join the rebellion against distracted driving!"

Physical discomfort may also keep sleepy drivers awake but few drivers want to create an uncomfortable seat position or turn on the air conditioner to the point of shivering. Brief exercise such as getting out of the car and walking around for a few minutes, or listening to the car radio may help some. Talking on a cell phone might be presumed to help but has been associated with increased crash risk.

That advice might have prevented a recent accident when a truck driver caused a fatal accident in Tennessee. The National Transportation Safety Board (NTSB) announced on October 4, 2016, that a semi-tractor-trailer driver's fatigue contributed to a 2015 multi-vehicle crash near Chattanooga, Tennessee, in which six people died and four were injured.

Despite the truck driver having an opportunity for overnight rest before the crash, he went without sustained rest for 40 hours prior to the accident. He did not respond to slowed traffic caused by a lane closure in a road construction work zone. He maintained a speed of 78-82 mph before slamming into the rear of a car. The truck continued forward and collided with seven additional vehicles, forcing them into subsequent collisions. A post-crash fire consumed one vehicle. Reducing fatigue-related accidents is one of the priorities identified on the NTSB's 2016 Most Wanted List.

A recent study of teen-age crashes caught on camera was published in June 2016 by the AAA Foundation for Traffic Safety entitled "Using Naturalistic Driving Data to Examine Teen Driver Behaviors Present in Motor Vehicle Crashes, 2007-2015." The survey covered drivers aged sixteen to nineteen in eight states. Some 8,228 crashes were culled and 2,229 were studied in depth. Crashes involved 51.3% of male drivers and 48.5% female. What happened during the six seconds before the crash? Those distractions ranked highest were: talking to a passenger, adjusting a radio, eating or drinking, talking on a cell phone, reading text/e-mail, and sending text/e-mail.

There were fewer crashes with passengers in the car during 2015 than in 2007. More crashes (71.5%) occurred during the week rather than on the weekend. More crashes occurred from 3:00 p.m.

to 6:00 p.m. (26%) followed by 6:00 to 9:00 am (18.8%)—rush hours. In 2008, 83% of those had a basic cell phone. In 2015, 92% had a cell phone and 76% had a smartphone with e-mail capability. More were looking at and touching their cell phones to send and receive text in 2015 whereas in 2007 they were mainly talking and listening to a cell phone. The issue of drowsy driving occurred more with those teenagers alone in their car. Researchers keep concluding that driving alone is more dangerous than driving with a companion.

Car movies have shown changes through the years. A Stephen King 1983 horror movie called *Christine* depicted a nerdy teenager who becomes the coolest guy around as he restores an old 1958 Plymouth Fury. When a bully defaces Christine, the car exacts its revenge. Thus responsibility for the car's harm to others was transferred away from the teen onto the evil car. That is not the right message for a teen who must bear responsibility for what his car does.

Sleep and Danica Patrick

One young woman began her driving career at the age of ten while racing go-karts with her sister. Danica Patrick continued to race and won numerous titles including World Kart Association Grand National Championship at age 12, 14 and 15.

As a child, Danica dreamed of animals with claws chasing her and moving too fast for them to catch her. Speed became her goal. She dropped out of high school in her junior year and moved to England to learn stock car competition. Danica Patrick was the first woman race car driver in NASCAR's 64-year history. She won the 2008 Indy in Japan, was 3rd in the 2009 Indianapolis 500, and 8th in the 2013 Daytona 500.

This beautiful young woman uses healthy smoothies and dishes to give her "go power" and rest between competitions. Her Breakfast Hash recipe provided by NASCAR is the kind of meal that could be eaten morning, noon or night (but not before driving). It has ingredients to trigger sleep-inducing melatonin production in the brain. She placed this recipe online.

Danica Patrick Breakfast Hash

2 sweet potatoes, diced
1 apple, diced
1 red bell pepper, diced
1 bunch kale, chopped
1 lb. lean ground turkey
1 tablespoon coconut oil
½ teaspoon dried sage
½ teaspoon dried thyme
1 teaspoon dried rosemary
½ teaspoon sea salt
½ teaspoon ground black pepper
Fried egg, optional
Sliced avocado, optional

Sauté the diced sweet potatoes in a pan with 1 tablespoon of coconut oil. Add sea salt. In another pan, sauté the diced apple and red bell pepper until slightly softened. Add the chopped kale and cook until it's wilted, then combine the mixture with the sweet potatoes. Re-use the pan to cook the ground turkey and season with sage, thyme, rosemary, sea salt and ground black pepper. Combine the meat with the potato mixture, stir and serve. Add the fried egg and avocado if desired.

Movies with car chase scenes may be of interest to car buffs but they neglect to say anything about sleep. The 1968 *Bullitt* starring Steve McQueen as a San Francisco detective shows him racing around Russian Hill and Pacific Heights in a 1968 Dodge Charger 440 Magnum and a 1968 Mustang. Don't even think of counting the accidents when John Belushi and Dan Akroyd are chased by cops in the 1980 hit--*The Blues Brothers*.

Sleep and Carroll Shelby

Carroll Shelby was a race car driver who designed the Mustang. He first invented the Cobra from a dream. Shelby dreamt that the name "Cobra" appeared on the front of his car. "I woke up and jotted the name down on a pad which I kept by my bedside—a sort of ideas pad—and went back to sleep," he said. "Next morning when I looked at the name 'Cobra', I knew it was right."

A heart defect treated with medicines that induce sleepiness caused Shelby to quit racing but he trusted other drivers to carry his cars to victory. In January, 1963, Cobras won first and second place at Riverside, beating the Corvette Stingrays. By March, 1964, Ford officials met with him to develop a big black Cobra. The Cobras won the 24 hour Le Mans in June, 1964. Ford asked Shelby to develop a high-performance Mustang fastback to challenge the Corvette. The first 1965 Shelby Mustangs were built and they won at Daytona that year.

Shelby held his first chili cook-off in 1965 at Terlingua, Texas, as well. Carroll's daughter, Sharon Anne Shelby, married Larry Lavine. Larry was so impressed by the chili cook-off idea that he created Chili's Restaurant. The first Chili's opened in 1975 one block from Presbyterian Hospital in Dallas on Greenville Avenue near my medical office and I was present at the opening. The restaurant had mostly stand-up counters to place your sandwich or chili and drinks, over a floor covered with straw. With few seats, people freely moved about the restaurant. It was a meet and greet place in the beginning. It opened with a limited menu of chili, burgers and condiments to go with them. Pictures on the walls showed the Terlingua, Texas; chili cook-offs attended by Sharon and Larry Lavine and put on by Carroll and his backers.

Carroll Shelby died in 2012 but his legacy lives on in the classic Mustang and the Chili's restaurants, now owned by the Norman Brinker firm who bought out Larry Lavine. Brinker was first married to tennis star Maureen Connelly who died of cancer. He later married Cindy Brinker whose cancer started the pink ribbon campaigns to bring cancer awareness. Brinker's company continued after his death to promote Chili's and all restaurants continue to display photographs from Terlingua and other chili cook-offs.

My son-in-law, Alan Cheney, Ph.D., who is serving as my co-editor, has been a psychologist and trainer for the Chili's Corporation in his capacity as an organizational psychologist. He and his lovely wife of some forty years, Deidre, had some of their first dates in that original Chili's Restaurant.

I knew Larry and Sharon Lavine during their time at the Greenville Avenue restaurant in Dallas during the 1970s. Here is Carroll's own chili recipe which contains a good amount of tryptophan to produce melatonin which will promote sleep. He used to pass this recipe around, but later the family made it into a chili kit which can be bought. Follow this meal with a Texas pecan praline for the sweet and you'll fall into a Texas twilight sleep.

Carroll Shelby Chili

¼ lb. suet or ¼ cup cooking oil
1 lb. beef round steak, coarse ground
1 lb. beef chuck, coarse ground
8 ounce can tomato sauce
12 ounces of beer
2 tablespoons crushed red chili peppers
2 medium garlic cloves, minced
1 small onion, finely chopped
1 ¼ teaspoons diced oregano (preferably Mexican)
½ teaspoon paprika
1 ½ teaspoons ground cumin
1 ¼ teaspoons salt
1/8 teaspoon cayenne pepper
¾ lb. Monterey jack cheese, grated

Melt suet or heat oil in a heavy 3-quart pot over medium-high heat. Remove the suet and crumble meat into the pot. Break up any lumps with a fork and cook, stirring occasionally, until meat is evenly browned. Add tomato sauce, beer, crushed chili, garlic, onion, oregano, paprika, 1 teaspoon of the cumin, and salt. Stir to blend and bring to a boil. Lower heat and simmer uncovered, stirring occasionally, for one hour.

Taste and adjust seasonings, adding cayenne pepper. Simmer uncovered one hour longer. Stir in the cheese and the remaining ½ teaspoon cumin. Simmer ½ hour longer, stirring often to keep cheese from burning. Serve the chili with sour cream and shredded cheddar cheese to garnish, and warm cornbread on the side. Serves six.

Sleep and Paul Newman

Paul Newman was an accomplished movie actor but also enjoyed driving race cars. He won four national championships in racing and won second place in the 24 hours of Le Mans in 1979. The actor participated in some other important competitions such as the 24 Hour Daytona in 1995. Newman competed into his 80s despite having much time consumed by his acting career and charity work. His son was injured in a motorcycle accident while under the influence of drugs and/or alcohol. The son died two months later at age 28 of a drug overdose of pain killers, narcotics, and booze.

Paul Newman created a treatment center for young people on drugs. By the time he died, through his food enterprise with author A. E. Hotchner, Newman had contributed $250 million to various charities.

Paul Newman liked racing but thought food and pictures were more thrilling. "With a film or a recipe, there is no way of knowing how all the ingredients will work out in the end," he said.

The 2006 animated movie called *Cars* used Owen Wilson's voice for a race car that damaged a town road while driving in a race. Sentenced to repair the road before he can leave the town, the car learns some life lessons from the Fabulous Hudson Hornet car using Paul Newman's voice. *Cars* was the last and highest-grossing movie of Newman's career.

Newman was known for his altruism and his wish to help teens learn safe driving. He came out of retirement to do a documentary honoring Dale Earnhardt who died on February 18, 2001, in the Daytona 500 final lap at age 49. Newman was posthumously inducted into the SCCA Hall of Fame in 2009 after his death at age 83. He also served as an ordained minister of the Universal Life Church. He liked hamburgers and followed by a bit of something sweet, a person might enjoy a good night's sleep. He had an interesting method of creating a hamburger.

Paul Newman Hamburger

Paul took ground chuck and formed it into hamburger patties by tossing meat from hand to hand to keep it fluffy. He never patted down the meat. He never put seasonings in the meat before cooking. He never added onions, eggs, bread crumbs, or any other ingredient like steak sauce. He greased the grill with vegetable oil and when hot, seared the burgers well on one side and then the other. Then he lowered the grill and never turned them again until they were seared enough to suit him. His hamburger was crisp outside and "tomato-red" inside.

One of the top stock car champions was Richard Petty, nicknamed the "King of Horsepower." Petty kept trim and slim by getting enough rest to avoid being sleep-deprived as so many racers were. This Petty recipe for a night-time treat gives you room for your own preferences.

Richard Petty Angel Food Cake

Make your favorite angel food cake but sift your all-purpose flour four times to make it really light. Then top the finished cake with smashed berries or fruit.

Ariana Huffington and Her Sleep Revolution

Greek American author and columnist Arianna Huffington of *The Huffington Post* has made great efforts to end drowsy driving. She wrote *The Sleep Revolution* in 2016 detailing her own problems with sleep deprivation when, despite lots of coffee, she got sleepy while checking e-mails and messages. She fell, breaking her cheekbone against her desk and damaging her face badly. Her book included recommendations to reduce sleep deprivation. She said: "After my own collapse from sleep deprivation, I became an all-out sleep evangelist."

In 2016, her company teamed up with Uber and Toyota to raise awareness of drowsy driving and help save lives. The *Huffington Post* article on April 5, 2016, cited research showing that crashes kill 8,000 people per year. They mentioned one study that found being awake for 17 to 19 hours causes cognitive impairment equal to having a blood alcohol level well beyond being legally drunk.

July 4 is the deadliest day of the year for driving-related fatalities. The worst year was 2013 when 32,894 people died in vehicle crashes in the USA, which was by far the highest rate of most countries in the world. Alcohol-impaired driving caused a third of the US crashes.

Furthermore, the USA has one of the lowest rankings for use of seat beats, with only 87% of car users using front-seat belts and 78% using rear-seat belts. The CDC estimated that 3,000 lives could be saved by increasing seat-belt use to 100%. They added that up to 10,000 lives could be saved by eliminating alcohol-impaired driving. The implementation of seat-belt laws that cover all occupants, publicized sobriety checkpoints, and lower limits for blood alcohol intoxication could lower deaths caused by traffic accidents.

Diane Holloway Cheney, Ph.D.

Sleep and Cole Porter

Popular music composer Cole Porter (1891-1973) and his millionaire wife Linda traveled about the world until he fell under his horse and suffered two terribly broken and damaged legs, requiring the amputation of one leg. Following that surgery, he never wrote another song and lived on alcohol, narcotics, and sleeping pills until his death. But during his musical career, he was gay and wrote about the fast life including fast cars. In his song, *Anything Goes,* he had the following lines:

Anything goes.
If driving fast cars you like, If low bars you like,
If old hymns you like, If bare limbs you like,
If Mae West you like, Or me undressed you like,
Why, nobody will oppose. Anything goes.

In his song, *I Get a Kick Out of You,* he wrote about getting a kick with champagne, cocaine, on a plane, and this was typical of his fast life in 1920s and 1930s high society. Often, censors changed the words of his songs and they extracted the word cocaine from these lyrics:

Some get a kick from cocaine, I'm sure that if I took even one sniff
That would bore me terrific'ly too, Yet I get a kick out of you!

He also wrote a song called *I Sleep Easier Now* featured in the 1950 musical *Out of This World.* It was to be sung by an aging female who described how she used to be younger, cuter, prettier, but in old age she sang "I sleep easier now!" This recipe, probably prepared by his cook, provided a tryptophan meal. It could be followed with a sweet that produces melatonin for a good night's sleep.

This recipe was in the 1942 book *Sincerely Yours,* with recipes collected by Bess Borden. I own one copy of this very rare book from the 750 copies made, with proceeds going toward war relief. It was published by Grabhorn Press which ceased to exist in 1965.

Cole Porter Kedgeree (Fish Dish)

1 cup boiled halibut or codfish
2 tablespoons rice, cooked
4 hard-boiled eggs
2 tablespoons of butter
1 teaspoon chopped parsley
Salt and pepper to taste

Break fish in small pieces, chop up the eggs, put the butter in a saucepan. When melted, add all the other ingredients. Simmer for ten minutes and serve.

Drug Abuse Testing of Drowsy Drivers

New challenges for police officers have created new methods to prevent impaired driving. The number of drivers involved in fatal motor vehicle crashes who tested positive for drugs increased from 28% in 2005 to 32% in 2012. Why?

First, the U.S. population is aging and becoming more dependent on prescription medicines which can impair drivers. Second, more states have legalized cannabis for medical or recreational purposes. The National Highway Traffic Safety Administration reported that the rate of THC (tetrahydrocannabinol—the ingredient of marijuana that gives the "high") in drivers almost doubled from 7.8% prior to cannabis legalization in Washington State to 18.9%, one year after legalization.

Drivers under the influence of cannabis tend to think they are better drivers because they drive more slowly; however, their reaction time is also affected. Cocaine and amphetamines may sharpen the reaction time of drivers, but those substances increase high-risk behavior such as speeding. Pain medications such as hydrocodone and oxycodone can cause drowsiness, especially at the beginning of treatment cycles.

Law enforcement jurisdictions have responded by developing screening kits to identify drivers and collect biological specimens for laboratory testing. They are using a cheek swab to verify oral fluids. This is far less intrusive, dangerous, and painful than blood testing. This type of testing was legitimized under the Fourth Amendment wherein a person's identity through DNA testing is a legitimate police-booking procedure. On-site oral fluid testing is now recommended to replace blood and urine testing, since those tests require a warrant.

Driving Nuclear Bombs Across America

We do not want drowsy drivers carrying military weapons across the country on our roads. However, President Donald Trump has asked Congress to approve a remarkable increase in military weapons. Atomic weapons are hauled in unmarked trucks across the United States every day. They carry warheads from missile silos and bomber bases to nuclear weapons labs operated by the U.S. Department of Energy under the Office of Secure Transportation. This agency operates 42 tractor-trailers guarded by armed couriers as they pass through our cities—without any incidents, so far. Many of these special drivers and guards served in the Iraq and Afghanistan wars.

This brief history of the agency shows a problem in need of more answers. The agency has been dealing with forced overtime, high driver turnover, old trucks, and poor worker morale. The Soviet Union break-up in 1991 diminished the threat of nuclear attack. The U.S. reduced its nuclear stockpile and the budget was lowered. Despite staffing shortages and aging trucks, accidents have not occurred. However, long working hours led to morale problems and management inadequacies.

The agency is undermanned and more than one-third of the workforce has been putting in more than 900 hours a year of overtime. In 2010, the Energy Department inspector found widespread alcohol use and 16 alcohol-related incidents over three years. Half the trucks are over fifteen years old and were designed before current terrorist threats.

Despite these problems, each weapon requires routine inspection, testing, and maintenance, and that is accomplished by bringing the weapons to the workers who perform those services. So, the weapons are transported to the Pantex Plant near Amarillo, Texas, from 450 silos across the country. From there, pieces are taken to various other plants for work and then returned to Texas and finally returned to their silos.

The trucks contain thick walls and axles designed to explode to prevent a trailer from being towed away. The security officers in front and behind such trucks must pass yearly psychological and medical evaluations. The work is tiring, involving long hours on the road under a constant state of high alert. Tensions mount and a 2014 report showed that a supervisor had been involved in seven verbal and physical incidents with uncontrolled anger and aggression toward fellow workers.

Thus far, the agency request for an increase in funds was not approved and their funding is very limited. New trailers are not expected to be available until 2023 and this disturbing information illustrates, among many things, the great need for adequate sleep by employees who bear such a large responsibility for the safety of our country. Of course, the worst-case scenario would be a terrorist group hijacking a truck and obtaining a multi-kiloton atomic bomb. The responsibility of these drivers, and all drivers, is to be sure that they do not cause accidents and harm.

Should Others Suffer from Your Sleep Problems?

Humorist Will Rogers said, "When I die, I want to die like my grandfather who died peacefully in his sleep. Not screaming like all the passengers in his car."

Those who transport others must consider their precious cargo in addition to themselves. The National Sleep Foundation conducted a poll in 2012 of pilots, truck drivers, train operators and taxi/bus/limo drivers. The majority (80%) were white males between the ages of 26 and 78 (average age forty-nine to fifty years). The study included 202 pilots, 203 truck drivers, 180 train operators, 164 bus drivers, and 46 taxi drivers.

Some 23% of the drivers believed that sleep affected their job performance at least once a week! Some 11% reported a "near miss" due to sleepiness, 20% reported serious errors at work due to sleepiness, and 6% reported having had a car accident going to or from work due to sleepiness.

Who are the villains? They are those of us who ignore the responsibility to convey people safely. If we give ourselves excuses to do unjust things, we must expect blame. It is human nature to be angry at the perpetrator when a driving accident has resulted in harm to others.

Will Electric Cars Reduce Drowsy Driver Accidents?

Hal Lind is a local celebrity and designer of military radios and satellite communications, a chief scientist for Hughes Communications Division, a team member of the GM SunRaycer solar car project in Australia, and consultant for the GM-Chevy Racing Team. He contributed this information to our understanding of electric cars and drowsy drivers.

The automobile has been important to the United States since its origin. It gives us freedom, fun, power, and helps us view the magnificent parks and sites in our country on vacations. Cars introduced more rapid transportation than we had before them and they are affordable. The newest cars have sensors that adjust speed based on the traffic in front of them. In fact, the car may slow down, brake, or change lanes to avoid collisions in one 2017 Mercedes-Benz model.

As we move into the future, some cars will emit warnings when they detect, by cameras or sensors, that a driver is getting sleepy.

Future cars might take over for drowsy drivers and pull to the side of the road and shut down. If a car senses that a driver's eye-blinking increases, or respirations and heart rate change dramatically (such as in a heart attack or unconsciousness) it could even shift into self-driving mode.

Until new innovations and safer driverless cars evolve, drivers must heed warnings, use rumble strip vibrations to increase alertness, pull over when sleepy, and get rides from taxis or UBER or LYFT or friends instead of driving. Responsible drivers will consider themselves, those they transport, and those on the road who could be impacted in a crash.

Electric cars (self-driving cars) have more limited mileage than gas cars so drivers may have "range anxiety." They may wonder "how far can I go before it runs out of power?" The cars of 2017 can go 200 miles so range anxiety has been reduced. They are much cheaper to operate than gas-fueled cars (four cents a mile for electric). Self-driving cars could reduce our dependence upon foreign oil by 30 to 60 percent. They could lower the carbon pollution from the transportation sector by as much as 20 percent, say some.

Sleep deprivation can cause small or large accidents where hundreds of people, pets, or other creatures on the road can be affected, in addition to gigantic costs for repairs and insurance claims. Sleep loss is so important that laws and requirements have been passed in the last ten years affecting many who operate dangerous machinery. The next chapter summarizes some of the largest catastrophes where all or part of the accident came from sleep deprivation and resulting fatigue.

Chapter Ten
CATASTROPHES AND SLEEP DEPRIVATION

A number of catastrophes have been blamed on sleep deprived workers. The problems of sleep deprivation affect so many people and so many parts of life. What can be learned about sleep deprivation so that we can prevent disasters that have occurred in the past? Certainly, all human errors occurring in these incidents did not result only from lowered alertness or inattention due to sleep-related processes. But it appears that the serious accidents were made worse by inadequate human response at times when sleepiness would have been greatest.

The following descriptions of major catastrophes have been widely publicized and some of them were experienced by television viewers. These terrible accidents help us understand the role of sleepiness when complex machinery must be manipulated by human workers.

Three Mile Island Nuclear Reactor 1979

On March 28, 1979, employees at Three Mile Island Nuclear (TMI) reactor near Middletown, Pennsylvania, failed to notice loss of coolant in the early morning at 3:56 a.m. The crew was confused by some readings and it took the next work shift coming on duty to identify the problem. By the time they discovered that the problem was a stuck valve, half the nuclear reactor's core had melted. Cleanup took twelve years and cost one billion dollars. This was the worst nuclear disaster in the United States to date and had many consequences.

Hundreds of people reported metallic taste, hair loss, skin redness/rash, nausea, vomiting, diarrhea, death of pets, animals and plants. In the beginning, they were told that these were symptoms of psychological stress. However, the fear of possible cancer caused the Pennsylvania Department of Health to monitor 30,000+ people within five miles of TMI for eighteen years. By the end of the study, no evidence of health problems was reported and the amount of radiation received was never admitted. TMI was restarted in 1985 without using the bad unit. A new training program, accident scenarios, event reporting, discipline, teamwork and communications were stressed.

Despite these improvements, in 1987 two TMI shift operators were fired for sleeping on the job. In 1988, more employees were fired for drinking and doing drugs on the job. Another employee was fired July 31, 1990 for sleeping on shift and being inattentive to his duties. By June 1991, Columbia University published in the *American Journal of Public Health* that cancers in the Three Mile Island area were four times the number before the accident. Dot after improbable dot connected.

The plant owners had paid $40 million in medical claims for people, pets, animals, plants and $1.2 million for one child born with Down's Syndrome. Legal battles continued for years.

Rancho Seco Nuclear Reactor

On December 26, 1985, the Rancho Seco nuclear reactor near Sacramento, California, automatically tripped after power to the control system was lost at 4:14 a.m. It became the third fastest shutdown in United States reactor history due to a control circuit malfunction. The sudden temperature change could have cracked the reactor vessel and led to a meltdown. Sacramento residents called for a study of the safety of Rancho Seco.

The board convened to investigate and chose their words carefully, mindful of how many people would see their report. They wrote: Rancho Seco was "mismanaged, mismaintained, and misoperated" since its beginning. Two Rancho Seco workers were fired for drug use. Sacramento Municipal Utility District (SMUD) claimed there was drug abuse throughout the plant. The Chief of Nuclear Operations was fired in 1987 and Rancho Seco was shut down in 1989.

Space Shuttle Challenger 1986

On January 28, 1986, the Space Shuttle Challenger was launched from the Kennedy Space Center. The huge crowd grinned as they watched the launch. The Shuttle exploded 73 seconds after lift-off at 11:39 a.m. killing seven crew members. Mouths dropped, tears ran down faces. More people than usual (17% of Americans) were watching on television because school teacher Christa McAuliffe was going to teach some lessons from space to students. The astronauts weren't robots to those watching—they were vulnerable humans.

The last word recorded on the crew voice recorder was astronaut Mike Smith saying "Uh-oh!" The astronauts did not die immediately because some of them activated their oxygen packs on the final plunge. It was assumed that all were killed upon capsule impact with the ocean.

There had been work problems earlier. In 1984, 117 incidents occurred at the Kennedy Space Center and 51.3% were termed human error. In 1985, 147 incidents occurred and 56.5% were attributed to human error. On January 6, 1986, three weeks before the Challenger launch, a near-catastrophic launch of the Shuttle Columbia occurred when console operators at Kennedy Space Center inadvertently drained 18,000 pounds of liquid oxygen from the shuttle tank within five minutes of scheduled launch time. The liquid oxygen loss went undetected until the mission was cancelled only 31 seconds before liftoff. Operator fatigue was reported as one of the major factors contributing to this incident. The operators had been on duty for 11 hours. It was their third day of working on a 12-hour night shift.

The Challenger explosion was caused by O-rings that became brittle under colder than normal night temperatures in Florida on that fateful January morning. At the point of breaking the sound barrier, hot gas escaped from the booster impinging powerfully on the strut connecting the booster and the rocket. Hydrogen gas streamed from the fuel tank as the explosion ripped the capsule from the rocket.

The omission of temperature checks and discussions of postponing the launch to re-check O-rings at the colder temperatures were critical factors. Those omissions cost the lives of the crew, a loss of millions of dollars, and delayed space projects for three years. Condensation had been noted to issue during previous tests but was over-looked because nothing critical happened, and there was a "Go mentality!"

Was there sleep deprivation? The 40-hour week plus 20-hour overtime limit was exceeded 480 times by Thiokol employees and 2,512 times by Lockheed employees. There was no system at Kennedy for monitoring overtime from the safety perspective. Examples of employees who worked consecutive 12-hour days were rampant. Many of these were shift employees despite the fact that shift changes often take employees a week to adjust to the new times.

The 1988 report of the Presidential Commission on the Space Shuttle Challenger Accident under human factors stated that "The willingness of NASA employees in general to work excessive hours, while admirable, raises serious questions when it jeopardizes job performance, particularly when critical management decisions are at stake." They concluded, "An evaluation by National Aeronautics and Space Administration (NASA) of the consequences of work schedules should be conducted as part of its effort to reform its launch and operation procedures."

Christa McAuliffe continued to touch futures as her students at Concord High School class of '86 petitioned the Obama administration to have a national holiday named for McAuliffe and the Challenger crew. Concord, New Hampshire, a city of about 42,000, built and named a planetarium for McAuliffe, 37 when she died. It was later re-named the McAuliffe-Shepard Discovery Center, recognizing native son Alan Shepard, the first American in space. Just a few years ago, the city of Concord named an elementary school for Christa.

The city has been low-key on marking Challenger anniversaries as families of the victims in Concord grew up. Today, both Christa's children are educators with children of their own. She inspired generations of classroom teachers and students, and her death focused public attention on the critical importance of teachers to our nation's well-being.

Chernobyl Nuclear Reactor in the Ukraine 1986

Three months after the Challenger disaster, the worst nuclear disaster ever occurred in Chernobyl in the Ukraine in its secret Mayak plutonium manufacturing site. On April 26, 1986, a sudden surge of power during a systems test destroyed a nuclear reactor at 1:23 a.m. This caused a fire that released radiation into the environment. Thirty workers died and 300,000 were evacuated. Engineers who had been working 13 hours were running the plant at low power and failed to coordinate the systems tests with other safety personnel.

On a trip to Budapest, Hungary, two weeks after Chernobyl, my husband and I learned from many Hungarians how worried they were about the radioactive fallout on crops. We purchased strawberries from a local market and got on the bus eating them when the driver said: "No, no, you need wash them. Zey haf poison!. You vill glow in ze dark!"

Our guide said that his wife was pregnant and they were very worried about whether their child would suffer from the radioactivity that had spread across all of Europe. The initial plume on April 29-30, 1986, drifted toward Hungary and the last release during May 5-7, 1986, was directed to Romania, Bulgaria and Greece. The contamination of soil surface and vegetation were strongest in Budapest. One of the worst consequences was the contamination of the Techa River. Many villages had to be evacuated and the entire flood plain became an unintentional laboratory for long-term radiation exposure in animals and humans.

Ten years after the event, a Budapest Chernobyl Day commemoration gave citizens the opportunity to reflect upon the event and how the air they breathed, the food they ate, and the water they drank was a major threat. It caused a collapse of everyday life. They vowed "No more Chernobyls!" Fifteen years later, the isotopes were still higher than normal in that area.

The tragedies caused by sleep deprivation are serious, indeed. So many lives lost, so much damage, such huge expense. To swallow all this, we will insert moments of relief which were not afforded to victims. At the harshest moments in our lives, humor and distraction give a needed rest before proceeding since a bit of levity heightens one's sense of survival and preserves one's sanity.

Hungary was the birthplace of beautiful actresses Eva and Zsa Zsa Gabor. Eva was the aristocrat on the *Green Acres* TV series with Eddie Albert years ago. Zsa Zsa is most famous for her nine marriages, which included her favorites, British actor George Sanders, and hotel magnate Conrad Hilton. Both show-business sisters had goulash recipes but we are choosing Zsa Zsa's. Conrad Hilton was the great grandfather of media star Paris Hilton.

I saw Zsa Zsa having dinner at a Hilton Hotel in Dallas, Texas, in 1996 at the next table to me. The word "bling" must have been created for her. Her unknown male companion was considerably younger, but she looked extravagantly done up for the dinner.

She died in 2016 at age 99, and said her goulash was the dish she used to catch a man. She claimed it was for ten hungry Americans or eight dieting Hungarians but we cut her recipe in half. Did Zsa Zsa know that her dish contains the ingredients for a good night's sleep if followed by some little sweet. One of her special goulash ingredients were bits of ginger snaps.

If you make it with a Hungarian red wine, even Hungarian actor Bela Lugosi (who played Dracula in movies) would enjoy it. Of course, cooking the wine takes out the alcohol. Let us, however, remember that Dracula and Lugosi had a lot of trouble sleeping.

Zsa Zsa Gabor Goulash

Her idea was to slow boil for 1 to 1½ hours chopped up onion, pork, beef, maybe even a little sausage, sauerkraut, caraway seeds, Hungarian red paprika, olive oil or butter, salt and pepper, and red wine. At the last, drop in broken bits of ginger snaps and swirl in some sour cream in serving bowls.

Sleep and Human Errors Societies 1986

Two months after Chernobyl, the annual meeting of the Association of Professional Sleep Societies was held in Columbus, Ohio, on June 15-22, 1986. They decided to form a committee to review the role of human sleep and brain clocks in the occurrence of medical and human error catastrophes. The results of their discoveries are described in "Catastrophes, Sleep, and Public Policy: Consensus Report" by Merrill M. Mitler and colleagues published in the academic journal *Sleep* in 1988.

One major discovery by the committee was that there was a diminished capacity to function during certain early morning hours (2-7 a.m.) and to a lesser degree, during a period in the mid-afternoon (2-5 p.m.). This came from observations of those falling asleep at various times of day by Carskadon and associates. They found that even brief episodes of sleep produce inattention, forgetfulness, and performance lapses, particularly during early mornings and afternoons.

They also learned that more deaths occur between 4 and 6 a.m. and a smaller peak between 2 and 4 p.m. This was based on 50 studies by Smolensky and associates and Mitler and their associates with a total of more than 437,000 deaths due to all causes. This information caused researchers to study circadian sleep rhythms in more detail than earlier.

Exxon Valdez Oil Tanker 1989

Three years after Chernobyl, the *Exxon Valdez* oil tanker ran aground in Prince William Sound, Alaska, on March 24, 1989 at 12:04 a.m. A crewman fell asleep at the controls after working 18 hours. The spill killed 200,000 birds, 2,800 otters, 300 seals, 250 bald eagles and still leaves a mess despite clean-up. The final report was published by the State of Alaska in February, 1990. The report described a pizza party with much drinking the night of the disaster. Captain Joseph Hazelwood was so impaired that he did many things against the rules. Such attitudes by the upper echelon of command become infectious and contagious.

The third-mate who was asleep at the controls was to have been relieved but didn't wake up his crewmate, feeling sorry that the mate had little rest. There was an abundance of ineptitude then "poof", the moment to correct controls vanished!

The tanker carried 6.3 million barrels of oil and the spill has impacted tourism and livelihoods in addition to wildlife. None of the 42 crew members died but several people died and thousands were sickened by breathing toxic fumes in the clean-up. That clean-up still continues as the Alaska Oil Spill Commission tries to monitor and save various animal species and handle the remaining oil to this day.

Texas City BP Explosion 2005

On March 23, 2005, a terrible hydrocarbon vapor cloud exploded at British Petroleum (BP) in Texas City, Texas. Fifteen were killed and over 170 injured. Employees had not recognized that the vapor feed was entering their tower for three hours. One of the deceased was Eva Rowe, and her parents were very upset at the small settlement offered by BP. Ed Bradley of *CBS Sixty Minutes* publicized her case on television on November 9, 2006.

The James Baker Panel (Baker had been United States Secretary of State) was established to study the explosion. To cut costs, BP was working people for 12 hours in a 24-hour period for 29 consecutive days at the time of the accident. Employees would go home (45-60 minutes each way), take care of business and children, get 5-6 hours of sleep and return. Many did not take rest breaks at work and ate at their monitors through their shift. These problems had been communicated to Canada and London BP officials but substantive changes had not occurred.

Baker's panel noted that sleep deprivation and employee fatigue degraded their judgment and problem-solving skills. The panel described how fatigue makes people more rigid in thinking and they have greater difficulty responding to changing or abnormal circumstances. They develop a kind of fixation or tunnel vision of possible actions to be taken in emergencies.

In addition to faulty mechanical operations, Baker's panel revealed a weak safety culture without any fatigue policies, and therein lay the main problem. They recommended limiting the number of working hours in a 24-hour period and the number of consecutive days at work. The details of this event can be found in the U.S. Chemical Safety and Hazard Investigation Board Investigation Report: *Refinery Explosion and Fire*. 2007. BP was found at fault in many areas, which led to larger settlements, and finally to the sale of the refinery by 2013.

Texas food is famous because of beef but there are other Texas dishes that the Baker panel and British Petroleum employees would have eaten during their time in Texas. One of those dishes is a Texan version of yams by an old-time silent actress, known as the "orchid of the screen." Her voice did not transfer well to talk movies so she left Hollywood and married a wealthy football coach.

Corinne Griffith Texas Yams

12 cooked yams
1 ¼ lb. melted butter
1 cup brown sugar
½ cup brandy.

Slice yams. Cream the sugar and butter. Add brandy to the mixture and spread on yams in a pan. Place in 375 degree oven for 15 minutes. If you prefer crisp potato patties, roll mashed yams in chopped black walnuts, then fry patties in a skillet with just enough lard or butter to cook. Don't have greasy yams.

USS Port Royal 2009

On February 5, 2009, *USS Port Royal* ran aground in Honolulu. The Navy Safety Investigation Board reported that Captain John Carroll had slept only 15 hours in the last three nights before the accident. In addition, he had returned to his command after a five-year break from sea duty. Other problems involved broken equipment so that location and depth were unknown, alarms were ignored, and those who were supposed to be on watch were serving food due to manpower shortages. The 9,600-ton cruiser was stuck for days and the damage to the Honolulu port cost $8.5 million and ship repairs cost $40 million.

Bronx Train Derailing 2013

On December 1, 2013, a Metro-North train in the New York City's Bronx derailed killing four people and injuring more than 70 others. The sleep-deprived engineer nodded off at the controls just before taking a 30 mph curve at 82 mph. The decision was not to charge engineer William Rockefeller in the deadly crash because his sleepiness was due to undiagnosed sleep apnea and a drastic shift in his work schedule. The National Transportation Board said the railroad lacked a policy to screen engineers for sleep disorders. Furthermore, they said had a system been in place to automatically apply the brakes when an engineer nods off, the crash would have been avoided.

Diane Holloway Cheney, Ph.D.

Amtrak Crash in Philadelphia 2015

There was an Amtrak crash of a train on May 12, 2015, in Philadelphia on its way from Washington, D.C. to New York City. Engineer Brandon Bostian was distracted by radio transmissions or fatigue, and lost situational awareness. He had finished one run from New York City to Washington, D.C. but equipment had not worked properly so he had to spend over three hours carefully monitoring speed and controls. That delayed him by some 30 minutes. This erased the time he would ordinarily have for a sandwich or phone calls. When he arrived to get his assignment, an Amtrak worker said he looked "frazzled."

He got into the train, checked controls and departed at the approved time of 7:10 p.m. This was a new assignment of only a few weeks for Bostian who very much desired this extremely busy route. The train approached a 50 mph curve at 102 mph, and crashed at 9:23 p.m. Of the train's 258 passengers and 8 employees, 8 people were killed and 200+ injured.

The final results by the National Transportation Safety Board was that the accident was preventable if a planned train control device had been installed, but its installation had been delayed. The engineer had suffered a concussion but later recalled pushing the throttle to speed up only to realize the curve was coming. He realized the crash was happening and applied the brakes too late.

In seeming retaliation, the day after the crash, the U.S. House Appropriations Committee cut Amtrak's budget by $260 million from $1.36 billion for the next fiscal year.

In March, 2016, the U.S. Department of Transportation's Federal Motor Carrier Safety Administration and the Federal Railroad Administration announced that they were seeking public input on whether commercial motor vehicle drivers should be screened for obstructive sleep apnea. They cited Bronx 2013 accident described above as the reason they were considering whether to screen, evaluate and treat federal rail workers and vehicle drivers.

Commuter Train Crash in New Jersey 2016

On September 29, 2016, a train of commuters from New York to Hoboken, New Jersey, slammed into the historic station, flying up from the tracks and causing a collapse of the depot roof onto the train wreck scene. The trip began at 7:30 a.m. in New York and crashed in Hoboken at 8:45a.m. The train held 250 passengers and 108 were injured, requiring medical treatment. The one fatality was a young woman who was hit by falling debris while waiting on the platform to catch the train.

Fabiola Bittar de Kroon, a beautiful 34-year old lawyer and mother of a 1 ½ year old little girl died at the scene. Rahman Perkins, 29, rushed over to her and stayed with her until police arrived. He explained that he didn't know where all her blood was coming from and just told her to breathe, focus on your family and loved ones, and promised he wouldn't leave her. He didn't.

Fabiola's husband, a Dutch man named Daan de Kroon, was contacted and told of his wife's demise. He rushed to pick up their toddler at a daycare past closing time, and begged the daycare manager to tell him how to explain to their child that she would never see her mother again. The victim's mother prepared to send Fabiola's body to Brazil where she was born. Governors Andrew Cuomo of New York and Chris Christie of New Jersey announced a joint investigation into why the train did not slow down. Liberals and conservatives alike fixed on the urgent need to prevent such accidents.

Fabiola came from Brazil, home of the famous soccer player Pele. His favorite dessert was fried plantains and it may have been hers as well. The same recipe could be made with bananas if plantains are not available where you live. If they are, get the blackest ones you can find to fix this delicious evening sweet for a good night's sleep.

Pele Fried Plantains

1 plantain per person, sliced across or lengthwise as you please

Fry in oil until golden brown and then drain and cool

Place sugar and a little cinnamon in a sack, then drop the pieces of plantain in the sack and shake so the plantains are somewhat sweet.

The result of the investigation of the New Jersey crash revealed that engineer Thomas Gallagher had undiagnosed sleep apnea. This disorder robs its victims of rest because they are repeatedly awakened as their airway closes and their breathing stops, leading to dangerous daytime drowsiness. Gallagher had been cleared for duty after a physical 11 months before the accident. It wasn't clear how he passed the sleep apnea screening program. The Federal Railroad Administration said it would issue a safety advisory to push railroads to address worker fatigue and accelerate the installation of inward- and outward-facing cameras.

The Federal Railroad Administration issued a safety advisory December 2, 2016, calling for mandatory sleep apnea screening and treatment. It required that engineers with severe sleep disorders should not be allowed to operate trains until they are treated. The agency also urged railroads to install inward-facing cameras in passenger train cabs to record engineers' actions and aid crash investigations. Passenger and freight rail traffic already face a December 2018 deadline to install positive-train controls. These include GPS-based technology designed to automatically slow or stop trains that are going too fast. The system can take over control of a train when an engineer is distracted or incapacitated.

Sleep problems have been found in several specific occupations and those receiving the most press coverage are usually airplane crashes. These accidents are the most closely monitored in the last 40 years because of the large number of potential victims and because of the creation of recording devices in the cockpit. Earlier pilots used their own methods of fighting off sleep problems which will be examined next.

Chapter Eleven
AVIATION AND SLEEP DEPRIVATION

Nearly a century ago, brave aviation pioneers dealt with sleep deprivation as they tried to fly long distances and set records. The probabilities of flying like birds seemed almost impossible. Those early aviators would probably be shocked to see what happened to air transportation a century later.

The first funeral I ever attended was a friend of my father who crashed in his yellow Piper Cub while flying in Tulsa, Oklahoma. I had never seen a dead person before. He was lying in a casket and Dad reached me up. I put my hand on the man's forehead and it was cold. He no longer had that big smile on his face.

William Piper had a dream in 1937 for all people to fly, or so my father told me. Dad's friend spent hours after work flying about in his 4-seater plane. In 1947, he and my father invited me to fly with them one day. I fell in love with flying. The wind in our hair, the view of land below, and the wooshing sounds were all so exciting. It was like being God and looking down upon the earth and all its beauty. This nice man showed me the controls and let me push or pull on one. Only two weeks after that flight, the man died. Dad said he heard that his friend came home, had supper and a drink, and went out to fly the plane in the evening, perhaps under the influence of alcohol. In later years, I marveled that the man's face (I can still picture it) remained intact despite the crash.

Charles Lindbergh's Sleep Deprivation

The most famous aviator of nearly 90 to 100 years ago, was Charles Lindbergh who was the first to fly from the United States to Europe. He became an international celebrity when he flew from New York to Paris, France, on May 20, 1927. Lindy took off at 7:52 a.m. with 450 gallons of fuel. As he flew through the day and night, the skinny pilot wanted to stay warm but had to keep his window open so the cold air would keep him awake. Lindbergh would fall asleep for seconds, sometimes minutes, and fought very hard to stay awake over the ocean.

Lindbergh recorded these (abridged) memories of the flight: Describing his eyes, he wrote:

My eyes feel dry and hard as stones. The lids pull down with pounds of weight against their muscles... The very exertion of staying awake exhausts. Nothing is more desirable than sleep...Not even life itself. [After being awake for 39 hours straight, he thought] "I've lost control of my eyelids. Every cell in my body is on strike...in protest, claiming that nothing, nothing in the world could be worth such effort."

He began to hallucinate. "Ghostly presences" filled the cabin behind him. Lindbergh reported: "I feel no surprise at their coming." They spoke to him in human voices. They commented on the flight and how he was handling it. They gave him messages of importance and Lindbergh felt one with them. "I'm on the borderline of life and a greater realm beyond...The feeling of flesh is gone...I'm almost one with the vapor-like forms behind me." Lindy broke an ammonia capsule (smelling salts) and brought it to his nose but sensed nothing--no sting, no tears.

Suddenly the dawn light alerted him and despite 24 hours in the air he felt a little less fatigued. Charles Lindbergh described green turf below: "I've never seen such beauty before, field so green, people so human, a village so attractive. I know how the dead would feel to live again." By the time he landed at 5:22 p.m. the intrepid young pilot had flown 33 hours and 30 minutes and been awake fifty-five hours. Determination was his special gift. Paris and, later, New York threw huge parades and celebrations for him.

Many songs were composed about Lindbergh; so many that one was called "This Song Is Not About Lindbergh." But here is part of one written by Howard Johnson and Al Sherman named "Lindbergh, the Eagle of the U.S.A." included in my book about *American History in Song*.

> In a mighty aeroplane flew a boy in search of fame,
> Far across the bounding main.
> Lindbergh! Oh what a flying fool was he
> Lindbergh! His name will live in history.

Charles Lindbergh trained himself to be as fit and healthy as possible. His relish recipe for a tryptophan meal of hamburgers, hot dogs, pork or cold beef is quite interesting and can be found on the Internet.

Charles Lindbergh Relish

½ head green cabbage
2 carrots
1 red pepper
1 green pepper
3 medium onions
2 tablespoons pickling salt
¾ cup white vinegar
1 ½ cup sugar
½ teaspoon celery seed
½ teaspoon mustard seeds

Grind all vegetables to relish-sized bits. Place in a large bowl with pickling salt. Mix well. Let sit 2 hours. Drain liquid off by squeezing out well. Add spices, seeds, sugar and vinegar. Place in jars in the refrigerator until used. Makes 10 helpings.

Charles taught his wife, Anne Morrow Lindbergh, to fly and she loved it. They both flew about the world, interacting with leaders and royalty. Lindbergh made everybody interested in airplanes. There were air shows with pilots doing fantastic stunts, wing-walking, diving, and doing loop the loop maneuvers. Some died, especially some who flew in early airplane movies, when there was little safety in making a movie exciting.

Howard Hughes and Sleep

Howard Hughes made one of the biggest-selling movies about planes in 1930 called *Hell's Angels*. It starred pilots, actors, and Jean Harlow who went on to some fame but died young of kidney failure. This very long movie with an intermission included 25-30 airplanes in a scene, and some crashing into a dirigible. Three pilots and one mechanic died during filming, so pilots who worked on the film in the last months of production wanted protections. Hughes hired Pancho Barnes (who won Powder Puff Derbies and broke Amelia Earhart's air record) to fly and to organize a union for pilots so they would help him finish the movie.

Barnes' grandfather, Thaddeus Lowe, had begun the first military aircraft unit with balloons during the Civil War. Pancho became famous because she opened the Happy Bottom Riding Club, a dude ranch and restaurant, which catered to pilots. It was located near the Edwards Air Force Base in Antelope Valley, California. She was a friend of Chuck Yeager, Gen. Jimmy Doolittle, and Buzz Aldrin. Pancho promised pilots a free steak dinner when they broke the sound barrier. She was featured in *The Right Stuff,* a movie about the first team of astronauts that were specially trained for missions in space.

Howard Hughes set many air records. He was also known for his Hughes Tools, Hughes Aircraft Company, and his famous medical center in California. Despite several aviation movies, his most famous movie was *The Outlaw* with Jane Russell showing her cleavage in provocative poses.

Hughes wanted to be famous as both a billionaire and for his aviation career. Although he was a womanizer, he admitted to Russian actress Alla Nazimova that he took momentary pleasure in bodies. However, he added that when such short-lived pleasure was over, he preferred to sleep alone.

Sleeping with someone rarely meant actual sleep, but instead meant sharing a bed to have sex. Nazimova was an actress playing vamps who slept around with men starring in silent movies. She made *Camille* in 1921 with Rudolph Valentino. Nazimova was intimate with women and enjoyed a "lavender marriage." That phrase indicated a sham marriage wherein at least one spouse had relations with the same sex outside of marriage.

She helped silent film starlet Edith Luckett (Nancy Davis Reagan's mother) get into a 1917 Broadway show. She called Edith "Lucky" and Edith asked the Russian actress to be Nancy's godmother. After Edith met prominent neurosurgeon, Dr. Royal Davis, she retired from movies but continued her relationship with Alla Nazimova who died in 1945. Ronald Reagan had stayed in Nazimova's hotel, Garden of Allah, where he claimed to have slept around after he left Jane Wyman and before he met Nancy Davis. But, as Reagan might have said at the end of his movie career: "I'll be back!"

Howard Hughes married the beautiful actress Jean Peters. Theirs was an unusual relationship with very little time together because of Hughes' gradually increasing mental illness. Hughes was born in 1905 and died in 1976. He worked for days without sleep, became emaciated from diet and drugs, and moved from place to place in luxury hotels. Jean died in 2000 at age 74. When they did spend nights together, she was kept awake, according to her obituary notice in *The Telegraph*, by the clicking of the uncut toenails of husband Hughes.

Hughes deteriorated in health and cognitive ability in later years and finally lived in the dark. In his final illness, he was reported to have said: "I sleep. In this room. In the dark. I have a place I can sleep...It's beautiful."

Wiley Post, Will Rogers and Sleep Deprivation Tricks

Early pilot Wiley Post flew his Winnie Mae airplane around the world on July 5, 1931, with navigator Harold Gatty. They stopped 11 times for fuel, food, and a little sleep but were the first to circle the earth. It took them 8 days and 51 minutes.

Wiley had only one eye due to an oil field accident with a metal fragment. He used his financial settlement to buy his first plane. He wore a patch over his eye and worked very hard to overcome his lack of distance perspective because of his one-dimensional vision. He and Gatty wrote a book about their flight. *Around the World in Eight Days*, with a preface by Will Rogers. Among Rogers' introductory words were these:

Post piloted the plane on the whole trip. He was raised on a Texas "Norther" and weaned on an Oklahoma "Cyclone." So, a little thing like fog looked like a clear day to him... Now this Gatty he is an Australian. That's where they stand on their tail and kick you with their hind feet.... These Birds stayed awake over seven full days out of eight. There must be no worse torture and misery in the world than to have to keep going, when it looks and feels like you can't possibly hold your eyes open, and how wide theirs had to be open? We can all make some kind of a one big effort, but we can't sleep an hour and then get up and make another one just as big, and keep it up for over a week. Well, that was about the most sustainingest effort that was ever sustained!

Post described his sleep preparations for the trip. For the greater part of the winter before the flight, he never slept during the same hours on any two days in the same week. Breaking himself of such common habits as regular sleep hours was far more difficult than flying an airplane, or so he said.

Unfortunately, many criticized Post saying that he was uneducated and that Gatty did all the important work. So, Post decided to make a solo trip around-the-world in 1933 to receive full credit. He cut 21 hours off their first flight, making the trip in seven days, 18 hours, and 49 minutes. The first leg was a phenomenal 26-hour flight from New York to Berlin on July 15, 1933. He set a record that would only be broken by Howard Hughes, who flew with four other men in 1938.

Post practiced for his one-man flight by going long periods of time without sleep. He also designed a trick for waking himself if he fell asleep. He tied a string around a finger attached to a heavy tool, and flew holding the tool in his hand. If he fell asleep, it would drop and tug on his finger waking him up.

He was best friends with fellow-Oklahoman and actor Will Rogers, a columnist, humorist, and one of the world's greatest trick ropers. They died together in a plane crash on August 15, 1935, at Point Barrow, Alaska, in bad weather conditions.

Will Rogers had a radio show and in a broadcast about politicians said: "Why sleep at home when you can sleep in Congress?" A phrase he used frequently was: "I never met a man I didn't like." Well, he said he never met a meat sauce he didn't like, but this was the best. For a nice tryptophan meaty meal, this dish followed by a little sweet will yield a good night's sleep.

Will Rogers Meat Sauce

He boiled up some ketchup, a little A-1 steak sauce, Worcestershire sauce, brown sugar and a pinch of chili powder. He thought that went with most cuts of beef.

Amelia Earhart and Sleep Deprivation Remedies

Amelia Earhart set several aviation records. She was the first woman to fly across the Atlantic Ocean, and she did it twice. First, she was one of a three-member crew in 1928. On May 20, 1932, she flew alone from Harbor Grace, Newfoundland to Londonderry, Ireland, for 15 hours. She didn't like tea or coffee so kept herself awake with smelling salts. Her diet consisted of a thermos of soup and a can of tomato juice. She was awarded a Distinguished Flying Cross by Congress.

On April 20, 1933, she was dining with First Lady Eleanor Roosevelt and others. Eleanor Roosevelt (1884-1962) served as the First Lady for longer than any other presidential spouse in history. Eleanor was orphaned at age nine when her father died in a drunken fall. She described weeping at bedtime as a child, and dreamt about the world she wanted to live in.

Eleanor and Amelia had a spirited conversation about women's rights and flying. Despite being dressed in long gowns and high heels, Earhart invited Eleanor to fly with her over the Capitol. They left the dinner party and had a delightful time. They took turns at the controls in their flight from Washington, DC, to Baltimore, MD. Mrs. Roosevelt shared with her that she was studying for a student pilot's license.

When they returned to the White House, Eleanor asked the chef to make them a special dessert. She called it Pink Clouds on Angel Food Cake, symbolizing flying through clouds. A bit of this recipe could provide the evening sweet to produce melatonin.

Eleanor Roosevelt Pink Clouds on Angel Food Cake

1 cup sifted cake flour
1 ¼ cup egg whites (10-12 eggs)
1 ½ teaspoon cream of tartar
1 ½ cup sugar

1 teaspoon almond flavoring
¼ teaspoon salt
For Pink Clouds:
1 pint fresh strawberries rinsed and drained
½ pint heavy cream, whipped
½ cup sugar

Sift cake flour at least twice and set aside. Beat egg whites with beater until foamy. Add cream of tartar and one cup only of the sugar gradually. Continue beating until egg whites stand up in peaks. Add almond flavoring. Sift the remaining ½ cup of sugar with salt and flour. Slowly fold the flour mixture into the egg whites. Bake in an ungreased tube pan at 375 degrees for 30-35 minutes. Remove from oven and invert upside down to cool completely. Run a knife carefully around the sides to remove cake from pan.

Prepare the pink clouds by crushing all berries but one or two with the sugar. Let stand 30 minutes. Carefully fold crushed berries into whipped cream. Spoon on top of angel food cake. Garnish with a slice of strawberry and serve.

Nicknamed Lady Lindy because the willowy Earhart resembled Lindbergh, she inspired little girls and women to take up aviation. Shirley Temple sang the song "Good Ship Lollipop" in the 1934 movie *Bright Eyes* with music by Richard Whiting and lyrics Sydney Clare:

I've thrown away my toys, even my drum and train.
I wanna make some noise with real live aeroplanes.
Some day I'm going to fly, I'll be a pilot, too.

Earhart set another record by flying from Honolulu to Oakland, California, on January 11, 1935, in 18 hours. Ten other pilots including

214 | *Diane Holloway Cheney, Ph.D.*

three women had died trying to make that flight. Air travel became more personality-focused like sports. Lindbergh and Earhart were superstars. Everything they did was news.

Amelia attempted still another world record to circle the earth along the equator. Her luck ran out when she and navigator Fred Noonan crashed into the sea after 40 days of no more than five hours sleep a night. They died on July 2, 1937. In papers found after she died, there was a message from Eleanor Roosevelt saying that she recently had acquired her student pilot permit, but Franklin would not grant her permission to fly.

Enola Gay

On August 6, 1945, pilot Paul Tibbetts dropped the first atomic bomb on Hiroshima. A little over one hour prior to the drop, a weather pilot named Claude "Buck" Eatherly flew over the target and seeing very little cloud cover, cleared it for Tibbetts' mission. Eatherly was 300 miles away back at Tinian Island by the time it exploded and Tibbetts crew was 11 miles away but saw and felt the extraordinary blast.

Tibbetts' flight took only 12 hours and 13 minutes. He landed back at Tinian and was greeted as a hero. Enola, his mother's name, was "alone" spelled backwards. Paul Tibbetts was in the spotlight. The next atom bomb was dropped at Nagasaki on August 9, 1945. These bombs caused Japan to surrender and World War II ended.

Tibbetts' never expressed guilt over his role. President Harry Truman, who had ordered the bombs to be used, never expressed guilt over his decision. However, two other people have made news because they claimed to have sleepless nights over the people who were killed in the two explosions—Claude Eatherly and J. Robert Oppenheimer. Both men suffered from sleep problems the rest of their lives. However, Eatherly's story was a bit different.

He was jealous of Tibbetts' success and left the military as a major in 1947. He returned to his home in Texas where he drank, gambled, robbed post offices, wrote bad checks and committed numerous forgeries. He carried out one hold-up with a toy gun. He treated his wife and children badly and the marriage cratered. He attempted suicide several times. He was hospitalized at the Waco VA Hospital where psychiatrists treated him with Thorazine, a major tranquilizer used for people with psychoses such as schizophrenia.

One of his psychiatrists (Oleinick Pavlovitch Constantin) told the press that he claimed guilt for Japanese victims. That made news all over the world. Another psychiatrist (Dr. Ross) noted that he had no moral feelings toward wife or children, or toward any human being. He pleaded insanity to avoid prison and spent much of his last years in the old red two-story VA Hospital in Waco, Texas.

One of the psychiatrists who reviewed his case and believed he needed psychiatric hospitalization was my boss, Dr. William A. DeLoach, who later became chairman of the Department of Psychiatry at the University of Texas Health Science Center.

The story of Major Eatherly ended badly when he died in 1978 of throat cancer at the age of 49, after four years of sleepless nights in pain and suffering. His life and supposed guilt was praised by those who wanted to "ban the bomb." They felt he struck a blow for ending nuclear war. Famous English philosopher Bertrand Russell and European authors who were unaware of his true character praised him for objecting to nuclear weapons. When Russell led the Easter 1958 "Ban the Bomb" march down Oxford Street in London, I ran out and joined when I heard the commotion and saw the signs. I learned later that Russell spoke at Trafalgar Square extolling Eatherly before the march began.

Movies, Pilots, and Sleep

General Charles (Chuck) Yeager was the first man to break the sound barrier and did so when his experimental X-1 rocket-powered aircraft was dropped from a B-29 bomber at 45,000 feet over the Mohave Desert on October 4, 1957. Several had died trying to accomplish that feat when their planes broke apart. But Chuck did it and celebrated by going to stunt pilot Pancho Barnes' Happy Bottom

Riding Club, where she gave him a free steak dinner. He described how he broke the barrier the month after his accomplishment.

He said he went horseback riding the night before and fell off his horse breaking two ribs. He had a bad night's sleep from the pain in his side, but also from the indecision about whether to fly the mission incapacitated. He finally decided that if he could get into the pilot's seat he could fly. Ignoring his safety belt regulations, he did it unstrapped. He said when he broke the sound barrier there was no buffet, no jolt, no shock and he was alive.

Yeager served in WWII as a pilot testing many aircraft. He commanded fighter squadrons in Germany and Southeast Asia during the Viet Nam War. He commanded the USAF Aerospace Research Pilot School in 1962 which produced the first astronauts. He was not able to be an astronaut because he had only a high school education. He muscled his way to break the sound barrier in 2012 on its 65th anniversary when he was 89 years old. He had courage and heart that showed when he had to overcome deficits and adversities.

He was featured in the movie *The Right Stuff*. His role was played by actor Sam Shepard. Chuck Yeager was actually in the movie playing the role of a waiter at Pancho's Restaurant where pilots hung out. He contributed his grandmother's 1880 recipe for cornbread whenever people asked him for a recipe. This recipe on the Internet plus some sweet jam will make melatonin in the evening.

Chuck Yeager Cornbread

1 cup white cornmeal
3 tablespoons all-purpose flour
½ teaspoon salt
½ teaspoon baking soda
1 tablespoon bacon grease or vegetable oil
Buttermilk (lots for crispy, less for not crispy)

Preheat the oven to 450 degrees. Combine all ingredients well, adding enough buttermilk to make a smooth batter. Bake in a greased cast-iron skillet for 45 minutes or until brown. 6 servings.

During the Vietnam War, my friend Lt. Col. Edward Carr flew the C-133 called "The Widowmaker." It had two pilots, a navigator, two flight engineers, and a load master. It carried military cargo and ballistic missiles about the world mainly from 1961 to 1967. It was noted for crashes and Carr, now retired, described losing four aircraft in his squadron. Two were on take-off and two were at about the top of the initial climb. These occurred at Wake Island, Dover Air Force Base, Travis Air Force Base and the ocean near Japan. Many pilots did not want to fly this gigantic Cargo Master because of its record of crashes.

"The C-133 standard crew duty day was 24 hours with two pilots or 27 hours with three pilots," said Carr. "As the war wore on, we were all tired but training and crew standardization avoided most accidents. We had two bunks which allowed for short two to three-hour naps. When the Tet offensive happened in 1968, all crew rests were reduced. There was a lot of 'getting away with it' in those days."

In the last 40 or more years, the National Transportation Safety Board has produced many important reports and recommendations for every form of transportation. One of their first important reports was *Review of Flightcrew-Involved Major Accidents of U.S. Air Carriers, 1978 through 1990.* They found 37 accidents and learned that half the captains had been awake more than 12 hours prior to their accidents, and half the first officers had been awake more than 11 hours.

The most accidents occurred around 9:00 a.m. and 6:00 p.m. but several were around 2:00 p.m. and 8:00-10:00 pm. Most (19) occurred in approaches and landings but ten occurred at takeoff.

The Safety Board recommended to the U.S. Department of Transportation: (1) Expedite research on the effects of fatigue, sleepiness and sleep disorders, (2) Disseminate educational material regarding shift work, rest schedules, and proper regimens of health, diet and rest, and (3) Upgrade regulations governing hours of service for all transportation modes with the latest research on fatigue and sleep issues.

On August 2, 1981, President Ronald Reagan blocked a strike by air traffic controllers and his strong stand made history. He threatened to fire some 12,000 air traffic controller strikers because their union had become so strong that they were going on strike too often. He had led his actors' union (SAG) on a strike in the movie industry. He took a terrible chance that air traffic would come to a halt, but it continued despite shortages.

Kalitta Crash at Guantanamo Bay 1993

The first aviation accident in which the public learned of pilot fatigue and sleep deprivation cited as a cause was in 1993. The Kalitta International DC-8-61F crashed at Guantanamo Bay on August 18, 1993, at 4:56 p.m. with a crew of three who survived the accident.

The crew's extremely long day began in Dallas at 11 p.m. on August 17, 1993. They landed first in St. Louis, then flew on to Detroit landing in Atlanta, Georgia. They were to be relieved but were summoned to fill in for a cancelled flight to pick up freight at Norfolk, Virginia, fly it to Guantanamo Bay in Cuba, and ferry the plane back to Atlanta, Georgia where they were off-loaded from Cuba.

Thanks to cockpit voice recorders, the following airplane crash shows the deterioration of thinking and planning of pilots under the effects of sleep deprivation. In no other profession are we likely to have the actual words and attitudes reflected as clearly as in these comments by various crews. The accidents that occurred claimed many lives and details of survivors and some who perished are included to remind us of the dreadful consequences of sleep-deprived pilots. Pilots are trained to learn routines so they perform safety checks but these routines don't keep them thinking.

The First Officer later said the crew discussed that they might be "pushing" the edge. He described the company's attitude "If the trip was legal, you better really be tired" to refuse it. None of them had flown to Cuba so they went over flight plans while waiting and were happy to read that there was a strobe light that would help them find the right runway. They departed Norfolk at 2:13 p.m. At 4:34 p.m. they saw the Guantanamo runway, and contacted the tower where they talked with a new employee who did not know the strobe light wasn't working. They then looked for the strobe light. The nose pitched down as the plane flew lower, striking the ground. Several fires erupted from the crashed plane. All three crew members were seriously injured. The crash occurred at 4:56 p.m., at the end of the afternoon.

The captain flew the approach in a manner that placed the airplane in a dangerous flight regime despite warnings from other crew members and the stall warning stick shaker. The strobe light wasn't working but the crew was never told that by the air traffic controller. Cockpit conversation just before the crash was helpful in seeing how limited the fatigued captain was viewing his options.

Flight Engineer: (Expletive), we're never goin' to make this.

Captain: Where do you see a strobe light?

First Officer: Right over there.

Captain: Where's the strobe?

First Officer: Do you think you're gonna make this?

Captain: Yeah, if I can catch the strobe light.

First Officer: Five hundred (feet). You're in good shape. (Stall warning)

Flight Engineer: Watch the... keep your air speed up. (Stall warning)

Captain: I got it. (Stall warning)

Crew: There it goes. There it goes. Oh, no. (Scream)

Once they recovered, the 54-year old captain, 49-year old first officer, and 35- year old flight engineer were questioned at length during the investigation. The captain had been awake 23.5 hours and stated: "All I can say is that I was—I felt very lethargic or indifferent... So it's frustrating...to think of how you could be so lethargic when so many things were going on, but that's just the way it was." The first officer had been awake 19 hours and said he "accepted the trip to fly to Guantanamo." The flight engineer had been awake for 21 hours. The Kalitta CEO said that to remain competitive, the company must often assign long duty times. He indicated that this practice was "common" in the air freight industry. We are, after all, a competitive society.

AA Crash in Little Rock, Arkansas, 1999

The next flight where sleep deprivation played a part was a short hop from Dallas to Little Rock, Arkansas. On June 1, 1999, American Airlines MD-82 from Dallas/Fort Worth crashed upon landing at Little Rock, Arkansas, at 11:50 p.m. Eleven of the 145 aboard died (the captain and ten passengers). The pilot duty time was 14 hours so far for the day and had to fly out by 11:16 p.m. to comply with rules about rest time needed by pilots. They received word of bad storms so flew quickly to beat the storm headed for Little Rock and tried to land quickly as well. They failed to check the pre-landing checklist, failed to arm the automatic spoiler system, failed to set the braking system, and failed to set landing flaps. Wind at 11:49 p.m. was 25 knots which exceeded the 20 knot crosswind limit for landing on wet reduced visibility runways.

The 48-year old pilot and 35-year old first officer had been awake 16 hours--not that stressful for pilots but the crash occurred two hours later than their usual bedtimes which makes some difference in fatigability. The crew never considered aborting the landing despite fierce deteriorations and poor visibility in the storm at Little Rock airport. They exhibited "get there-it-is" as one observer called it. Details of the crash and cockpit conversation were reported by the National Transportation Safety Board Report entitled: Runway Overrun during Landing AA Flight 1420, June 1st, 1999. The crew's behavior was more characteristic of pilots who are fatigued and considered only their original mission rather than variations according to the severity of conditions as shown by their cockpit conversation for the last two minutes.

Captain: This is a can of worms. I'm gonna stay above it a little.

First Officer: There's the runway off to your right. Got it?

Captain: No.

First Officer: I got the right runway in sight. You're right on course. Stay where you're at.

Captain: I got it. I got it.

First Officer: Five hundred feet (altitude).

Captain: Plus twenty.

First Officer: Aw (expletive) We're way off course. We're way off.

Captain: I can't see it.

First Officer: Got it?

Captain: Yeah, I got it.

First Officer: Hundred feet. Above. Hundred. Fifty. Forty. Thirty. Twenty. Ten. We're down. We're sliding.

Captain: (Two expletives)

First Officer: ...on the brakes. Oh sh... Other one, other one, other one. Aw (two expletives)

Impact noise (expletive). Several impact noises. Fires began to rage everywhere as the plane broke apart into several sections.

The plane slid down the runway into the building that housed the runway lights crushing the plane's nose and first two rows of coach seats. It broke into several large sections.

Passengers tried to escape from the plane and the fires. Among them were 25 members of the Ouachita Singers from Ouachita Baptist University in Arkadelphia flying home from giving a singing tour in Eastern Europe. Singer James Harrison, 21, kept rescuing people and going back for more and finally succumbed. Rachel Fuller, 14-year old daughter of the choir director who was traveling with his wife and daughters, could not recover from her burns and died later. Trudging about in the dark of night through water, wreckage, and fire, the singers and other passengers worked to save each other. The Ouachita singers began to comfort people quoting the 91st Psalm in the American Standard Version of the Bible, 1929, which described the security of those who trust in God.

On the tenth anniversary of the crash, the Ouachita Singers survivors met to thank God for protecting them during the plane crash. They sang the songs they had sung on their trip.

Corporate Airline Crash in Missouri 2004

The next American incident involving sleep deprivation occurred on October 19, 2004, when Corporate Airlines Flight 5966 bound for Kirksville, Missouri, crashed at 7:37 p.m. hitting trees as it approached the runway. Kim Sasse, 48-year old pilot, and co-pilot, Jonathan Palmer, 29 years old, began duty at 5 a.m. By the time of the crash, they had been on duty 14+ hours and Kirksville was their 6th landing of the day in challenging weather. FAA regulations permit 16 hours of duty but American Airlines permits 14 hours of duty and Corporate Airlines was a subsidiary of American.

The passengers were mainly osteopathic physicians who were flying to Kirksville's Osteopathic Hospital for a conference. The plane came down about a mile south of the runway hitting trees and breaking apart. All crew and passengers died in the fiery crash except two—Dr. John Krogh fell into some trees and his assistant Wendy Bonham was wandering around when rescuers arrived. The two escaped from a hole in the fuselage after it broke open before fire reached that part of the plane.

The Jetstream 32 twin-engine turboprop plane departed St. Louis at 6:42 p.m. During the last thirty minutes of the flight, the cockpit conversation was extremely unprofessional with 45 expletives, and making fun of the passengers enjoying themselves noisily. They crew joked and criticized things, airline employees, and passengers. In fact, it almost sounds as if the captain was criticizing the First Officer for comments when he called him the "director." There was much yawning, humming, and chatter distracting themselves from watching their instruments and going through usual checking procedures. The last minute of the cockpit conversation demonstrate their distraction and their lack of ability to see the runway:

Pilot: When we get within a hundred feet if you'd uh, arm that uh...

First Officer: Disarm it?

Pilot: Director again, yeah, uh, altitude.

First Officer: Oh for altitude, okay.

Captain: C'mon, go down there.

First Officer: Five hundred, four hundred feet to go.

Mechanical voice warning: Five hundred.

First Officer: Thirteen twenty.

Captain: What do you think? Thank you. I can see ground there.

Mechanical voice warning: Minimums, minimums.

First Officer: I can't see (expletive).

Captain: Yeah, oh there it is. Approach lights in sight.

Mechanical voice warning: Two hundred.

First Officer: In sight. Continue.

Captain: We get rid of the director.

Captain: Getting a little slow.

First Officer: Flaps thirty-five?

Captain: No.

Mechanical voice warning: Sink rate (which means prepare for sudden landing)

Captain: No.

First Officer: Trees.

Captain: No, stop

Sound of impact.

Captain: Oh, my God.

Sounds of numerous impacts

First Officer: Holy (expletive)

The choice was up to the pilots. And it was simple. When the mechanical voice warned 200 feet, they could have taken the plane back up. Hindsight is always easier than being there, of course.

Ten years after the crash, the two survivors, emergency

responders, faculty, staff and students and the Kirksville community gathered to remember those lost. Dr. Krogh told those assembled at the A. T. Still University campus he dealt with a severe case of survivor guilt and many times I wished I had died. To this day, Krogh wonders if he could have done more, despite being told that if he had spent any time trying to pull bodies from the wreckage, he would have been killed by the fire that soon took over.

European Pilot Fatigue Recommendations of 2005

The European Organization for the Safety of Air Navigation (Eurocontrol) produced a booklet in 2005 for air traffic controllers (not pilots) called "Fatigue and Sleep Management: Personal Strategies for Decreasing the Effects of Fatigue in Air Traffic Control." They described the symptoms of sleep deprivation: longer reaction times, decreased attention, decreased memory and mood deterioration. These symptoms would be nearly the same in air traffic controllers and pilots.

Those with sleep deprivation become more withdrawn, overlook task elements, preoccupy themselves with a single task, have reduced audiovisual scans, are less aware of their poor performance, are worse in recalling information and events, forget tasks, are more irritable, develop a "don't care" attitude, are more distracted by their discomfort, are less likely to converse, and choose to perform low-demand tasks more than high-demand tasks.

Their booklet advised that sleep comes with warm temperatures, low social stimulation and interaction, dim lighting, little physical activity, low noise levels, and passive monitoring work. Sleep deprivation effects occur such as: micro-sleeps, failure to respond in a timely manner, impaired short-term memory, reduced communication, choosing options requiring less effort, loss of situational awareness, doing new tasks slower, lower morale, and lower motivation. The booklet included methods for air traffic controllers to use in getting more sleep and changing their work environment for the better.

Comair Crash in Kentucky 2006

The next American flight where sleep deprivation was a factor occurred on August 27, 2006. A Comair jet crashed when pilots went down the wrong runway and hit a berm, a fence, trees, and terrain. The berm tossed the plane up in the air some 20 feet and it hit a tree and broke, catching fire. Only the co-pilot survived when the pilot, attendant and 47 passengers died in the fiery crash. The air traffic controller on duty that night was alone and did not watch the plane as it took off, or he might have alerted them to depart on another runway.

Two days before the accident, the pilots had a six-leg trip. The day before this flight, they checked in at 5:10 p.m., departed Cincinnati, Ohio to Minneapolis and back to Cincinnati. Then they flew to Lexington, Kentucky. The pilot's family drove several miles to pick him up for dinner at 4:30 p.m. and to spend the evening with him before they returned home. He awoke in his hotel the morning of the accident at 4:15 a.m. and was on duty by 5:15. The pilot and first officer checked in at 5:15 a.m. casually conversing.

They boarded the *wrong* airplane and started up its power unit. A ramp agent notified them and they shut down and proceeded to the correct plane. This error is a possible result of their fatigue. It underscores the maybe/maybe not process of sleep-deprived thinking.

The pilot's duty time the day of the accident was 12 hours and 26 minutes before his take-off. His probable fatigue was further compounded by the air traffic controllers fatigue. The tower controller had worked two complete 8-hour shifts with only 8-hours between. He had only two hours of sleep during the last 24 hours and was slowed in reaction time, vigilance, and had a lowered task performance. Had he been watching the plane's departure, he would have realized the plane was on the wrong runway before clearing it to take off.

During the last few minutes of their fatal flight, it was pre-dawn dark. There was considerable non-pertinent conversation regarding job opportunities and family which diverted attention from checking the runway surface markers and other procedures. There was also some yawning during the short taxi stretch. There were told to take Runway 22 but they turned down a short Runway which is not used for take-offs. We pick up their comments about how many children they would like six minutes before the crash.

Captain: Yeah, I like two years apart basically and that's kinda what we were going for. My wife wants four, I, I, I'm, I was good at one.

First Officer: She wants four.

Captain: Yeah.

First Officer: It'd be like honey... Yeah, it's especially being on reserve, it it's gotta be tough being away.

Captain: Ah, tough on her, oh my God. That's why she came down yesterday. She's like, I just need to get out of this house.

First Officer: Yeah, I bet.

Captain: I'm like I understand. I, I told her, why don't you just spend the night. She said, well, if you're gonna get up at oh dark thirty and she said you'll end up waking the babies. I'm like yeah, you're probably right.

First Officer: Yeah, it would just be like being at home.

Captain: Yeah, she's like you know, I don't know, she's like I'll...

First Officer: Instead of having her rush back and drive...

Captain: And we got a dog.

Ground: Lexington tower roger, hold short.

First Officer: Aah, trust me. The dog...be on the slim-fat diet for a night. Laughter. Uh, parking brake.

Captain: That's on.

(They continue their taxi checks and we resume three minutes before the crash.)

First Officer: Yeah, I know three guys at Kennedy. Actually two guys, uh, (name omitted) he went but he didn't get past the sim [simulation test].

Captain: Oh, really.

First Officer: And the um, a First Officer from Cinci...got through the second part. What do you do the uh, these tests...and he didn't, and that's as far as he got. And then he actually got offered the position.

Captain: Did he take it or...

First Officer: Yeah.

Captain: Ah, okay.

First Officer: Hydraulics check, APU's on, FMS we got runway two two out of Lexington up to six. Thrust reversers are armed, auto crossflow is manual, ignition is off, altimeters three triple zero across the board, crosschecked. I'll be in the back.

Captain: Got one.

First Officer: Pre-takeoff, complete cabin report received CAS.

Captain: Checked and clear.

First Officer: (Whispered) six seven.

Captain: Oh.

First Officer: Oh yeah. I'm looking at it 'cause like, okay I see seven but it's...

Captain: Yeah, there's a green extra one there but... (both pilots are confused by what they see)

First Officer: uuuh, cabin report's received, CAS clear. Before takeoff check's complete, ready.

Captain: All set.

Tower: Comair one ninety one, Lexington uh, tower, fly runway heading, cleared for takeoff.

Captain: And line-up check. Throw that bad boy on.

First Officer: Transponder's on, packs on, bleeds closed, cleared for takeoff, runway heading. Six grand.

Captain: All right.

First Officer: Anti-ice off, lights set, takeoff config's okay, line-up check's complete.

Captain: All yours, Jim.

First Officer: My brakes, my controls. Set thrust please.

Captain: Thrust set.

First Officer: Dat is weird with no lights. (The runways should be lit at night.)

Captain: Yeah. One hundred knots.

First Officer: Checks

Captain: V one, rotate. Whoa. (expletive) Sound of impact.

The First Officer, Jim Polehinke, was pulled out by a rescuer who burned his arms in the process. Jim was badly injured and unable to remember the wreck for some time. He lost the use of both legs and one was amputated at the knee. He took months to heal and now uses a wheelchair.

In 2012, a documentary of sole survivors in crashes was made by CBS and aired. Jim was one of the 14 who were described in the story. He discussed his hazy memories and his guilt about being at the helm of the plane in a crash ruled as being caused by pilot error. He thinks about the crash daily, said the documentary producer, and occasionally ventures into a "dark place" in his mind. He found therapy in skiing and religion, and hopes to use his story as inspiration for people in similar difficulties.

Two Pilots Fell Asleep and Overflew Hilo in 2008

The next American flight situation is totally the result of sleep deprivation. On February 13, 2008, two pilots fell asleep on a flight from Honolulu to Hilo from 9:16 a.m. to 9:40 a.m., cruising past their destination for 18 minutes before waking up and returning safely to Hilo. They had flown 8-leg flights for three arduous days before the incident beginning at 5:40 a.m. each morning.

Flight 1002 was run by Mesa, Arizona, Go! Airlines and had 40 passengers and three crew. The 53-year old captain first lied about being on the wrong radio frequency but, in a brief moment of reflection, decided that he and the 23-year old co-pilot who also slept should remove themselves from duty.

The captain said that he was feeling burned out from because of less time off and schedule changes. He admitted that he usually napped once a week for 20 minutes on flights. He was found to have obstructive sleep apnea. Both pilots were fired and each was suspended from flying for a few weeks by the Federal Aviation Administration.

The U.S. National Transportation Safety Board recommended working hour limits for flight crews, aviation mechanics, and air traffic controllers. With greater investment by an airline come higher expectations of pilots. It mattered little to this airline how much sleep the pilot got until he napped during a flight.

Colgan Crash in Buffalo, New York, 2009

The next American airplane accident due to possible sleep deprivation and fatigue is notable because the pilots were talking about their futures and minutes later they had no future. On February 12, 2009, a Colgan Air passenger flight with 45 passengers and four crew left Newark, New Jersey, at 9:18 p.m. They flew into Buffalo, New York, and crashed at 10:17 p.m. The pilot lost control of the plane and both he and his female co-pilot did the wrong maneuvers at the last minute so it crashed into a house near the runway killing one person on the ground but other inhabitants of the house survived. All on the plane were lost.

Both pilots were at Newark airport overnight and all day before the 9:18 p.m. departure. The voice recorder indicated unnecessary conversation in violation of federal rules banning nonessential conversation and not paying enough attention to instruments.

The plane was on autopilot for most of the journey. Earlier in the conversation between 47-year old Captain Marvin Renslow and 24-year old Rebecca Lynne Shaw, she described head and nose congestion and not feeling well. Their final moments were captured on the flight recorder and went thusly:

Shaw: "In the past I would have freaked out" about the ice conditions. "I would have like seen this much ice and thought, oh my gosh, we were going to crash." (Relevant conversation)

Shaw: "No, but all these guys are complaining. They're saying, you know, how we were supposed to upgrade by now and I'm thinking, you know what? I really wouldn't mind going through a winter in the Northeast before I have to upgrade to captain. I've never seen icing conditions. I've never de-iced. I've never experienced any of that. I don't want to have to experience that and make those kinds of calls. You know I'd've freaked out. I'd have, like, seen this much ice and thought, oh my gosh, we were going to crash."

Renslow: "Oh yeah. I'm so glad...I mean I would have been fine. I would have survived it. We never had to make a decision that I wouldn't have been able to make but...now I'm more comfortable. Gear down. Loc's alive."

Controller at Buffalo. "Colgan 3407 contact tower 1205. Have a good night."

Shaw: "Over to tower. You do the same, 3407. Gears down."

Renslow: "Flaps fifteen before landing checklist."

When the turboprop flew too slow for safety, the crew received a stall warning known as a "stick shaker."

Renslow: "Jesus Christ!"

Shaw: "I put the flaps up. Should the gear up?"

Renslow: "Gear up. Oh, (expletive)! We're down!"

Shaw: "We're (scream)!"

Investigation revealed that Renslow had not admitted to Colgan Air that he had failed five performance tests and mentioned only one many years earlier. So without checking further, they hired him.

Other items explored were how very far each pilot had flown to get to this job and how the pay was so low ($16,000 per year) that they could not afford to stay in a hotel or proper place to sleep before the flight. Among items mentioned in the final report were red-eye commutes, and lack of places for pilots to sleep created the risk of dangerous fatigue at the regional airlines. Inattentiveness, failure to perform correctly and fatigue were three of the main four conclusions by the National Transportation Safety Board. Such pilots used "crash pads" where a cheap bedroom with bunk beds and tight sleeping quarters serves as many as ten pilots.

One passenger on that fatal Colgan journey was Beverly Eckert who had just been honored by President Barack Obama six days earlier. Her husband, Sean Rooney, was killed when airplanes deliberately flew into the Twin Towers of the World Trade Center eight years earlier at New York City in 2001. Beverly worked tirelessly with other families to establish the 9/11 Family Steering Committee and to develop a memorial to those who died.

She declined to accept the $1.8 million award for her husband's death claim and wrote an article on September 19, 2003, saying that she wanted to know why two 110-story skyscrapers collapsed in less than two hours and why escape and rescue options were so limited.

Hudson River Landing, New York 2009

Captain Chesley "Sully" Sullenberger was interviewed after this crash. He said he was convinced that "had we been tired, had we not gotten sufficient rest the night before, we could not have performed at the same level...I may not have been able to perform as well." He was referring to his miraculous landing of an airplane with no injuries on January 15, 2009, in the Hudson River after a flock of geese flew into the engines. Sullenberger said pilot fatigue is an industry-wide problem. The industry has called for improved and regulated sleep scheduling to ensure pilots are properly rested before taking off with an airplane full of passengers.

After the tragic 2009 crash of Colgan Flight mentioned earlier, pilots of passenger planes were limited to flying either eight or nine hours, and airlines were required to provide pilots with a minimum of ten rest hours in the Safe Skies Act. On April 14, 2016, Captain "Sully" called for one level of safety for all pilots along with Senators Amy Klobuchar and Barbara Boxer in Washington, D.C. Pilots of cargo planes were left out of the Safe Skies Act but this loophole was closed by the 2016 FAA bill. Sullenberger brought enhanced visibility to the changes needed for safer flying.

A movie featuring Tom Hanks as "Sully" was made and the retired captain said he was not a hero but he was using his publicity to help the airlines and the public prevent these terrible accidents. As the movie pointed out, there are two elements of flying that pilots can control—their attitude and their decisions.

Air India Crash in Mangalore in 2010

On May 22, 2010, the pilot of another Air India plane that crashed killing 158 people, could be heard snoring on the cockpit voice recorder shortly before the incident. The Boeing 737-800 overshot a runway at Mangalore and plunged down a ravine. The Serbian captain was asleep for more than half of the three-hour flight from Dubai and was disoriented when he attempted to land the plane. Zltko Glusica awoke before the crash but was believed to have "sleep inertia." Only eight people survived after leaping from the wreckage before it burst into flames.

The court of inquiry found that Glusica actually landed the plane at Mangalore's airport in heavy rain but unsatisfied with their location, he and the co-pilot attempted to take off again but failed to gain height and the plane plunged off the edge of the runway into jungle below. Investigators concluded that had Glusica applied emergency brakes he could have stopped the plane in time. The cockpit recorder picked up the co-pilot repeatedly warning the captain to abort landing saying there was not sufficient runway to land. Just before the crash both men are heard saying: "Oh my God."

Survivors must deal with the hand they are dealt as they lose loved ones, and those can be dreadful. Three months after the crash, some families had been paid $160,000 because they had higher salaries whereas some women, children and poor people with lower salaries resulted in families receiving amounts like $20,000.

Air Traffic Controllers and Sleep Deprivation

In April 2011, FAA Administrator Randy Babbitt told a hearing of the House Appropriations Committee's transportation subcommittee that an air traffic controller went to sleep for five hours on February 19, 2011, at the Knoxville, Tennessee, airport during the midnight shift. Disciplinary hearings to terminate the employee were underway. While the controller (who was to handle regional approaches) was sleeping, the tower controller landed seven planes at Knoxville and worked the radar position at the same time. That required him to switch back and forth between monitoring radar and visual observation. Controllers are only supposed to work one job at a time.

In March 2011, an air traffic supervisor acknowledged that he dozed off while two airliners carrying 165 people landed at Washington's Reagan National airport. That supervisor was the lone controller working the midnight shift in the tower. A series of six incidents where air traffic controllers fell asleep caused the Federal Aviation Administration (FAA) to undertake a comprehensive study of air traffic controllers.

In April 2011, a US air traffic controller was suspended for watching a Samuel L. Jackson film. That incident happened in Oberlin, Ohio, where an air traffic controller decided to watch a movie. All the pilots flying overhead could hear from the control tower was a scene from the thriller movie *Cleaner* starring Samuel L. Jackson, Ed Harris and John Cusak. Incoming calls to the air traffic controller were blocked by the transmission. Finally, an Air Force pilot contacted the tower and the controller was confronted by another employee. The relationship between pilots and air controllers is pragmatic and built almost entirely on the proper performance of the duties assigned to each of them.

The FAA's 2011 report was described in "Air Traffic Controllers Suffer Scary Sleep Deprivation" by John Johnson published August 10, 2015, was shocking to the public. The article showed the following results about air traffic controllers:

(a) About 20% of controllers committed serious errors on the job in 2010 such as bringing planes too close to one another and about half blamed fatigue

(b) About 33% of controllers deemed fatigue a "high" or "extreme" risk

(c) More than 60% say they dozed off or zoned out while driving to or from the late-night shifts, those that typically run from 10 p.m. to 6:00 a.m.

(d) While controllers averaged 5.8 hours of sleep per night in a work week, that figure dropped to 3.25 for some of the more grueling shifts.

(e) Chronic fatigue may be considered to pose a significant risk to controller alertness, and hence the safety of the air traffic control system. Researchers closely examined the "rattler" schedule in which they cram five eight-hour shifts into four 24-hour periods. Others work six days a week for a stretch of several weeks. Controllers told the Associated Press that such shifts were still in use years after the study was completed.

Deborah Hersman was the face of the National Transportation Safety Board (NTSB) from 2004, then in 2009 she became their chairman. The decisions about the cause of crashes was overseen and shaped by her leadership before she resigned on March 11, 2014. As chairman, Hersman broadened the board's mission to transportation risks such as drunk and drugged driving and fatigue across various modes of travel, rather than just responding to accidents. She intended to improve the safety landscape with the employees of the National Safety Council, another organization dedicated to saving lives and preventing injuries.

The National Safety Council is located in Itasca, Illinois. It was formed in 1913 to partner with business, government, elected officials, and the public to impact: distracted driving, teen driving, workplace safety, prescription drug overdoses and safe communities.

Actor Harrison Ford 2015 Crash and 2017 Errant Flight

On March 15, 2015, movie star Harrison Ford crashed on Penmar Golf Course in Venice, California, breaking his pelvis. Ford has been an avid aviator since the 1960s and owns several planes. He has provided emergency helicopter service to rescue a Boy Scout once and a dehydrated hiker elsewhere. In 2004, he became chairman of the Young Eagles of the Experimental Aircraft Association replacing Chuck Yeager who retired from the Board.

The crash of his two-seat open cockpit 1942 airplane occurred when the engine lost fuel within a minute after takeoff and he attempted to return to the airport runway. His plane was coming down steeply, clipped a tree, and crashed on the golf course. Nearby were physicians and EMTs golfing and they ran quickly to assist him. Later, determinations by the NTSB showed that a shoulder harness which he added to the antique plane, was improperly installed which caused Ford's injuries to be more severe. He had slept well the night before and had done mountain biking the morning of the crash which occurred at 2:10 p.m.

This evening meal was prepared as a breakfast starring Ford in the movie *Morning Glory*. This amazing actor built his own house, flies his own planes, and cooks his own food. The frittata includes proteins and high-tryptophan cream, vegetables, eggs, and cheese and can be seen as you watch *Morning Glory*.

Harrison Ford Frittata

4 eggs
¼ cup cream
1 cup cut up vegetables (like mushrooms, broccoli, green onions, green peppers)

½ cup parmigiana reggiano cheese
2 tablespoons olive oil
1 tablespoon butter
Salt and pepper

Sauté vegetables in hot oil and butter. In a bowl, mix eggs, cream, cheese, and add to cooked vegetables. Cook without stirring until bottom is golden. Pop pan into hot oven (375 degrees) for 5-10 minutes until set. Slice into wedges. "The key is a very hot pan" he said.

Ford was in another, his fourth, errant flight on February 14, 2017. He was coming into the John Wayne Airport at Santa Ana, California, and flew low over a 737 American Airlines plane as it taxied for takeoff carrying 110 people and a crew of six. His flight can be seen on the Internet. The 74-year old man was recorded as getting his landing directions mixed up. There are penalties for such actions, and he did not have to yield his pilot's license.

Preventing Fatigue in Pilots and Air Traffic Controllers

A recent study of Brazilian air traffic controllers was reported in 2016. Rotating shiftwork is common for air traffic controllers and usually causes sleep deprivation. This study identified physical inactivity, overweight, excess body fat, low scores for physical and social relationships, and sleep deprivation in all four work shifts. They suggested the need for more rest time before working night shifts and adding work environments that stimulated physical activity and healthy diets.

Many good aviation improvements have occurred in the last ten years. As long as human beings are pilots, fatigue will be a critical safety issue that demands our attention. The [NTSB] board has long advocated for science-based regulations to address the complex nature of fatigue.

Captain C. B. "Sully" Sullenberger has stressed that fatigue is insidious, it's cumulative, it's predictable and it's getting worse. He emphasized that we're flying farther, faster and through more time zones than ever before, so pilots should include two nights a week of uninterrupted sleep to catch up from sleep deficits.

He also recommended to pilots eating light, even if it's just a snack such as a high protein food to promote awareness and physical activity. He suggested switching to high carbohydrate, low-protein foods after the flight and before resting to promote normal circadian sleep by raising serotonin levels. Healthy snacks such as carrots, yogurt, nuts, fruit and peanut butter on celery sticks can boost energy and alertness.

In addition, scientists recommend that travelers stop drinking caffeinated beverages at lunch or by early afternoon to get a good night's sleep. But when trying to stay awake, coffee can be used. It takes 15 to 45 minutes for caffeine to take effect but it can prevent you from sleeping for up to eight hours. Caffeine is a diuretic and too much dehydration can make you moody, irritable, and jittery as well as contributing to insomnia.

In addition to caffeine, pilots can use physical exercise before the flight and stretching or isometrics during flights or waypoint by waypoint navigation logs to boost alertness. Conversation, especially work-related, during a mission can help as well. But staring all night at the screens can lull one to sleep.

To calm our uncertain nature, philosophy offers Socrates' phrases to which anyone can relate: "I know one thing; that I know nothing!" Is there any fact in the aviation world about which we can be certain anymore? Well, maybe one: Sleep deprivation is deadly!

Sleep can affect those professionals whose business is to stay more fit than almost anybody else. How do athletes, firefighters, and police officers handle sleep since their lives are dominated by quick decisions and reactions, often with little sleep? How are young business people being affected by working twenty-four hours a day in our world? What are the costs of sleep deprivation for the fittest of the fit in society today?

Chapter Twelve

SLEEP IN THE FITTEST: ATHLETES, FIREFIGHTERS AND POLICE

Employees and employers are beginning to pay much more attention to sleep and the effects of sleep deprivation. Even the field of sports is realizing the need to study sleep in athletes. Other professions where fitness must be maintained include firefighters and police officers. Sleep deprivation by those employees could cause life-threatening injuries to them and to the public. What kinds of sleep issues have been seen with sleep among these public servants?

In the early years of my career, it was my job to test people who applied to the Dallas County Sheriff's Office to serve as deputies. Later, I was chosen to develop the first assessment center for the uniformed services (police and fire) in Dallas, Texas. Candidates for higher positions had to undergo various tests which were watched and judged by high ranking officers whom we flew into Dallas and trained. In addition, I was hired by the Dallas Fire Department Union to perform a morale survey of all 1,400 members which was presented to their chief, with positive changes resulting.

In addition, I had to select special chauffeurs for millionaires (like developer Trammell Crow) and others who had threats made against them. When the Mayor and Police Chief selected me as the Drug Czar of Dallas, it was necessary to consult with law enforcement agencies at all levels to develop a cadre of 53 agencies to deal with the "war on drugs." These experiences gave me a great appreciation for these special people who lay down their lives for us.

The most physically fit people in our world are athletes, firefighters, police officers, and those in the military who must withstand all kinds of abuse to their bodies and their minds. We have to admire the hard work they put in to develop their special capabilities.

In prehistoric times, physical fitness and sports were as bloodthirsty as war. The Olympics date back to the 8th century B.C. and were held in Olympia, Greece, west of Athens and northwest of Sparta, in the Peloponnese Peninsula.

Mesoamerican ball courts were popular 3,000 years ago about the same time as the Greek Olympics. More recent ball courts were built in Arizona at Wupatki, Pueblo Grande, and Casa Grande. That bloody sport (sometimes to slay opponents) has physical connections to football, because they are both played on wide surfaces of ground with seats for spectators.

Baseball-type sports came mainly from the British Isles and Europe, as did tennis. Golf stemmed from the special development of sticks and balls on the terrain of Scotland and may be related to cold weather games on ice such as hockey and lacrosse. Basketball is not even as old as movies. It was created in 1891 and was played in college in the early 1900s. Professional baseball teams have played for over 100 years.

Sports Team Travel and Time Zones Crossed

What has travel to play teams across the country done to athletes, sleep, and the way each sport is managed? A recent survey of travel by basketball, football and hockey teams gives us some ideas. Five years of regular season games in the NBA, the NFL and the NHL were studied to investigate the effects of travel and the number of time zones crossed for every game. The results showed an advantage in more points scored in all three sports by teams traveling from west to east.

National Basketball Association teams traveling from west to east had a winning percentage of 45.38% compared to 36.23% for teams traveling from east to west. National Hockey League teams traveling from west to east had a winning percentage of 47.62% compared to 42.48% for teams traveling in the opposite direction. National Football League teams traveling from west to east had a winning percentage of 46.54% compared to 37.98% for teams traveling from east to west.

Sleep physicians are advising East Coast teams to travel to the West Coast a day ahead for every time zone they cross. It takes one day of acclimation to adjust to moving one time zone away, according sports therapists. So, if an East Coast team is traveling across three time zones to the west, the team should arrive three days early. Tom Brady, Super Bowl quarterback, has made a point of discussing how his improved sleep habits have helped give him a winning edge in the lead up to the 2015 Super Bowl. Las Vegas odds have been shown to favor professional west coast teams when they go east over east coast teams when they go west to play.

Individual circadian rhythms are being studied by professional teams to help athletes schedule games that suit their peak performance times. If an athlete's sleep rhythm creates his peak performance time in the afternoon, he should be scheduled then instead of in a night game. Athletes are also being trained about sleep. Athletes who slept less than seven hours had a 1.7 times greater chance for injury than those who had a good night's sleep. Acute injuries may be caused by a mistake in thinking, due to a lack of sleep. Chronic injuries may not heal quickly because the athlete isn't getting enough sleep.

Adolescent athletes, who sleep eight or more hours each night, are 68% less likely to be injured than young athletes who regularly sleep less. Also, the higher the athlete's grade level, the greater the likelihood of injury—2.3 times greater for each additional grade in school. Adolescents may benefit from additional sleep as they get older to help reduce the risk of injury during sports.

More and more, young people find their heroes in sports. If those athletic superheroes want to inspire them, they could display healthy fitness training, diet, and sleep habits. Derek Jeter, a shortstop and record-breaking batter for the New York Yankees, was one such person.

After retiring, Derek set up Jeter Publishing Company with Simon and Schuster Books for Young Readers to expose youth to good morals. He also set up an organization to fight cyber-bullies called Turn 2 Foundation. In his spare time, Jeter cooks up some good dishes. Here is his idea for pancakes.

Derek Jeter Game Day Pancakes

Use your regular pancake mix but substitute buttermilk for the milk. If you don't have buttermilk add a tablespoon of lemon juice or vinegar per cup of milk and it will have the same effect as buttermilk. Also beat the pancake batter to get more air into it so you will have fluffy pancakes.

Sports figures must work on their fitness and bulk up but with healthy foods. They need a good night's sleep before a game and former Dallas Cowboys' end Jay Novacek had his own idea for S'Mores.

Jay Novacek Indoor S'Mores

Pick out a cereal like Golden Grahams and put some in a bowl. Melt some marshmallows, corn syrup, margarine, and chocolate chips in a little saucepan. Stir in a bit of vanilla and pour the stuff over your cereal in the bowl, mixing it all up. Then butter a regular baking pan. Put everything in that buttered pan and let sit or refrigerate until it's firm. Then cut it into squares to eat. Be careful how much you eat after supper so it doesn't keep you awake since it has chocolate.

Jamaican runner Usain Bolt has been timed as the fastest man ever. Bolt can run 27.78 miles per hour. He was the first man in history to win six Olympic gold medals in sprinting and the first person to hold 100-meter *and* 200-meter world records. He's been quoted saying "Sleep is extremely important to me—I need to rest and recover in order for the training I do to be absorbed by my body."

Some football teams such as the Arizona Cardinals really believe in naps. Their owner built the Cardinals a $15 million Tempe training facility adding a "Rest and Recovery Room." Team president Michael Bidwell wanted his players to have enough rest to play well. The room has three bed-like tables that offer a very gentle massage in a dark, cool, room that players love. Cardinals star player Larry Fitzgerald said he tries to get ten hours of sleep during the season with nine at night and a mid-day nap. Cardinal's quarterback Carson Palmer told a reporter that sleep is brought up in meetings, after practice and you hear it from trainers, the weight-room guys, the head coach, and all the other coaches.

The San Jose Sharks players are encouraged to drink chamomile, lavender and tart cherry juice, a melatonin producer, every night since they are recommended for sleep. A Stanford University researcher found that free-throw shooting improved by 11.4% and three-point shooting improved by 13.7 % when players increased their nightly sleep from 6.5 to 8.5 hours.

Larry Fitzgerald has his own recipe for a protein and sweet smoothie. Fitzgerald has been a wide receiver for the Arizona Cardinals football team in Phoenix for 15 seasons. He has equipped over nine schools with needed equipment for students to access technology and participated in missions to support economic development in Africa, India, the Philippines, and Eastern Europe. While taking time out from those activities and his two sons, he often uses this smoothie in the morning or the evening.

Larry Fitzgerald Protein Smoothie

2 scoops 100% Whey Protein Powder
8 ounces almond milk
1 tablespoon peanut butter
1 cup ice

PGA pro golfers travel extensively, often competing in back to back tourney miles apart; i.e., ending play on a Sunday in Hawaii and starting the next on Thursday in California, even traveling from one country to another within a week.

Young elite golf prodigy Jordan Spieth's trainer has revealed the daily diet for the young champ.

Jordan Spieth Snacks

Baked sweet potato with ¼ cup pecans and 1 tablespoon honey
Snacks of grain-free granola (no oats, just nuts, seeds, fruits, and spices)

Businesses with Sleepy Young Employees

Sports organizations are not the only ones to see the value in rest. Many companies are forcing workers to use time off. Human resources officers are telling employees that constantly being available on-line translates into more work hours. That intrudes on your personal life, can cause burnout, and lead to a variety of physical and mental health issues. In fact, the U.S. Travel Association took action when it discovered in 2013 that only 19% of its employees were taking all their vacation time. The number soared to 91% the next year when they offered a $500 bonus to employees who used all their days. The company has seen a dramatic drop in health care costs, sick days and turnover.

Labor advocates in the United Kingdom, France, and Germany have been addressing this issue with employees and the United States could be next in ensuring that employees take their earned time off.

The new workplace epidemic threatening American employers and the productivity of their employees may be sleepy workers. Businesses lose $63 billion in productivity each year from sleepy workers. Accountemps reported that 74% of U.S. workers say they work while tired, and nearly one-third say they do so very often. More than 1,000 employees surveyed by Accountemps cited being easily distracted (52%), procrastinating more (47%), being grumpier (38%), and making more mistakes (29%) as consequences of their sleepiness.

Younger workers are more likely to be tired on the job. Workers aged eighteen to thirty-four admitted to being sleepy at work more than people aged thirty-five to fifty-four. Only half of respondents ages fifty-five and older claimed to be tired on the job. More than half of workers said they would use a nap room if their employer offered one. Google, Apple and AOL are known for their nap rooms. Bill Driscoll, district president of Accountemps suggested implementing flexible work schedules and telecommuting options.

On March 2, 2016, *Employer Benefit News Magazine* outlined how American employers are developing more awareness of the sleep epidemic leading to absenteeism, on-the-job accidents, vulnerability to infections, cardiovascular disease, and jitters. They are challenging the macho view that sleep isn't necessary if you're tough. Fitness programs, meditation programs, and much media discuss how sleep hygiene practices are conducive to good sleep. Sleep problems and sleep deprivation are more important to some professions than others. Those who are charged with protecting the public must be sure they are protecting themselves, first of all.

Firefighters and Sleep Needs and Health Problems

Drowsiness and sleep were discussed by fire chiefs on the International Fire Chiefs Association web site in June, 2016. They compared policies about how many hours firefighters could work to avoid fatigue problems. There was a variety of duty hours but all were trying to avoid sleep deprivation and fatigue.

An Illinois chief said members in his district will not work more than 56 consecutive on-duty hours and must be off duty at least 16 hours before working again. A Michigan chief said no employees will be allowed to work more than 72 consecutive hours without an eight-hour break in between unless emergency or disaster conditions prevail. An Idaho fire chief cited their union policy that no 56-hour member can work more than 52 consecutive hours without a 12-hour time off period unless authorized by the Fire Chief or his designee for emergencies.

A New Jersey chief noted their policy of 24 hours on, 72 hours off, and no more than 24 hours in a row without a ten-hour break in between unless there is an emergency. He commented that studies have shown that stress, associated with long hours of limited sleep and fatigue, decreases our decision-making capabilities and can expose our firefighters and the public to greater risks. An Ohio fire chief mentioned that personnel aren't allowed to work more than 48 consecutive hours without specific approval by the chief. A Florida fire chief wrote that no employees could work more than 48 hours without a minimum of twelve hours off unless there is a declared disaster, late calls, or when awaiting relief by oncoming personnel.

Around 2002, firefighters in Kern County, California, developed the 48/96 schedule because their commutes to and from work were so long. Various other California departments tried out the schedule and began to find unexpected advantages. When firefighters finish their 48-hour shift, they are free to be with family, do other projects or have extra jobs. Their other jobs do not usually involve the intense readiness needed in life or death emergencies.

They save money on driving to and from work less often in a week. Spouses are usually happier because of more family time except for when their 48 hours are on Saturday and Sunday from time to time. Many fire chiefs say the new schedule improved morale and decreased sick leave, which in turn cut overtime costs. But they worry that extended shifts will cause fatigue and mistakes.

On February 1, 2012, *Fire Engineering* wrote about the enthusiastic reception of the 48/96 schedule by fire districts in other California areas and other places such as Lakewood, Colorado. Employees are often unaware of their own impairment, don't recognize their mistakes, operate with eyes open but little cognizance, and have more accidents the longer they are sleep-deprived.

Chief Rob Biscoe of the North County Fire and Medical District of Arizona has been using the 48/96 schedule in his District since January, 2012. "There are only three fire districts in Maricopa County that have not adopted that schedule," he said. "We have not seen a down-side and one of our firefighters is happy that he now can live farther away in Flagstaff. We continue to test our system with pilot trials of 24 hours on and 48 off. We do that because sometimes there is a lot of coming and going by the ambulances and we want to be sure they get enough rest."

Chief Biscoe has led his department to become the first Arizona fire district to acquire an Insurance Services Office (ISO) rating of One (out of ten), which places them at the top one per cent of the nation's 49,000 fire departments. They have also achieved CFAI accredited agency status, and are notable as a Heart Safe Community and a Premier EMS Agency.

They have recently hired a nurse-practitioner who will be able to do personnel physicals, make house calls, and do basic treatment of those who do not need to go to crowded emergency rooms. This forward-thinking district has annexed one fire district and has worked out a Joint Powers Authority with another Fire Department—a new way to reduce costs for personnel and create cost-effective joint purchases. Working with another fire district, employees are shared and do not get overworked and sleep deprived, and districts save money by sharing chiefs and fire marshals.

Firefighters with Sleep and Health Problems

An important study of sleep deprivation in firefighters was undertaken by the International Association of Fire Chiefs and the U.S. Fire Administration in June 2007. They stated that firefighters and EMS responders are charged with the immediate care of our 24/7 society. While compressed work-weeks may have advantages for this profession, chronically sleep-deprived people make increased errors in tasks requiring alertness, vigilance, and quick decision-making.

Some 7,000 firefighters in 66 fire departments were examined in 2014 for obstructive sleep disorders, insomnia, restless leg syndrome, and shift work disorder. Using interviews and documented traffic accidents they found that 37% of the firefighters screened positive for at least one sleep disorder (usually obstructive sleep apnea). Unfortunately, fewer than 20% had been diagnosed and sought treatment.

Those with a sleep disorder were about twice as likely to have a motor vehicle crash, to nod off while driving, and to have cardiovascular disease or diabetes. They were more than three times as likely to suffer from depression and anxiety. Researchers concluded that 60% of firefighter deaths are caused by heart attacks and traffic accidents. They recommend reducing sleep disorders to better preserve the lives of firefighters.

Sleepy Firefighters May Commit Suicide

An *On Scene* newsletter published by the International Fire Chiefs Association in 2016 brought a sobering realization of the role sleep plays in mental health. In 2015, 90 firefighters and 24 EMS personnel committed suicide. The Firefighter Behavior Health Alliance has identified the top five warning signs that lead to suicide.

1. Recklessness/Impulsiveness: Riding reckless or charging into burning buildings against procedure.
2. Anger: Seemingly minor issues may produce explosive anger.

3. Isolation: Becoming distant from firefighters and family members
4. Loss of confidence in skills: An experienced firefighter who can't remember how to put an engine in gear to pump is an example.
5. Sleep deprivation: Loss of sleep can indicate stress, anxiety, or post-traumatic stress issues.

The newsletter recommended that "If you see someone struggling or just off their game: Be proactive, be direct, ask direct questions, be compassionate, take discretionary time to talk, walk the walk, and take care of your brothers or sisters out there."

Firefighters and Alcohol

Alcohol use in career firefighters has been reported in several studies. Some 160 London firefighters completed on-line health assessment surveys. About 89% stated that they consumed alcohol and approximately one-third reported having a drinking binge in the past 30 days. White respondents were 4.5 time more likely to binge drink than non-white respondents. For each year of service, firefighters were slightly less likely to binge drink. Researchers noted that firefighters drank more alcohol than the general adult population, including college students. Thus, firefighters were an at-risk drinking group and sleep disruptions due to alcohol use needed assessment.

A study of 656 firefighters from career and volunteer U.S. fire departments in 2012 found that 58% of career and 40% of volunteer firefighters averaged three or more drinks and more binge drinking on the days they consumed alcohol. Nine per cent of career and ten percent of volunteer firefighters admitted driving while intoxicated in the previous 30 days. Given the high rates of heavy and binge drinking, efforts to increase the surveillance of drinking behavior among firefighters and prevention methods are critically needed.

Driver Engineers of big fire vehicles might benefit from some new inventions to track eyelid movement. Employers could install eyelid tracking options to aid drivers and alert them.

Sensor technologies inside a truck as well as a fire vehicle can track eyelid closure, head positions, nods, steering wheel grip and so on. To be functional in monitoring driver drowsiness, a device must be portable and able to produce feedback to the driver before drowsiness reaches the level of accidents. Eyelid frequencies of 2 or 3 per minute would indicate marked drowsiness. Alarms could alert the driver regarding his impairment.

Firefighters and Healthier Diets

Health is being promoted by many fire districts in recent years. Some chefs have learned the physical demands of firefighters and designed special meals for them. Chef Marshall O'Brien has developed a list of healthy meals for the Minneapolis Fire District. Sweets which hasten the sleep hormone should be small but citizens bring in donuts and cookies especially at holidays. Perhaps they could be coaxed to bring in nuts and cheese instead. Chef O'Brien offered this recipe as an example of healthy food for a fire department.

Minneapolis Firefighters Salmon, Potatoes and Green Beans

Salmon:
4 six-ounce salmon filets
2 tablespoons olive oil
Salt and pepper to season filets

Relish for salmon:
2 tomatoes, diced
1 avocado pitted, peeled and diced
½ cup onion, diced
2 tablespoons fresh cilantro, chopped
1-2 tablespoons fresh lime juice, or to taste

Garlic Potatoes:
2 cups red potatoes, quartered
4 cloves garlic, chopped
2 tablespoons olive oil
Salt and pepper to taste

Lemon Green Beans:
1 pound green beans, frozen
2 tablespoons olive oil
2 teaspoons lemon juice (about ½ lemon)
Salt and pepper to taste

Preheat oven to 350 degrees. Usually feeds the whole fire station.

Tom Ansell, member of the International Association of Fire Fighters submitted a plan for firefighters to improve their food choices to help their sleep and health. His choices decrease Sweets, White food (flour, potatoes, rice, pasta), Oils (except olive oil and coconut oil), and Processed foods which contain MSG, so he calls it SWOP. He recommended cooking foods at moderate temperatures rather than high heat which damages food and makes it unhealthy. He said once he started this diet, his "food cravings disappeared, energy levels improved, he slept better, and woke feeling rested, thought clearer and felt in control of his health again.

Firefighters and Tobacco

Smokeless tobacco and cigarettes are used by many firefighters but little study of their use prompted researchers to investigate in 2013. In a group of 478 male career firefighters from many fire districts, 13% reported using smokeless tobacco and 2.6% used both smokeless tobacco and cigarettes. Binge alcohol drinking and high dietary fat consumption were associated with those who used smokeless tobacco (chewing tobacco, dip or snuff). As a result, firefighters using smokeless tobacco had more significant health risks. Almost all smokeless tobacco users were white adults, who used more alcohol, and were more likely to do risky behavior such as not wearing their SCBA (breathing apparatus) during a fire.

Dual use of cigarettes and smokeless tobacco was very high (2 to 4 times higher than national data) in this cohort. Almost half of the dual users reported using smokeless tobacco only after joining the fire service. They concluded smokeless tobacco intervention programs should be specifically developed and tailored for this occupational group.

Recommendation for smokeless tobacco intervention programs for firefighters was even stronger in more recent studies due to the many health problems (cancer, less sleep by tobacco users, more meat consumption, etc.) that have been uncovered.

Female Firefighters and Sleep

Gender comparisons of firefighters were studied in 2012. Out of 300,000 paid firefighters, only 3.7% were women despite the International Association of Fire Fighters and the International Association of Fire Chiefs promoting a diverse work force. That low number is well under law enforcement figures where 13% of police officers are women. Compared to male firefighters, females are less obese and in better health. However, some 11% use smokeless tobacco (and more use cigarettes) which far outweighs the use of smokeless tobacco by American women but is similar to females in the military. Rates of their alcohol use were higher than the general population with some binge drinking.

These high-risk behaviors of firefighters can be modified, of course, but they appear to be part of the social bond that creates brotherhood among employees. Sleep patterns are disrupted because of the duration of shifts and the unpredictability of emergency calls. Substance use (alcohol, nicotine, caffeine) may provide relief from the demands of the job or may be an acceptable norm of social bonding. That social bond might be used to help fire departments take a more active role in helping firefighters improve their health.

Wildlands Firefighters and Sleep

Wildlands firefighters generally work in more perilous surroundings trying to put out wildfires before they reach homes and businesses. Nineteen wildlands firefighters lost their lives together on June 30, 2013, when fighting a fire near Yarnell, Arizona. The Granite Mountain Hotshots had done non-stop firefighting for 28 days on duty. Their group of hotshots started in 1946 and was a close-knit team.

They were to have two days off and began their brief holiday on June 29th when some of the Hot Shots went to a bar in Prescott, Arizona. They had just come off a 12-hour shift and the owner gave them a discount. They had some drinks. All were in bed in various places only to be awakened early on June 30 because a fire had broken out from a lightning strike near Yarnell, a community of some 700 persons.

They rushed to the area where they were told to climb up a hill carrying their equipment. A witness saw them hiking up the trail at 9:18 a.m. "What I saw was a group of men who were totally spent. They looked like they were tired. They weren't somebody you would want to fight a fire. They needed rest."

Their spotter, the only one of the 20 to survive, was just contacting them that the wind had changed direction and was coming toward them. It was too late for them to do more than descend slightly into a canyon and don their fire sacks. They all died and their charred remains were found inside each sack.

Autopsies showed alcohol in 13 of the 19 bodies, and one firefighter had a number of drugs in his system. He had taken several narcotics, a tranquilizer, and a stimulant which may or may not have been prescribed for pain, but alcohol was not found in his body. One of the men had a tattoo that said "Dream as if you'll live forever. Live as if you'll die today!" It was surmised that their fatigue and weary thinking ability sorely impaired their activity that day. This was the worst firefighter tragedy ever in Arizona and was the 6th worst in the country.

Post-Traumatic Stress Disorder in Firefighters

Emergency workers, such as firefighters, are routinely exposed to potentially traumatic events. The role of multiple traumas that produce post-traumatic stress disorder, depression, sleep deprivation and alcohol misuse was assessed in 488 current firefighters and 265 retired firefighters in Australia in 2015. Among their current firefighters, rates of post-traumatic stress disorder were 8%; and some 4% reported consumption of more than 42 alcoholic drinks per week. The more fatal incidents experienced, the higher the rates of post-traumatic stress disorder, depression, sleep deprivation and heavy drinking.

The occupation of firefighter is associated with danger, uncertainty, and unpredictability. The notion of "waiting" (prepared readiness) is one of the central factors in a firefighter's working life. They must hold themselves ready to respond from the instant they start a shift until it ends. When the station alarm system sounds, lights come on and sirens alert firefighters to cease activities, put on their protective clothing, and move to their vehicles. In this way, they become conditioned and hyper-vigilant to changes in light and sound intensity.

This hyper-vigilant response extends to off-duty time as well. A light turned on by a spouse may trigger a response. Since firefighters sleep during nightshifts in departments across the world, knowing that they may be wakened does not improve the quality of sleep. Obviously, this is likely to enhance fatigue.

Most firefighters use some black humor in the mess room to release upset feelings and build unity in stressful times. However, grief and emotional shock of exposure to accident trauma persists. One firefighter admitted, "When I went to my first motor vehicle accident, I could not talk about it for two years afterwards. My wife noticed something was wrong when I came home that night, but she didn't ask once I said I didn't want to talk about it."

Firefighters run upon scenes where people were incinerated, or the Jaws of Life had to be used as people were dying. The sights and smells prevail and they often smell the burnt flesh even when the event is over. Certain scenes such as watching a child catch on fire and scream and die, but being unable to reach them remain in memory and disrupt one's life. Once they keep it inside, they must rely on more experienced firefighters to help them talk about it and help undo the trauma. Driving by the same scene or seeing a child of the same age may trigger reactions. Finding a body in a hundred pieces is a trauma that is relieved only by horrible jokes about death. Some people become more callous, others are too devastated and become helpless, and there are those who develop symptoms of physical and emotional dysfunction.

Trauma Screening

Some 5,656 firefighters involved with the World Trade Center were studied for post-traumatic stress disorder. They were assessed six months after the 9/11/2001 event and at three to four years after the event. At six months, 15.5% of the firefighters had symptoms of post-traumatic disorder. Nearly three years later, 11.1% still had such symptoms. Nearly half of all the post-traumatic stress disorder symptoms occurred much later, and many were associated with functional impairment in their work and life.

A basic Trauma Screening Questionnaire (TSQ) was developed by C. R. Brewin and colleagues in 2002. It is recommended that the TSQ be offered 3-4 weeks post-trauma to those who have been in a potentially traumatic event, to allow time for normal recovery processes to take place. If at that point, an individual has six or more YES answers, a referral to a behavioral health practitioner is indicated. A YES answer should be scored if the event happened at least twice in the past week. Sleep is often impaired for some time after a traumatic event. The Trauma Screen Questionnaire includes:

1. Upsetting thoughts or memories about the event that have come into your mind against your will.
2. Upsetting dreams about the event.

3. Acting or feeling as though the event were happening again.
4. Feeling upset by reminders of the event.
5. Bodily reactions (such as fast heartbeat, stomach churning).
6. Difficulty falling asleep or staying asleep.
7. Irritability or outburst of anger.
8. Difficulty concentrating.
9. Heightened awareness of potential dangers to yourself and others.
10. Feeling jumpy or being startled by something unexpected.

If therapy is recommended for a person with the symptoms above, it must be developed in a relationship that creates a sense of safety. A distressed individual should be calmed using a bedside manner and connected with whatever support services fit the situation and the individual. Physical and psychological evaluations will be performed and re-measured at the end of the therapy program. A desensitization program will be developed so that over a 2-3 weeks program of three or four visits, the person will become much calmer and able to overcome most of the mentioned symptoms.

At the end of the program, questions should be asked of the individual. What was our (your) mission? What went well? What could have gone better? What might we (you) have done differently? Who needs to know and what should they know (other employees, superiors, the station, the battalion chief, the chief, others)?

Sleeping with a Firefighter

An article was on the Fire Engineering web site by the wife (Anne Gagliano) of a fire captain. It can be found on the Internet under "How to Sleep with a Firefighter" posted January 6, 2015. Anne said that in addition to getting along with each other during the day, firefighter couples have to get along with each other when their spouse works a 24-hour shift. She said that often a firefighter is wired and tired when he comes home—kind of like a two-year old. They are in perpetual hyper-arousal because of the fight-or-flight response of the body. When the station bell rings, they must be ready.

She gave spouses some advice. Offer your mate some hot milk and a warm bath to relax. Get rid of all light and forget pretty curtains in favor of complete dark. Your spouse may talk in his sleep or move about because he is hyper-alert, and he may fall asleep in the middle of your conversation about the day. Don't be offended if he falls asleep while you talk. And if he has things on his mind, he may want to scribble them down next to the bed without getting up. A "to do" list is better than getting up to do something in the middle of the night. Anne has been married to Captain Mike Gagliano in the Seattle Fire District for 29 years so she speaks from experience.

Linda Willing worked as a career firefighter and fire officer for 18 years. For more than 15 years, she has provided support for fire and emergency services through her company, RealWorld Training and Consulting. She said, "It is surprising how little attention has been given to the role of sleep for firefighters." She referred to a 2014 study of 7,000 firefighters where 37% screened positive for at least one sleep disorder. Some 80% of those with a sleep disorder were undiagnosed and untreated. She described her early years sleeping in large open dorms with poor ventilation on old saggy beds that often smelt of cigarette smoke and after shave. Station personnel resisted improvement saying, "We're not paying you to sleep." Now many fire dorms are split into separate sleeping cubicles for men and women.

She developed seven steps for better sleep in the fire service. First, departments must recognize that adequate sleep is a wellness and performance issue. They should evaluate sleep and make cheap and expensive changes from installing fans or white noise generators to renovating dorms into sleeping pods. Assess sleep fitness by gathering data anonymously to get a picture of how members manage sleep on and off the job. Allow naps on duty. Make resources available for those with sleep disorders. Reconsider shift schedules and overtime rules to diminish sleep deprivation effects on emergency responders. Look at new technology to manage sleep and performance. She ended "Assuring quality sleep for firefighters is a health and wellness issue whose time is long overdue. Lives depend on it!"

Firefighters and Suicide

Suicide is known to be a problem for police officers but many people don't realize that it is also prevalent among firefighters. The Installation Remarks of Chief John Sinclair, upon becoming the President and Chairman of the Board for the International Association of Fire Chiefs (IAFC) on August 22, 2016, made it clear that he wanted reduce that problem:

> "We are facing significant challenges in the fire service and I want to shine a light on some of them. We are learning more and more about PTSD (post-traumatic stress disorder) and behavioral health issues facing firefighters. Firefighter suicide is a trend we must reverse."

Firefighter suicides in the United States have risen over the past several years. In 2012, there were 81, in 2013, there were 70, in 2014, there were 112, and in 2015, there were 132 firefighters and EMT suicides. Suicide is the tenth leading cause of death in the United States with 13 suicides per 100,000 people dying annually. The rates of suicide among the protective services (firefighters and police) was 34.1 per 100,000 people, which puts them 6th highest for males and 14.1 for women—the highest suicide rate for any female occupational group.

This highlights the importance of crews watching out for each other and being aware when one of their own is having a problem

Firefighters Must Help Each Other

One of the most recent female suicides was Nicole Mittendorf of Fairfax County, Virginia, in April, 2016. This beautiful firefighter and paramedic was put on a male employee's Facebook in a lewd way.

That site criticized her and other female employees using terrible insults and accusations by male co-workers. She talked with her husband about those Facebook comments before her death and told him that she had decided to just ignore them. However, perhaps she could not. She had been sleepless and restless for days. She called in sick on April 13, and her husband could not find her. A search party was sent out. She was found April 23 near her vehicle where she had hanged herself.

She left a suicide note. Steve, her husband of four years, said it helped him "to get a better idea of what she was going through." Five months after her death, the Fairfax Fire Department held a 5K walk in Fairfax to bring attention to suicide prevention. It was publicized as an "Out of the Darkness Walk" because her death was called "a fire bell in the night."

Fire Chief David Dangerfield of Florida committed suicide October 15, 2016, after leaving the following note on his computer which is shown just as he worded it:

> PTSD for firefighters is real. If your love one is experiencing signs, get them help quickly. 27 years of deaths and babies dying in your hands is a memory that you will never get rid of. It haunted me daily until now. My love to my crews. Be safe. Take care. I love you all.

Dangerfield had married Leslie, a teacher, in 2002. They soon had son Bryce and Leslie already had an older son. She described disturbing experiences for her husband: "A few years ago there was a shark attack. A boy went in the water. They found his bathing suit and portions of his body. It's haunting. There are nightmares." Later David had to recover the body of a small boy who drowned. About four years before his death, Leslie told David to see someone for help because he was having so much trouble sleeping and worrying. She thought he matched the symptoms of PTSD but he said, "No, that's for veterans, the military." She said, "David, this is you."

He began working with a psychiatrist and was on various medicines. Things were better for a while, but gradually he no longer seemed like his old self to his wife. A few months before his suicide, they separated. Leslie said: "I knew every night when I got home... who is going to be there when I get home? Which David? The David I fell in love with? Or am I getting the PTSD David?" She asked for a separation because he seemed so different.

On the evening of his death, he was returning 14-year old Bryce to his mother after having him for the weekend. He had called Leslie crying and saying "I can't do it anymore." She said, "You can't do this to the boys, you can't leave them, please don't leave them." As he left the house, he had dressed in his best uniform. Young Bryce said, "Why are you all dressed up?" His father said, "I'll be back. Don't you worry about it." When Bryce saw his father's wallet on the table after he walked out to his vehicle, the boy ran after his dad with it. "Daddy, you left your wallet." Chief Dangerfield answered, "I don't need it. See you in a little bit, buddy."

He then drove to an off road and contacted dispatchers to tell them where they would find him just before he shot himself.

We mentioned these tragedies in detail because some of the main symptoms of post-traumatic syndrome disorder are sleep disturbances and nightmares. These symptoms can alert family members and fellow employees to help them get help. *News of these two cases drew attention to the shocking fact that there were more suicides in the fire service than deaths by fire personnel on the job.*

Police Officers and Sleep Deprivation

Police officers, detectives, undercover cops and police personnel frequently have irregular hours. They have trouble sleeping and the coffee pot is always going at the station. Furthermore, their jobs expose them to the worst side of human behavior that is hard to forget when they try to sleep.

The fictional story of detectives was perhaps best told by Sir Arthur Conan Doyle (1859-1930) creator of Sherlock Holmes. Doyle was a physician who specialized in eyes and finally retired to develop detective stories with exceedingly astute eyes. Doyle wrote in *A Scandal in Bohemia* published in 1891, "It is a capital mistake to theorize before one has data. Insensibly, one begins to twist facts to suit theories, instead of theories to suit facts." Being a man of science, he made evidence replace superstition and guesses.

Holmes was a supposed truth-seeker, often pictured with a magnifying glass to see even better. He might even have said: "You can't handle the truth!" if anyone denied his findings. He might carefully deduce that cookies produced by the following recipe could help even the guilty fall asleep.

Sherlock Holmes Thumbprint Cookies

Make a spot of herbal tea to sip on whilst you compose these cookies. Make your favorite cookie dough and shape the dough into one inch balls. Place them two inches apart on a baking sheet. With your thumb, make an imprint in the center of each cookie. Allow the swirls on your finger tip to show so that even Dr. Watson can detect just who made the cookies. Bake those 11 to 14 minutes. Now, the problem is to hide your fingerprint so nobody can find you out. Spoon ½ teaspoon of jam into the center of each cookie. Cool completely.

Be careful when eating these cookies not to drop any crumbs on your clothes or Sherlock will have his magnifying glass out to detect just what you've eaten, as well as when and where you were when the hound of the Baskervilles was howling.

Don't eat too many of those cookies. Tom Wickman, Chief of Police in Frisco, Colorado, wrote about the poor diet and physical problems of police officers. He commented that approximately fourteen police officers are lost in the line of duty every year to heart attacks. A lack of exercise, poor sleeping habits, and diets heavy in fats all contribute to the deteriorating function of the human heart and circulatory system. He ended his article in *The Police Chief Magazine* of June 2016 by encouraging police officers to spend 20 minutes of cardiovascular exercise three times a week, committing to one meatless day a week, and eating mostly plant foods.

The Fatigue Factor in Police Work is Immense

A study of critical incident exposure on sleep quality in police officers compared police against non-emergency workers. Police officers reported significantly worse sleep quality and less sleep time than most other people. Incident exposure created nightmares, and sleep disturbances were strongly associated with post-traumatic stress symptoms. Researchers commended police departments who have added critical incident debriefing to their services for impacted officers.

Studies have found that police officers have increased rates of cardiovascular and gastrointestinal disorders, divorce rates twice the national average, and suicide rates three times the national average. In addition, their immune system is reduced, their circadian day-night rhythms are abnormal, and their heart rate variability and psychomotor performance are impaired.

Dr. Bryan Vila's research has shown that officers on night shifts have much higher rates of accidents. In addition, officers working on 12-hour shifts had lower levels of alertness at work, and reported being sleepier than officers on 8-hour shifts. There was a loss in concentration and cognitive processing accompanied by fatigue, sleepiness, slower reaction times, and high numbers of citizen complaints.

Vila served as a police officer for 17 years. He explained his predicament in June 2011. "I was working up to 80 hours of overtime a month...No matter my intentions, I found myself becoming easily frustrated and unable to remain calm in situations because I was so tired." Because of this, Vila developed programs promoting officer safety by managing fatigue and work hours.

In his 2002 publication *"Tired Cops: The Prevalence and Potential Consequences of Police Fatigue,"* Vila commented that sleepy fatigued officers use more sick leave, practice inappropriate uses of force more frequently, become involved in more vehicle accidents, experience more accidental injuries, have more difficult dealings with community members and other law enforcement agencies, and have a higher likelihood of dying in the line of duty.

A survey of 4,957 U.S. and Canadian police officers found that 40.4% of the officers screened positive for at least one sleep disorder, with obstructive sleep apnea being the most common. That study was published in *SLEEP* Vol 39, 2016, and added that 21% of police officers reported use of sleep-promoting drugs or medicines that listed sleepiness as a side-effect. These drugs were significantly associated with motor vehicle near misses or actual errors.

While these daunting statistics suggest many problems, there is a new culture of crash prevention coming to the fore of police leadership. It shows up in many ways. Kirk McLean, Captain in Prince George's County of Maryland Police Department, framed it well. He wrote in March 2017 in *The Police Chief:* "Creating a culture in law enforcement where all members of the agency take an active role in education, awareness, and prevention of crashes is paramount to saving lives, including those of police officers." His department decided to seek a commitment from 100 percent of the personnel to use their seat belts. They found that the key ingredients to their success in this initiation were incentives and positive peer pressure. The program motto was: "Buckle up, slow down, pay attention, arrive alive!"

Most Police Officers Work Overtime and/or Off Duty

Chief Deputy (retired) A. Jay Six, Jr. served as a police officer for two years at the University of Texas in Arlington, 24 years as a police officer and lieutenant at the Arlington Police Department and 14 years as Chief Deputy of Patrol at the Tarrant County Sheriff's Office. Six said "My observation is that many, many officers work off-duty jobs. Officers who don't work off-duty are rare, and for the rest, it's a near necessity— if not an obsession. Our local football and baseball teams pay $75/hour and double that on holiday games. Thus, officers time off, even where work is limited by department standards, is often consumed with off-duty work."

He added, "Where part-time work once represented a subtle way for employers to augment police salaries without having to raise taxes, it has become a culture all its own. Cops sacrifice sleep to work off-duty. And talk about a sacred cow—just try to tell a law enforcement officer that he has to curtail off-duty work."

Six currently teaches police supervision and ethics at The Center for American and International Law in Plano, Texas. He also serves on their advisory board as well as the Institute of Law Enforcement Administration.

The Chicago Police Department was battling in 2013 over hiring more police instead of paying some $93 million in overtime to police officers. The City argued that hiring more officers involved taking on additional costs such as medical, health insurance, and the huge retirement funds that grow with a larger force. However, the Union felt that their people were overworked to the point of exhaustion. San Jose, California, went through the same problems in 2016. Officer fatigue from overtime was occurring because officers were quitting and too few were filling open slots.

Doug Wyllie, a police trainer, wrote how lack of sleep may cause deadly police errors. He described studies where fatigued officers chose to shoot more often than well-rested officers, and they took longer to decide on appropriate actions when faced with ambiguous situations. He concluded the article with the recommendation that "fatigue-mitigating measure can be enacted using simple adjustments, such as on duty nap periods for fatigued officers, circumscribed overtime rules and total work hours, and less frequent shift rotations."

Night Duty and Mae West

Back in the 1920s and 1930s, one sexy lady kept a lot of police officers awake at night with her performances. Mae West (1892-1980) was a vaudeville actress who wanted to be a Broadway star. She wrote plays such as her bawdy 1926 play called *Sex*. New York's deputy police commissioner raided the theater and Mae spent ten days in jail for lewdness. Her first theatrical smash was *Diamond Lil* where she played a fancy 1890s saloon hostess. Within a few years, she became one of the biggest movie stars of the era, with one sexual hit after another. Hollywood censors waged war against her and she became a favorite of audiences and many police officers. Her buxom figure caused inflated life preserver vests to be called Mae Wests.

Mae had so many famous lines. A coat check girl admired her diamonds saying, "Goodness. What lovely diamonds." Mae responded, "Goodness had nothing to do with it!" She was also the one who said, "Is that a gun in your pocket or are you just glad to see me?" She kidded people saying "When I'm good, I'm very, very good but when I'm bad I'm better." With lines like that, most guys would stay awake if they slept with her. Now, Mae won't mind if you substitute some other healthy fruit in her compote, since she's in the "big sleep" now.

Mae West Fruit Compote

Her recipe had one chopped apple, pear, and banana but you could have strawberries or blueberries. She threw in 2 or 3 chopped almonds and a few raisins. All this is topped with a mixture of 2 tablespoons of milk with a teaspoon or so of honey to taste.

Mae West, Gypsy Rose Lee and Sally Rand all knew each other. I discovered this one day in Texas. I was in Galveston visiting the Medical School and received an invitation from the Commander of the Blue Angels to see the aircrafts perform. While there, he said his wife had not accompanied him and he invited me to go to a nightclub where Sally Rand was doing her fan dance. He was a proper gentleman so I accepted. We were ushered in behind Sally's stage by the club owner. The lady wore nothing but the fan in front of her which shielded her, yet tempted her audience. We saw the back of her and the 68-year old lady still had a great body.

The next day, the commander called saying he had an interesting psychological study for me. Sally Rand called him, asking for a ride to the Houston airport where she could fly to California for an emergency. Lucky to be invited to "analyze" her, I found her most delightful. On the ride, she described her good relationships with Mae and especially Gypsy. They all had so much in common as early burlesque queens.

Sally kindly gave me a gift of some fuzzy hair rollers after we talked about the difficulty of sleeping with rollers on your head. She gave me hers saying she had another set and she included her card signed "Your fan, Sally Rand." When the commander asked for my analysis as we drove back to Galveston, I said "After knowing Sally Rand, I think I'll sleep better!" So, let us return to the jobs of those poor policemen who had to make a tough living enforcing laws.

Research by Dr. John Violanti (see his book *Dying for the Job*) noted that people in the general population live seven years longer than police officers. There is more cardiovascular disease among officers due to the physical strain placed on them with heavy equipment to carry coupled with sudden tasks like foot pursuits, running up steep inclines, engagement of defensive or arrest tactics, and additional stress. Violanti described an increase in suicide among police officers caused by chronic stress, a lack of coping skills and exposure to traumatic situations in policing. The book strongly recommended that strategies must be developed to deal with wellness issues, stress, sleep disorders, fatigue, post-traumatic stress disorders, and suicidal thoughts.

The President's Task Force on 21st Century Policing of May 2015 emphasized more effective training to promote public confidence in the police and more effective policing. High on their list of priorities was crisis intervention, de-escalation training, bias awareness, and communication skills.

Police Officers and Suicide

Suicides among police officers kill almost as many police as deaths in their line of work. From 2010 through 2014, there have been 684 fatalities of officers being dispatched to a call for service which resulted in a line-of-duty death. An article in January 2017 issue of *The Police Chief* added that in the last five years, there have been around 150 suicides per year, which amount to more than line-of-duty deaths.

Ben Clark is chairman of Badge of Life, a group of active and retired police officers, medical professionals and surviving families of police suicides in the US and Canada. He said, "Officers face so many traumatic events...that officers fail to recognize the toll that it takes on them... We need quality peer support programs and strong leaders (chiefs) who believe that good mental health wellness requires training." Clark added that names of policemen who killed themselves would *not* be etched in the National Law Enforcement Officers Memorial Wall in Washington, D.C., because the foundation doesn't recognize suicide as an "in the line of work" death.

An example of one such case was a Charlotte, N.C. police lieutenant named Thomas Forbes. He was 52 and reported for work on Monday, June 6, 2011, and around 8:30 a.m. shot himself. His daughter, Lauren, described what she knew about his death. She said her father was an officer for 31 years and was stressed out. He told her the climate at his police department was "very political." He discussed leaving the department for the sake of his health. Two months before his death, he responded to a call for a deceased man who had killed himself and it troubled him greatly. He started having trouble sleeping and saw his primary doctor who prescribed sleeping pills. That was not sufficient to prevent his suicide.

Her father's triumphs were many as he came from a poor family and received an athletic scholarship to Eastern Connecticut State University. He married, had two girls, became a licensed pilot, a rescue diver, and trained hostage negotiator. "My father would bend over backwards for people. He loved to help people. He's never going to be honored the way he should be, and that was hard for my family." She grieved over the fact that he would not be recognized for the good he had done, but only for his final act.

Doreen Marshall, senior director of education and prevention at the American Foundation for Suicide Prevention, said "Suicide is about ending pain, physical or psychological. Often they believe their only choice to end that suffering is to take their own life. It's often hard for them to see that help is out there."

Lauren wished her father had received help when he had trouble sleeping and his physician offered nothing more than sleeping pills. Encouragement by the physician and his department to deal with his stresses might have been Forbes' his life saver.

Bryan Vila, mentioned earlier has said "Asking police officers if they've had enough sleep to safely perform their jobs is akin to asking drunks if they are capable of driving. People are lousy at self-assessing themselves." As a professor with the Department of Criminal Justice and Criminology and Sleep Performance Research Center with Washington State University health science, Vila tells officers: "You may be driving your patrol car while just as impaired as the last person you arrested for DUI."

In the May 2016 issue of *The Police Chief,* results of a survey were reported when chiefs were asked "What do you consider to be the most prominent safety risks for officers?" They responded:

1. Unsafe driving practices—29%
2. Poor fitness or cardiovascular health—27%
3. Emotional trauma or other mental health issue—18%
4. Shift work leading to poor sleep habits—10%
5. Not using protective gear—10%
6. Other—6%

In the same issue, Richard A. Ruck, Jr., Professor, Criminal Justice at East Stroudsburg University of Pennsylvania wrote: "Research has consistently demonstrated that the lack of sleep for various occupations results in a variety of primary duty, operation, and mission failures...as job demands and scrutiny of police increases, budgets shrink, and violence directed at police is not halted, sleep issues will manifest and result in a higher rate of line of duty injury and death."

We will end this chapter with a sweet, a small serving of Almond Parfait. Rex Stout (1886-1975) wrote detective stories featuring an orchid-loving gourmand sleuth named Nero Wolfe. Nero mentioned Almond Parfait in his book *In the Best Families* and you can use his idea for your own treat.

Rex Stout (Nero Wolfe) Almond Parfait

Make a nice vanilla pudding but finish it up by adding 1 teaspoon of almond extract and 2 tablespoons of minced almonds.

We come now to the profession that should have the best sleep of all, being noted for their study of the human body—the medical profession. However, we are in for a surprise and a real battle!

Chapter Thirteen
SLEEP IN THE MEDICAL PROFESSIONS

For 2,500 years, the Hippocratic Oath has required physicians to pledge about how they will treat the public: "I will keep them from harm." (Some people believe it says "First, do no harm.") People have come to trust that physicians and medical professionals will do no harm. Hippocrates wrote: "Leave nothing to chance. Overlook nothing. Allow yourself enough time." Above all, he stressed honesty. That was the key to the old philosophical adage "Physician, heal thyself." It took physicians an inordinately long time to realize they were jeopardizing their lives as well as those of their patients by sleep deprivation.

I was attracted to medicine since childhood when I came to appreciate those physicians and nurses who cared for me during my rheumatic fever illness. My appreciation of their profession was enhanced by visits and sleepovers with my grandmother who was "House Mother" for nurses in training at the Hillcrest Memorial Hospital in Tulsa, Oklahoma. These smart young women dressed in white were impressive and downright funny. They had parties that I witnessed with IV bottles, hot water bottles, enema tubes strung all over the room, crazy snacks like candy eyeballs and tongues, and feather pillow fights. I grew up wanting to be a nurse at that point in my life.

The Physician as a Role Model

I was learning along the way that the patient has as much to do with his or her own health and healing as the medical profession. Mark Twain understood the individual's partial control over their own body when he wrote in 1903:

> The power which a man's imagination has over his body to heal it or make it sick is a force which none of us is born without. The first man had it, the last one will possess it.

How could physicians and sometimes nurses forget that? Many thought they were gods, in charge of what the patient should or should not do. They could be very bossy. My parents disliked that and selected a doctor who was very down to earth. I would go in to see him to be checked for the rheumatic fever or my asthma. I'd say something like "I had a terrible cold and was coughing and sleepless and what should I do?" He said, "I had that last week and I just took good care of myself and got people to wait on me and had a good slug of whiskey from time to time, just like your father does. But you should skip the whiskey and here are some instructions for what you can do for yourself." He would hand me instructions and I followed them faithfully.

He usually had me in stitches but he gave me good advice so that I could learn to take care of myself. Sometimes he would sing a little song as he finished with me or as the nurse was giving me a shot. "Button up your overcoat when the wind is free, Take good care of yourself, you belong to me." His nurse would chime in with "Eat an apple every day, get to bed by three, take good care of yourself, you belong to me." Of course, they were singing from the 1926 song made famous by the singer Ruth Etting. Her life was portrayed by Doris Day in the 1955 movie *Love Me or Leave Me*.

Many patients thought that rapport was missing from the training of young physicians in their relationships with patients.

How could that best be learned? Canadian physician William Osler had an idea: Have physicians in training live, eat, and sleep close to the patients they were caring for. Then they will learn more about how to communicate with the patient as well as how to cure medical illnesses.

Sir William Osler Began Residencies

Sir William Osler (1849-1919) began the first residencies for medical students, interns, and residents in Johns Hopkins Hospital at the turn of the century. He had this to say about sleep and death. "Undress your soul at night--not by self-examination but by shedding, as you do your garments, the daily sins whether of omission or commission, and you will wake a free man, with a new life...To die daily...ensures the resurrection of a new man, who makes each day the epitome of life."

As he addressed young graduating medical students, he gave them a "way of life" speech. It included the following admonition: "The young man who feels on awakening that life is a burden or a bore has been neglecting his machine, driving it too hard, stoking the engines too much, or not cleaning out the ashes and clinkers. Or he has spent too much with the Lady Nictotine, or fooling with Bacchus, or, worst of all, with the younger Aphrodite." He was warning them to stay healthy, not use tobacco or alcohol, or not be loose in sex.

He also accompanied his graduation speech of 1899 with a recommendation to develop equanimity or imperturbability. A physician should be calm and in self-control in front of patients to foster their trust. Then physicians could say, "Trust me, I'm a doctor!" For many years, his speech was printed in a small document called "Aequanimitas" awarded to graduating United States and Canadian medical students.

Osler is known for his revolutionary changes in medical history. He said at his 1905 retirement speech that he started medical residencies after seeing something like it in Germany and Bavaria. After working at the medical school and hospital in Philadelphia,

Pennsylvania, he was given the administration of Johns Hopkins as it was being built. Mr. Hopkins' will required that his money be used for a medical school and hospital that would be located next to each other.

Osler set up the residency of fully trained physicians and those in training at the hospital to facilitate more interaction with patients. Osler's ideas spread to Europe and other areas after he developed the successful sleep-in residency at John Hopkins where staff physicians lived inside the hospital.

Sleep Versus Death with Heart Transplants

People's trust in physicians was sorely tested when the first heart transplantation took place in 1967. There had been no clear definition of life and death. For physicians, the deepest sleep is an irreversible coma. It was already a difficult decision to end a comatose person's life. But now came a new issue—ending a comatose person's life and retrieving body organs to place in another person. Many still believed that the heart, not the brain, was the seat of life so the idea of removing one's heart was like killing their soul. Surgeons knew that the seat of life was in the brain. They had been experimenting with heart transplantation in animals for at least 15 years by that time.

Christiaan Barnard performed the first heart transplant on December 3, 1967, in South Africa. Before that, he had been working with chimps until an event occurred which he described thusly:

> I had bought two male chimps from a primate colony in Holland. They lived next to each other in separate cages for several months before I used one as a heart donor. When we put him to sleep in his cage in preparation for the operation, he chattered and cried incessantly. We attached no significance to this, but it must have made a great impression on his companion, for when we removed the body to the

operating room, the other chimp wept bitterly and was inconsolable for days. The incident made a deep impression on me. I vowed never again to experiment with such sensitive creatures.

When Barnard performed the first heart transplant on Louis Washkansky, he inserted the heart of a young female in a man's body. The recipient lived only 18 days but the event was celebrated across the world. Immediately, Barnard wrote the details of his operation in a paper called "A Human Cardiac Transplant." But within two weeks, he performed another transplant on Dr. Philip Blaiberg who lived 18 months.

The issue became how to differentiate comatose sleep from death. In the United States, that definition involved medical rulings reviewed by the President's Commission for the Study of Ethical Behavioral Research. Those guidelines were concluded by declaring that a person in irreversible coma with lack of activity in all parts of the brain is dead. In the event of death by heart problems, a person could be defined as dead when there was no more circulatory action in the blood vessels and heart stoppage.

Poor Dr. Blaiberg's heart donor was a young man who died of a brain hemorrhage while swimming. The man was comatose but there were still some reflexes. The physician in charge of declaring him dead was a worried Dr. Raymond Hoffenberg. He spent a sleepless night because the transplant team for Blaiberg was ready all night to perform a heart transplant once a physician declared him dead. Hoffenberg held out until those reflexes stopped.

In later years, Dr. Barnard left surgery and pursued other tasks. One of his three wives prepared a beef stew recipe using what was known about heart-healthy foods at the time. The vegetable condiments served with this beef stew made it better than most beef dishes for health and for sleep ingredients. When we find beef, we have found a valuable source of tryptophan. That tryptophan can be escorted through the blood brain barrier to the hypothalamus by sweet condiments so that melatonin production can be increased.

Another cardiothoracic surgeon, Mehmet Oz, a Turkish-American, became famous through four or five seasons on the *Oprah Winfrey Show*. He now has the *Dr. Oz Show* on TV and is famous for looking into non-traditional or alternative remedies from time to time. His recipes on the Internet could also be used in place of, or after an evening meal, because they have sleep-inducing ingredients. He tries to share his recipes by making them in front of television audiences and by publishing them on his web site where these were found.

Dr. Oz Yogurt Smoothie

2 tablespoons peanut butter
8 ounces Greek yogurt
½ cup ice
1 banana
1 pinch cinnamon

Place peanut butter, yogurt and ice cubes in a blender and mix at high speed. Slice banana, add to mixture, and re-blend. Pour smoothie into two cups and serve. Sprinkle cinnamon on top for flavor. To make this more energy-boosting earlier in the day, add 2 tablespoons of cocoa powder. Serves two.

Dr. Oz Weight-Loss Smoothie

2 tablespoons cooked rice or protein powder
2 tablespoons ground flaxseeds
½ cup frozen berries
½ banana
1 cup unsweetened vanilla almond milk

Blend all ingredients together until you achieve the desired consistency. This can be a night time drink after a light dinner.

Physician Training and Sleep Deprivation

The extremely long working hours of those training to be physicians have met with much criticism. To understand this issue, we will examine the controversies from the famous Libby Zion case up to the present. Physician training hours are not as simple as some other professions where errors made by sleep-deprived pilots, truck drivers, firefighters and police officers mandated national changes.

The biggest controversy in medicine over the last thirty years has been about errors that sleep-deprived physicians made or could make in their care of patients. It began with the death of Libby Zion and became notorious through a lawsuit by her father—lawyer and journalist Sidney Zion.

Sidney Zion's career has received mixed acclaim. Four years after his daughter's death, Zion published *The Autobiography of Roy Cohn*. Cohn was a friend of Zion's and was reviled by many because he prosecuted Julius and Ethel Rosenburg, who were executed for espionage. Cohn also acted as chief counsel for Senator Joseph McCarthy during his Communist witch-hunt years. Although Zion was criticized for his defense of Cohn, he became a powerful ambassador for patients whose lives were ruined because of the sleep deprivation of their physician.

On May 4, 1984, 18-year old Libby Zion arrived at a New York City Hospital at 11:30 p.m. A college freshman, she arrived with a fever of 103 degrees, agitation, intermittent disorientation and strange jerking motions of her body. She said she was being treated for depression and was taking Nardil, a monoamine oxidase inhibitor pill for depression. She denied using illicit substances.

She was evaluated by an intern just eight months out of medical school and a resident with an additional year of training. They suspected it might be a viral syndrome with hysterical symptoms, suggesting that she was overreacting to a mild illness. Unable to diagnose her immediately, she was admitted for hydration and observation. Her father's physician was called and approved the decision to hospitalize her for work-up. She was given an injection of Demerol for pain, which is absolutely not to be used by someone taking Nardil. These days, computer alerts about adverse interactions by drugs might have prevented this fatal mistake.

Blood was drawn and urine collected but the results of the elevated white blood cells (seen in most infections) were apparently unheeded and other tests for infection were not carried out. She was hospitalized in a unit separated from where the intern was seeing 40 other patients. The resident left the intern in charge but was on call as he went to another building for a nap.

Nurses contacted the intern twice when Libby became more agitated through the night. He did not come to see her but ordered a stronger tranquilizer, Haldol, which was also not to be given to people on Nardil. After the second call reporting that she was flailing about, the intern instructed nurses to restrain her arms and legs to prevent her from hurting herself. Libby finally fell asleep. A nurse took her temperature at 6:30 a.m. and found it between 107 and 108 degrees. They called the intern and tried to cool her body down rapidly but she had cardiac arrest and died at 7:30 a.m.

Libby's autopsy showed pneumonia in her lungs and cocaine in her bloodstream. She had denied use of such substances and her urine had been clear of cocaine whereas it usually shows up in the case of recent usage. Cocaine also is not to be used in someone taking Nardil.

The intern called her parents and told them the doctors had done everything they could. Her heart-broken parents gathered information about her treatment, and they were shocked to learn that the intern had not slept in 24 hours and had little supervision. Furthermore, there were no other physicians to help tend the patient load. The intern was to call the resident if needed but did not call. Zion wrote in a *New York Times* article, "You don't need kindergarten to know that a resident working a 36-hour shift is in no condition to make any kind of judgment call—forget about life and death." He also criticized the lack of supervision of these physicians in training.

The trial took ten years and a televised trial resulted. Due to the prosecution blaming the patient for not admitting cocaine use, the judge awarded the family half the amount due—some $375,000. Mr. Zion had hoped for a front-page announcement that the hospital had done wrong in treating his daughter. That did not happen but it generated much media. A TV *60 Minutes* presentation on the Libby Zion case included an interview with one over-tired intern who forgot one of interviewer Mike Wallace's questions.

Changes in Physician Training to Reduce Sleep Deprivation

Following the media blitz about medical errors because of sleep deprivation, the New York State Health Commission established a blue-ribbon panel of experts headed by physician Bertrand Bell. They evaluated the training and supervision of doctors in New York. It culminated in 1989 with recommendations that interns and residents should not work more than 80 hours a week or more than 24 consecutive hours and that senior physicians needed to be physically present in the hospital at all times.

Some New York physicians and hospitals resisted changes. They said one could not become a qualified doctor without experiencing what happened during the first 36 hours of a patient's illness.

Troyen A. Brennan and colleagues published "Incidence of Adverse Events and Negligence in Hospitalized Patients" in 1991. They defined adverse events as an injury caused by medical management that prolonged the hospitalization, produced a disability, or both. They reviewed 31,000 hospital records and found 1,278 adverse events and 306 adverse events due to negligence. The Harvard Medical Practice Study agreed with Brennan's recommendation of shorter hours and more supervision for interns and residents.

Nurses and Sleep Deprivation

The problem of sleep deprivation and fatigue was seen in nurses as well. In March 1991, a hospital-based survey on shift work, sleep and accidents was carried out on 635 Massachusetts nurses. Shift rotators had more sleep/wake cycle disruption and nodded off more at work than those working only day and evening shifts. Researchers concluded that a redesign of hospital work schedules would result in improved health and safety for nurses and patients.

Keith Wagoner, an R.N. in a Texas nursing and rehabilitation center, described his typical work week. He has two back-to-back 16-hour shifts before he goes back to 8-hour shifts and drives home nodding off from time to time. He is often assigned second doubles due to too few nurses and has discussed with other nurses how they have all had close calls going to and from work. They are vulnerable, he says, for making medication errors which he worries about.

Wagoner, like so many nurses, works more than one place. He treats home-bound quadriplegics and others who have numerous diseases and problems such as pressure ulcers, and various infections. The need for IV antibiotics at all hours of the day and night keep him busy when he is not at his rehab center, and sleep is a sometime thing. In today's world where he must support his family, unsteady shift work and additional patients become a way of life, leaving our nurses at risk for sleep deprivation.

Let's go back in time to look at what nurses were doing earlier. An English nurse named Florence Nightingale (1820-1910) was very influential. Dubbed "The Lady with the Lamp," she flitted day and night from patient to patient in the Crimean War, from her clinic in Turkey. She was so successful that her reputation spread. Then Union officers contacted her during the American Civil War for advice. She was told that more soldiers were dying from wounds, infections, and illnesses than from being killed by the enemy. She gave advice because she stayed up-to-date with Joseph Lister's germ theory and advised practices to reduce contamination.

Noting the English fondness for tea, she advised that after a sleepless night, patients should be given a hot or cold lemon drink with sugar instead of tea or coffee so they could rest. Caffeinated drinks, unfortunately, kept sick people awake.

A Canadian nurse and dear friend, Alexandra (Sandy) French loves her tea and chutney. She has nursed and done midwifery around the world. Sandy brought me a Christmas present of Mrs. H.S. Ball's Original Recipe Chutney which includes peaches and apricots along with other ingredients. The tang of the chilies makes an excellent evening snack on crackers, especially when a little cream cheese is spread upon the cracker. Any fruit chutney has the sweet needed for the evening conversion of tryptophan in meat into melatonin for sleep. Chutney, most popular in India, is also delicious in salads or on meats such as chicken in particular.

Chutney Basic Recipe

Add your favorite fresh and dried fruit (apples, mangos, apricots, peaches, raisins, etc.) to some sugar, vinegar and chilies with a little salt. Bring to a boil over high heat, stirring often. Reduce heat to maintain a lively simmer and cook until thickened, 30 to 40 minutes. To test doneness, put a spoonful of chutney on a plate and draw a spoon through the center. It if leaves a rut, it's just right. Otherwise, keep on boiling to dry it out some. Serve it on crackers covered with cream cheese for an evening treat.

The Cost of Sleep Deprivation Errors in Medicine

The costs of medical errors were estimated in a 1997 article about adverse drug events in hospitalized patients. Some 4,108 admissions to 11 medical and surgical units over six months were studied and compared with control cases in the same units. There were 190 adverse drug events of which 60 were preventable. The adverse drug event lengthened the stay by days and increased costs. They estimated that the annual costs in a 700-bed hospital for adverse drug events was $5.6 million and for preventable drug events as $2.8 million respectively.

An article in the *British Medical Journal* on July 17, 1999, grabbed attention. The article began with an announcement on an airplane where the captain said "I am pleased to report that you have a 97% chance of reaching your destination without being significantly injured..."

Would you stay aboard? The article referred to the improvements by the American Medical Association in forming the National Patient Safety Foundation and the Veterans Health Administration consortium to make changes to reduce medical errors.

"To Err Is Human: Building a Safer Health System" was published by the Institute of Medicine in November 1999. This landmark article described the large number of deaths each year as a result of medical errors that could have been prevented. What kind of errors? Those cited were improper transfusions, surgical injuries, wrong-site surgery, suicides, restraint-related injuries or death, falls, burns, bed sores, and mistaken patient identities. They estimated that additional care necessitated by the errors, lost income and household productivity and disability cost between $17 billion and $29 billion per year in hospitals nationwide.

The authors recommended a more extensive approach to achieve a better safety record such as:

1. Establish a national focus to create safety leadership and research
2. Develop a national mandatory error reporting system
3. Raise performance standards through oversight organizations
4. Develop safety systems and equipment so processes do not depend upon memory.

This article produced quick action from President Bill Clinton's administration. They appropriated $50 million to the Agency for Healthcare Research and Quality. That agency developed an action plan and booklet of practical tips for individuals.

The Resistance of Physicians and Hospitals
to Reduce Sleep Deprivation

Changes began to take place in hospitals across the country immediately after publication of that article. Articles appeared about surgery and internal medicine departments in hospitals who were cited for violations of new work-hour standards. Violations included doctors in training who often worked 36-hour shifts and 100-hour weeks.

The Accreditation Council for Graduate Medical Education (ACGME) reviewed 69 training programs in general surgery in 1999 and cited 25 of them for violations. If a training program loses its accreditation, it will lose some of its Medicare money and residents will shun the program. However, strict compliance with work-hour standards costs hospitals more because they rely on young doctors as a source of low-cost labor.

These conditions gave rise to the position of hospitalists, who worked an 8 or 12- hour shift to help hospitals comply with the new rules. They reduced medical errors more than doctors who saw patients all day and then saw their hospital patients in early mornings or late evenings. One hospitalist may work from 9 p.m. to 7 a.m. on certain days. Another may work seven nights then have a week off. It appeals to physicians who want more interaction with their children, more regular family vacations, and some who only want to work part-time.

An article in 2003 pointed out that the motor vehicle accidents of anesthesiologists leaving the hospital after long hours were twice the number of accidents compared to the general public. The European Union agreed to limit the work week for residents to 48 hours. In 1999, Israel had a longer residency with fewer hours enabling doctors to have time for their own needs and to provide compassionate care as a matter of habit. New Zealand residents could work up to only 16 hours consecutively with a weekly maximum of 72 hours. In Denmark, Norway and Sweden residents worked 37 to 45 hours per week. In the Netherlands, they were limited to 48 hours per week.

It was very slow going for physicians to comply with the new standards of reduced hours. In November of 2007, actor Dennis Quaid's newborn twins were among three patients accidentally given *1,000 times* the common dosage of the blood thinner heparin. Fortunately, none of the overdose victims had suffered any ill effects and hospital officials apologized to the families involved. The two-week old children were given a medicine to reverse the effect of the heparin and restore normal clotting so the children don't bleed to death through a wound. The news coverage kept the pressure up for more compliance by hospitals to limit training physicians' work hours.

Physician Burnout and Fatigue

A study of physician burnout showed dissatisfaction with long and hard work schedules. In September 2009, a study of 7,905 surgeons who had been in practice an average of 18 years found that 40% said they felt burned out, 30% had depression symptoms, and 28% were found to have a quality of life below the normal population. Only 36% felt their work schedule left enough time for personal and family life. Apparently, burnout was common among American surgeons at that time.

The standards for informed consent require that surgeons disclose to patients all issues that can affect the outcome of a planned operation. It might confuse and frighten patients immediately before an operation if a physician shares the number of hours he has worked before the operation. That is a time when patients are not well suited to receive new information and make a thoughtful, deliberate decision. Physicians have decided not to inform patients with such details.

On December 18, 2013, Dr. Perri Klass wrote "Getting Through the Night" in the *New England Journal of Medicine*. She described the excitement of sleep deprivation and her comments were similar to many who want no limit on their working hours. There is a kind of stupidity in staying awake when you can't think straight.

Some have studied the concern surgeons had about handing off sick patients to providers who are not familiar with their cases. A more recent article concluded that surgical leaders should focus on developing safe, resilient health systems that do not depend on overworked resident physicians. One article even stated that somebody should tell residents "We can take care of this case without you. Go home, see your family and come in fresh tomorrow."

Most researchers look at the cognitive losses of sleep deprivation without weighing the benefits of sleep. But a few decided to focus on why sleep deprivation is inconsistent with ethical standards and educational goals for medical training. Sleep deprivation results in the loss of sleep's benefits for memory and insight formation, the building blocks of learning, creativity, and scientific discovery. These losses are incompatible with health-providing goals and inconsistent with educational aspirations of residency training.

Sleep in Physicians Who Have Completed Training

Little attention had been paid to the work shifts of physicians who had completed training and were working in fields with risks of complications such as obstetricians/gynecologists and surgery. An ABC television broadcast on June 18, 2000, had Diane Sawyer interview a physician named Dr. Angela Nossett, a chief resident at UCLA Medical Center, who admitted falling asleep due to sleep deprivation while delivering a baby.

Pediatric neurosurgeon Ben Carson was the first surgeon who separated Siamese twins joined at the head. He also led teams to separate other conjoined twins. Ben (who ran for the U.S. presidency in 2016) worked long hours and described how he succumbed to fatigue in his 1990 autobiography *Gifted Hands*.

Christopher Massie reported about Ben Carson's sleep problems for *BuzzFeed News* on the Internet. In 1998, he was driving home after "a late night of surgeries" when he passed out at the wheel and was awakened by the "sound of the car's wheels on the shoulder." It scared him so badly that he wrote to the administrators of Johns

Hopkins to inform them that he could no longer perform surgeries so late into the night.

Carson explained that his superiors blamed the system where all the providers, hospitals, as well as doctors, are being squeezed harder and harder by the insurance industry that too often makes profits more important than quality health care.

While on the campaign trail for the presidency, Ben and Candy Carson appeared on Fox and Friends and cooked up the following dish on July 10, 2016. Ben held the pan while Candy cooked up this Coconut Spinach which has cashews, one of many good ingredients for producing melatonin.

Dr. Ben Carson Coconut Spinach

2 tablespoons coconut oil
¼ cup diced onions
1 pound frozen spinach
¼ teaspoon salt
½ cup chopped cashew nuts

Fry the onion in the oil, then add the spinach and salt.
Stir while cooking for 5 to 10 minutes then add the
cashews and serve.

What about physician burnout from sleep deprivation? A study in 2012 found that 45% of physicians felt they had burned out-- almost half of all physicians. This rate was much higher than other jobs in the general public. When asked why, physicians described excessive workload, loss of autonomy, inadequate time with patients, excessive administrative burdens, decline in the sense of meaning that drew them to medicine, and difficulty integrating personal and professional life with their practice. They tended to blame Medicare/ Medicaid services and major insurers because of their difficult demands upon physicians.

Sleep Issues for Female Medical Personnel

There may be some extra sleep problems for female nurses according to a study of 189,000 females, about 40% of whom were in the Nurses' Health Study which began in 1988, and the rest began the study in 1989. The women aged 25 to 55 at the start of one study had no coronary artery disease. During the follow-up period, there were 7,303 cases of coronary heart disease with problems like heart attacks, chest pain and bypass surgeries. The risk went up with the number of years the women spent covering night shifts but it went down as women quit working night shifts or retired.

One study compared burnout among European female physicians in 2016. The study revealed that sleep disorders are prevalent among physicians and especially females. The highest prevalence was among Spanish female doctors and was found to be 35 to 40%.

One study showed that the proportion of female physicians has been higher in Hungary than other European or North American counterparts since the 1950s. Hungarian female physicians have been working full-time and their workload has been equal to that of their male colleagues for almost seven decades. However, there was no division of labor at home and female physicians must come home and run families with little help from their spouses. They had more chronic diseases and reproductive disorders than in the professional control sample.

The study discussed the migration of physicians with data of 948 Hungarian physicians who applied for work abroad in 2014. A survey of why Hungarian physicians wanted to work abroad revealed that they wanted more salary, better quality of life, more health care coverage, better work conditions, more appreciation of the community and professional perspectives in their field of specialization. Overall, Hungarian female doctors reported significantly less leisure time than their male colleagues

Suicide among Medical Personnel

A shocking number of medical students have committed suicide in the last few years. There are approximately 80,000 medical students currently in a survey that found ten percent of them have had suicidal thoughts. According to the American Foundation for Suicide Prevention, the number of medical students suffering from symptoms of depression is 15 to 30% higher than the general population. The average number of physicians who commit suicide is 400 per year but that includes only clear and known suicides, but many physician suicides are hushed up, just as are many of medical students and residents. Why do they do it?

In 2015, the average U.S. medical school accepted just less than seven percent of applicants. The few who enter medical school must compete with other extremely bright students by learning at an impossibly fast pace, must pass multiple tests for licensing, must take out loans because over three-quarters cannot afford medical school, must deal with sick and dying patients whom they cannot help, are insulted and bullied by residents and physicians above them in the hierarchy of medicine, and endure sleepless nights due to studying and being on duty.

The first two years of medical school usually involve pass-fail grading which have been found to enhance well-being without affecting academic outcomes. Team-based learning and later team-based patient care is an emerging trend to prevent social isolation, as are wellness centers and healthy eating seminars. But what about counseling centers? The stigma of seeking help is so great that student's fear they will not pass or be admitted to residencies if it becomes known that they sought help. When they cannot find help, some medical students and physicians commit suicide.

One such case was Kaitlyn Elkins, a 23-year old student at Wake Forest Medical School who committed suicide on April 11, 2013. Her mother, a registered nurse, started a blog to alert others to the stresses on medical students. Tragically, Kaitlyn's mother ended up killing herself a year later. The medical school's summer 2016 issue of

Oasis, a legacy of writings by in-house communication, was labeled "Remembering Kaitlyn Elkins." One of her classmates wrote a moving story of how he did not reach out to her and now it was too late.

On January 31, 2017, the National Academy of Medicine published an article by Miguel Paniagua, M.D. about the number of admissions during 1999 in Seattle, Washington, during 100 days of rain. He became overwhelmed and overworked, and fell asleep during sessions with patients. He began to hope he was in a car accident severe enough that he wouldn't have to go on ICU medical rounds for a while.

He participated in the Global Forum of Innovation in Health Professional Education of the National Academies of Science, Engineering, and Medicine. They created a platform to assess and understand the underlying causes of clinician burnout and suicide, and advance solutions that reversed the trends in clinician stress, burnout, and suicide. They developed a brochure in 2016 showing a male and female with stethoscopes around their necks, and these statistics: "400 die by suicide each year, a rate more than two times the general population." Learn more about this at www.nam.edu/ClinicianWellBeing.

The President of the National Academy of Medicine is Victor J. Dzau, M.D. He announced his goals in the *NAM News* January 2017 by launching an Action Collaborative on Clinician Well-Being and Resilience to combat the nationwide burden of burnout and suicide among our health care workforce. This was a welcome message to the medical professions.

The *New England Journal of Medicine* responded to these pleas with articles in their March 23, 2017, issue. The first was entitled "Kathryn" written by David Muller, M.D. about a fourth-year medical student who jumped out of a window to her death. He concluded, after a gripping dissection of the stress of medical school, that the stigma of asking for help must be eliminated. He further recommended that the importance of MCAT scores and grade point averages in admissions should be minimized. This might reduce the pressures that begin even before reaching medical school.

290 | *Diane Holloway Cheney, Ph.D.*

I have known several doctors and nurses who committed suicide. In every situation that I can remember, sleep loss was one of the main things that had been noted just before the suicide. These are too painful to describe in much detail but their methods of death have left people forever changed, including me.

The Sleep of Hospitalized Patients

Let us look at the sleep deprivation of hospitalized patients. Physicians often pay more attention to treating an acute illness when a patient arrives at the hospital and less attention to the condition of the patient at discharge. Studies have found that nearly one fifth of Medicare patients discharged from a hospital have an acute medical problem within thirty days of discharge.

Hospitalized patients are enduring an acute illness, experience substantial stress, are commonly deprived of sleep, experience disruption of normal circadian rhythms, may be nourished poorly, have pain and discomfort, receive medications that can alter cognition and physical function, and become deconditioned by bed rest and inactivity.

Their sleep deprivation in the hospital adversely affects metabolism, cognitive performance, physical function, cardiac risk and jet-lag type disabilities. Commonly patients cannot take food by mouth due to tests (which are often delayed). Sedation can be disorienting, and schedules are unpredictable. A hospital room may be shared with another patient who keeps one awake or disturbed.

Finally, hospitalized patients commonly become deconditioned which places them at greater risk for accidents and falls. Their ability to comply with post-discharge instructions can be affected. Physicians should aim to reduce disruptions in sleep, minimize pain and stress, promote good nutrition, optimize the use of sedatives, emphasize physical activity and strength maintenance, and enhance cognitive and physical function.

Physicians should do no harm in the course of assisting patients who are acutely ill and expand efforts to reduce readmissions during this high-risk period by making hospitalization less toxic and promoting safe passage from acute care settings.

The timing of food also synchronizes with sleep so that circadian rhythms and food metabolism are inseparable. Hospitals must understand that sleep is as important as nutrition and exercise and they must do everything they can to help patients sleep.

There is data to support every opinion but the public's voice is louder than the physicians' voice. Increasingly the public feels that is has a right to understand and direct how people are trained as physicians.

Patients Are Becoming Active Participants with Physicians

In addition to this, the National Academy of Medicine issued a new perspective on the traditional role patients and families have historically played in their own health. They presented a new plan that is to have an active partnership between families and medical personnel. In this new culture, patients are not merely subjects but are active participants whose priorities are included in care planning. There is uncertainty about whether this will lead to better results but their Scientific Advisory Panel will compile important insights as they emerge.

Dr. Mark Gotfried, a trim, fit pulmonologist who not only treats patients with lung and sleep disorders, but does research on sleep problems, has a concern. "This information is helpful about the impact of sleep deprivation on the individual and society and I am intrigued by the food solutions. I am concerned about the unhealthy eating habits of many residents." He added that more attention should be paid to the health and diet of medical students and residents.

If the relationship between physicians and patients is becoming more participatory, the emphasis will be on more information about your physician. That will be gained by seeing him or her, and being able to gather information about your physician on computers. If they are role models for patients, as they have been in the past, they must reconsider their own health.

Gotfried's concerns are appropriate according to a study of 375 medical and surgical residents. Comparisons were made of their body mass index (BMI), blood pressure, eating habits, and physical activity during training in a residency after graduation from medical school. Nearly half (43%) of the overweight residents described themselves as having normal weight. When they began their residency, their vital statistics matched or were better than average persons. But during the three years of residency, they developed significantly more weight and health problems in that short time and they did not recognize it or denied it on questionnaires. This was particularly true for those who worked 65 or more hours each week.

Physicians who maintain a healthy lifestyle are more likely to identify which patients should receive counseling, and to provide accurate and consistent prevention counseling. Let physicians who want to motivate patients "practice what they preach" by adopting healthy diet, physical fitness and sleep habits for themselves.

A study of 104 medical residents in Boston, Massachusetts, area hospitals compared their activity with those in other professions. They found that physicians were expected to serve as role models for healthy lifestyles, but long work hours reduced time for healthy behaviors. Researchers concluded that a hospital-based physical activity intervention could improve physician health and increase healthier lifestyles among physicians.

The long hours, massive amounts of studying and high levels of stress make it difficult to start or maintain the good habits that will keep you healthy during your med school years. General tips for good sleep habits that med school students can follow include napping when the opportunity presents itself, not working in bed, maintaining a regular sleep schedule whenever possible and aiming for 7-9 hours of sleep a night. The Brody School of Medicine has put out this recipe for students and everyone to eat healthier. This is a nice evening treat to enhance a good night's sleep.

Brody School of Medicine Lime Dream Pie

2/3 cup boiling water
1 package sugar-free lime-flavored gelatin mix
Ice cubes
½ cup cold water
2 cups thawed fat-free whipped topping
1 ½ teaspoon lime juice
2 tablespoons lime zest
1 ready-to-use low-fat graham cracker crumb crust

Add boiling water to gelatin in large bowl. Stir with whisk for 2 minutes or until dissolved. Add enough ice to cold water to make one cup. Add cold ice water to gelatin. Stir until ice is melted. Stir in whipped topping, lime zest, and lime juice. Refrigerate 15-20 minutes or until mixture is thick and will mound. Spoon into crust. Refrigerate 4 hours.

Mehmet Oz, M.D., brings medical information to the public through his television series—*Dr. Oz*. He believes in changing the relationship between patient and physician to be more participatory. He has said "I want no barriers between patient and medicine. I would take us all back a thousand years, when our ancestors lived in small villages and there was always a healer in that village."

Now we come to professionals who must cross untold time zones in life-threatening peril with little control over their lives—the military. How are they coping with their role as protectors of all our people? Who is protecting them and how?

Chapter Fourteen
SLEEP AND THE MILITARY

Sleep deprivation occurs during military service, most especially in emergency and combat situations. This problem has been present since the beginning of time when sentries on duty and warring peoples have been unable to stay alert.

I tried to join the Navy in order to "see the world" at age 19. "You have severe myopia and your glasses could break and you'd be useless in an emergency" said the recruiter. So, I chose other ways to see the world. But I knew, dated, and married people who served in the military. Military experience changes people—sometimes for the better and sometimes for the worse.

Military Service Changes Sleep Drastically

Irving Berlin, a Russian-born America composer, served in World War I so he knew about sleep problems. In 1918, he wrote this great song about sleep and the military and got it right!

Oh How I Hate to Get Up In the Morning

Oh how I hate to get up in the morning.
Oh how I'd like to remain in bed
For the hardest blow of all
Is to hear the bugler call

"You've got to get up, you've got to get up,
You've got to get up this morning!"

Someday I'm going to murder the bugler,
Someday they're going to find him dead
I'll amputate his reveille
And stomp upon it heavily
And spend the rest of my life in bed!

Irving Berlin was still composing music for Americans and soldiers during World War II. He produced the patriotic musical *This Is the Army*. It became such a hit that General Dwight Eisenhower sent the group around the world as a morale booster. Berlin's popular song of the same name identified with the feelings of enlisted men. No matter one's station in life before entering the military, all were equal and nobody got special treatment.

This Is the Army

This is the Army, Mister Jones. No private rooms or telephones.
You had your breakfast in bed before
but you won't have it there anymore.
This is the Army, Mister Green.
We like the barracks nice and clean,
You had a housemaid to clean your floor
but she won't help you out anymore.

Even food and eating styles are changed by military service and war. KP (Kitchen Police) Duty was required of most enlisted soldiers and many spent hours paring spuds and washing dishes or trays. Military chow was C-rations (meat and beans, meat and vegetables, meat and hash); D-rations (quick energy pack of three chocolate bars made with raw oatmeal flour), and K-rations (food packaged in boxes instead of cans). The most notorious chow of WWII was Spam. One cook developed a variation on Spam. He told the mess sergeant: "I've got it! Something really different. We'll slice Spam lengthwise."

Here is a recipe from the *1945 Manual for Navy Cooks* which combines Spam with a little sugar. That sweet enables the tryptophan in meat to produce melatonin in the brain.

WWII Luncheon Meat *(1945 Navy Cook Manual)*

3 pounds luncheon meat (Spam)
3 tablespoons sugar
1 tablespoon mustard
¼ teaspoon cinnamon
3 tablespoons vinegar
3 tablespoons water

Score the surface of Spam with a knife. Mix together sugar, mustard, cinnamon, vinegar and water. Pour over meat. Bake 30 minutes in a 350-degree oven. Makes 10 servings.

Military Attitudes toward Sleep Differ

There was an attitude in the military spread by people like Lt. General George Patton that GIs should put service before sleep. In his stirring speech to the Third U.S. Army in 1944 he used the following off-color statements, but they made soldiers feel that he was one of them.

> A man has to be alert all the time if he expects to keep on breathing. If not, some German son-of-a-bitch will sneak up behind him and beat him to death with a sock full of shit. There are 400 neatly marked graves in Sicily, all because one man went to sleep on the job—but they are German graves, because we caught the bastard asleep before his officer did...

and you should have seen the trucks on the road to Gabes. Those drivers were magnificent. All day and all night they crawled along those son-of-a-bitch roads never stopping, never deviating from their course with shells bursting all around them. Many of the men drove over 40 consecutive hours... There will be some complaints that we're pushing our people too hard. I don't give a damn about such complaints."

Patton's men landed in Normandy in July 1944 and would play a key role in defeating the Germans. He was the kind of guy who might say to his enemies: "I'm mad as hell and I'm not going to take it anymore!"

Another general had a completely different way of looking at sleep. Major General Aubrey Newman said "In peace and war, the lack of sleep works like termites in a house: below the surface, gnawing quietly and unseen to produce gradual weakening which can lead to sudden and unexpected collapse."

Newman had preceded General Douglas MacArthur's return to the Philippines on October 20, 1944. When his men were pinned down by military fire, he said "Follow me" and bravely led his men to run down the enemy. He was very fit and competed in the 1928 Olympics pentathlon races while serving in the military. The Aubrey Newman award is now given to junior leaders who demonstrate a commitment to developing their soldiers.

The enemies of America during World War II were the Germans, Italians and the Japanese. The Italians and Germans were defeated first, but the Japanese were another matter. They had caused the United States entry into World War II by attacking Pearl Harbor in Hawaii.

In an article about how the Japanese fight, a Japanese officer said sleep is simply something to sacrifice for discipline. "During peacetime maneuvers, troops would go three days and two nights without sleep except for that which could be snatched during brief ten-minute halts and brief lulls. They already know how to sleep. We want to teach them how to stay awake."

The Japanese military view was that the high standard of living among Western people would produce softness. The strength of the Japanese lay in their fanatical obedience to authority. They thought that their perseverance at Pearl Harbor and afterwards with wave after wave of suicidal air attacks would leave the American soldiers exhausted, fatigued and unable to compete. It did not happen.

War Exposes the Problems of Insomnia

American soldiers found themselves fatigued and sleepless. Psychologists were used in World War II and they came up with training films called *Combat Fatigue Insomnia* and *Combat Fatigue Irritability* made in 1945 by the U.S. Navy.

Dick York acted in a film about insomnia playing the buddy of a soldier who couldn't sleep. The movie began with a Donald Duck cartoon about a duck unable to sleep, and shifted to a soldier who had unknown things on his mind that kept him awake. The narrator and Dick York did most of the talking and the film explained how to relax the body, one part at a time (progressive relaxation). The narrator added that if relaxation was unsuccessful, medicines could help. York was an actor who became best known for his television role as Darrin in the *Bewitched* serial where he was married to a witch, played by Elizabeth Montgomery.

Combat Fatigue Irritability is now called Post-Traumatic Stress Disorder (PTSD). The Navy training film, made to help servicemen understand the disorder, starred Gene Kelly, known for his films and his dancing. He played the role of a soldier with the disorder in a 30-minute movie. Kelly trained for the movie by going into a military hospital claiming he had the disorder, so he could learn more about symptoms and treatment.

He depicted a fear of harm and a guilty feeling that he let his buddies down when he was glad to be blown clear of his ship. These worries kept him awake at night. He went to a bar to drink, hoping to get a little sleep. The bartender threw the angry soldier out in the snow. He was edgy and haunted by dreams. Group therapy, individual counseling, and medicine helped him resolve his agitation. Gene Kelly was always very fit for his movies and his gymnastic dancing. He had a recipe that fit his persona.

Gene Kelly Greatest "Man-Sandwich" in the World

Kelly said: "Take yesterday's left-over mashed potatoes and spread on the bread as thickly as your mouth can get around. Salt and pepper heavily. Add thin slices of red onion or white onion, then your favorite mayonnaise. With these onions, be sure your wife has at least one bite. Reach for the nearest mug of beer. It's heavenly."

Audie Murphy, Most Decorated Soldier of WWII

One of the soldiers who suffered from the disorder that Gene Kelly portrayed was the most decorated American soldier of World War II. Audie Murphy (1925-1971) served in the Army and received every U.S. military combat award for valor available in the U.S. Army. He was five feet five inches and weighed 112 pounds when inducted. He was first shipped to Casablanca in Morocco, and also served in Africa, Europe, Tunisia, Sicily, Italy, the Rhineland, etc. This modest man went on to star in movies for 21 years before he died in a plane crash.

He said, "War is a nasty business, to be avoided if possible, and to be gotten over with as soon as possible. It's not the sort of job that deserves medals."

His "battle fatigue" (which we now call Post-Traumatic Stress Disorder) left him with trouble sleeping because of nightmares, headaches and vomiting. John Huston who directed him in *The Red Badge of Courage* commented that Murphy had much trouble sleeping because he felt he was back in the war shooting Germans.

Audie became addicted to sleeping pills and slept with a loaded pistol under his pillow, according to his relatives. I saw him several times in Dallas when he visited his niece, my best girlfriend, Donna Paxton.

Audie created a dish he called Beef Bandera. This meal was made for a friend, Scott Turner, who remembered the ingredients but not the amounts. Maybe you can figure it out because it has some ingredients to aid sleep. The ingredients are listed here with some guesses about amounts.

Audie Murphy Beef Bandera

Butter, 1 tablespoon
Onions, 1-2 chopped fine
Beef strips, I lb. skirt steak or other beef
Can of mushroom soup
Brown sugar, 1 tablespoon
Worcestershire sauce, 1 teaspoon

Melt butter in a frying pan and brown cut up onions in the butter When the onions are brown, add a can of cream of mushroom soup plus brown sugar, Worcestershire sauce, and let it simmer for about 3 minutes. Cut the beef into strips and brown them in a second frying pan. Then, add the beef strips to the mushroom mixture and cook on low for 10 minutes.

Actress Hedy Lamarr and Sleep

One of the problems in World War II was that Germans knew how to detect and destroy American torpedoes heading for German submarines and U-boats. Anti-Nazi Europeans united in many ways to defeat Nazis, but an unusual invention was created by French musical composer George Antheil and Austrian actress Hedy Lamarr. She came to the U.S. after leaving her munitions magnate husband.

She became a movie star after her nude scene in the 1933 movie *Ecstasy* and Hollywood wanted her. The incredibly beautiful woman first starred with Charles Boyer in *Algiers* in 1938. At that time, Boyer, who had a degree from the Sorbonne in Paris, was recruiting movie stars to defeat Nazis in Europe and Lamarr was enthusiastic. Hedy's Hollywood influence helped her to rescue her mother from Austria after the Germans invaded.

Hedy Lamarr had an interesting comment about the word "sleep." She said: "The ladder of success in Hollywood is usually a press agent, actor, director, producer, leading man; and you are a star if you sleep with each of them in that order." Something tells us that sleep had a very different meaning to Hedy.

She had scientific interests which may have exceeded her acting ability. She had first invented an improvement upon traffic lights and next invented a tablet which could be dropped into a beverage to turn it into a carbonated beverage—something like Alka-Seltzer. In fact, the company that made Bromo-Seltzer invented a fruit tablet called Fizzies later, but Hedy was first.

Next, Hedy chatted with composer George Antheil who wrote music for movies and knew something about hormones. She began by asking if hormones would help her breasts enlarge, but they wound up talking about scientific subjects. They teamed up to invent a radio guidance system for allied forces to use on torpedoes.

They applied for a patent for a "Secret Communication System" on June 10, 1941, in Los Angeles. They submitted seven diagrams involving carrier waves of different frequencies ("frequency hopping") useful in the remote control of torpedoes. It was hard to decipher but was easy to use based on player piano rolls consisting of 88 notes in random order. They expected their device to be used during World War II but it was not used until the Cuban Missile Crisis in 1962 under President John F. Kennedy. It was further used to develop GPS and Wi-Fi systems of communication, as well as cell phones.

Here is a sleep-inducing recipe from the Internet attributed to Hedy Lamarr. This could be an evening meal with tryptophan and a little sweet after the meal will promote sleep.

Hedy Lamarr Tuna Salad

She put a can of tuna fish, a chopped boiled egg, a chopped small apple, and a chopped stalk of celery together. She added not only mayonnaise but Greek Kalamata olives and capers. She mixed it and served it on lettuce leaves.

The Nazi Search for Drugs to Stay Awake

During World War II, the Nazis suffered sleep deprivation the same as all soldiers in war time. However, they took their search up several notches in 1944 as the Germans were becoming more desperate. Admiral Hellmuth Heye swore by a combination of cocaine, Pervitin and Eukodal. He sought these drugs to keep soldiers on solo operations awake and ready for deployment, and boosted the soldier's confidence in his reserves of strength. Pervitin was a methamphetamine and Eukodal was oxycodone, an opiate containing heroin. These three pills were tried on some pilots. These drugs were also used by Hitler, according to records found after his death.

The three pills were tried on others before being used by officers. Subjects who were previously fresh and rested displayed shaky hands during a brief euphoria, and those who were already tired complained of weak knees and tautness in the muscles. A general paralysis of the central nervous system set in, and decision-making power and intellect were inhibited. So Heye continued to search for something else that would allow pilots to stay awake four days and to take mini-subs to the Thames River in London and beaches of Normandy to blow up allied ships. They could keep pilots awake for two days and two nights but they never succeeded in keeping them awake for four days and nights and capable of conducting effective raids.

The use of methamphetamines for German citizens in the form

of chocolates and other edibles is described by Norman Ohler's remarkable 2017 book *Blitzed: Drugs in the Third Reich*.

Albert Einstein and Sigmund Freud communicated with each other in 1932 about the possibility of an atom bomb. They had met briefly in 1927 and Einstein admired Freud's principles. Einstein wrote President Franklin Roosevelt that a nuclear bomb could be created, and this inspired Roosevelt to have the United States Government begin a plan to build one.

A group of scientists were hired to develop a nuclear laboratory in the mountains above Santa Fe at Los Alamos, New Mexico. In 1942, they took over the Fuller School for Boys to develop Project Y of the Manhattan Project. Led by J. Robert Oppenheimer, they developed two types of atom bombs.

During their three years, scientists arrived from many countries. They developed unique recipes, entertainments, jokes, and tried to sleep at night despite intense emotions and crazy time pressures. Thanks to Oppie, as he was called, this conglomeration of different languages, interests, and parts of the project jelled. Both bombs they developed worked and shortened the war, which reduced American and Japanese military losses.

Parties and drinking helped relieve tensions on weekends. The wife of Dr. Frederick Reines (American physicist who won the Nobel Prize for discovering the neutrino) prepared a delicious banana nut bread. This bread has three ingredients that produce melatonin— bananas, nuts, and eggs.

Frederick Reines (Los Alamos Nobel Prize Winner) Banana Nut Bread

2 tablespoons butter
¾ cup sugar
1 egg
5 ripe bananas
Pinch of salt
1 teaspoon soda

2 tablespoons baking powder
2 cups flour
½ cup chopped nuts

Mix butter and sugar, add egg, mix well. Add mashed
bananas and dry ingredients which have been sifted
together. Add nuts. Bake about 45 minutes in a
350-degree oven.

After World War II, General George Marshall did not speak about
sleep but others who knew him well did. He was this nation's most
esteemed 20th Century military figure because he not only created
major awesome military power during World War II, but as postwar
Secretary of State and Secretary of Defense he created the Marshall
Plan to help Europe rebuild after their massive devastation. When
President Franklin Roosevelt had to choose someone to lead the charge
against the Germans on D-Day, he chose General Dwight Eisenhower
as Supreme Allied Commander instead of Marshall. The President said
"I couldn't sleep nights, George, if you were out of Washington."

MIT Professor Charles P. Kindleberger was involved in the
development of the Marshall Plan. He said of George Marshall that
he was a great man, funny, odd, but great—a man who would stay
up all night, night after night. Here again is the exhilaration from
working day and night that many explain as the attraction to this
work in the military. However, those who must stay awake often turn
to caffeine, drugs, smoking, and other substances to fend off sleep.

Effects of Wakeful Substances on Humor and Morals

Walter Reed Army Institute of Research studied drugs being
used to help the military combat sleep deprivation. One of their
studies in 2006 took 54 healthy volunteers ranging in age from
eighteen to thirty-six years who were sleep-deprived for 49 hours
before presentation of test material. They were divided into four
groups; those receiving 600 mg. of caffeine (equal to 2-3 cups of

coffee), 400 mg. of modafinil (a "go-pill" to combat fatigue), 20 mg. of Dextroamphetamine, or placebo. After sleep deprivation, they were presented with questions requiring quick physical responses, humorous cartoons and newspaper headlines choosing. Their task was to decide which was funnier. One example is: 1:"Veterinarian Investigates Failed Panda Mating," or 2: "Panda Mating Fails; Veterinarian Takes Over."

Humor appreciation is among the highest and most evolved of all human cognitive functions. It requires some learning and emotional intelligence. The conclusions were that all three stimulants resulted in faster response speeds than those taking the placebo. The Dextroamphetamine produced the fastest performance followed by modafinil, and last was caffeine. Modafinil enhanced the ability to detect humor in cartoons better than those on placebo or caffeine.

Another unusual study on sleep deprivation and moral judgments was published in November, 2006. Twenty-six healthy active-duty military personnel were tested with moral dilemmas at rest and then after 53 hours of continuous wakefulness. They found that the two-day/night sleep deprivation impaired or delayed reactions on personal moral dilemmas but those scores could be offset by those subjects with a higher intelligence score.

Researchers have studied a variety of sleep problems for those who serve our country. A 2008 study evaluated symptoms of sleep disturbance and insomnia in a group of 156 Air Force deployed military personnel. They lived in a tent city in Southeast Asia with loud construction noise, uncomfortable cots, aches and pains, worry about family back home, and heat over 120 degrees in the daytime. People queued up 30 to 90 minutes for Internet time. The average hours slept were 6.5. However, sleep efficiency was poor when it took 30 minutes to get to sleep, frequent waking, and difficulty going back to sleep. The 39 who worked the night shift had even more sleep problems and got 4.5 hours of sleep per 24 hours.

Researchers recommended that programs were needed to help deployed military members get more and better sleep, whether from pharmacological medications or cognitive behavioral treatment.

Mental Acuity and Sleepiness in the Military

About 4,000 active duty female military personnel were invited to receive treatment when they received a diagnosis of insomnia. Some 1,559 agreed to be treated for insomnia. Overall, more respondents rated cognitive behavioral therapy over medicine as an acceptable form of treatment (81.6% versus 55.2%) according to the 2016 report.

In July, 2016, the American College of Physicians endorsed Cognitive Behavior Therapy (CBT) for insomnia as the first line of treatment for the 24 million adults suffering from the condition. CBT combines sleep restriction, replacing negative beliefs with positive, and sleep hygiene. It may be done individually in four to eight sessions. This cuts in half the time it takes people to fall asleep or get back to sleep when they've awakened in the night. A variation of cognitive behavioral therapy is Mindfulness-based Therapy (MBT) which involves group therapy and guided meditation to undo the vigilance and thought rigidity in the mind of insomniacs. Usually an 8-week course changes the satisfaction with sleep though not always the length of sleep, and renders insomnia less problematic to those who have it.

A large study of 55,021 military people (called the Millennium Cohort Study) collected questionnaires from military records from 2001-2008. The presence of insomnia symptoms was significantly associated with lower health rates, more lost work days, higher odds of early discharge from the military and more health care utilization. Surprisingly, those reporting less than six hours of sleep *or* more than eight hours had similar findings. It seemed unnatural to find that under-sleeping and over-sleeping can both be problems. But it depends on what these troops need to do in their jobs.

The Impact of Sleep Deprivation on Moral Decisions

Another study tested decision making and adherence to a moral code. "The Impact of Partial Sleep Deprivation on Moral Reasoning in Military Officers" and was published in March 2010. Subjects included 92 first-year officer cadets at the Royal Norwegian Naval and Army Academies with an average age of twenty-four years.

Moral reasoning used the Kohlberg stage of cognitive moral development: People at Stage 1 are like infants—"I want what I want and I want it now!" Stages 2 and 3 pursue self-serving ends based on egocentric and opportunist outlooks (i.e., "what's fair is what serves my personal interest best"). Those at Stage 4 use rules to guide behavior choices; i.e. Ten Commandments and rules in home, school, or work settings. People at Stage 5 and 6 required decisions or actions where one must violate a rule such that one might have to decide something without any support from others.

The moral decisions were presented after resting to one group, and after two combat simulation training exercises giving cadets an average of 2.5 hours of sleep per day for five days for the other group. The only moral choices that showed effects from sleep deprivation were in the highest decision-making level--stages 4 through 6. Sleep deprivation affected tasks where flexibility, innovation, or plan revision was required. There was a tendency to use "group thinking" or "pressure to conform".

Some moral impersonal dilemmas proposed that the subject authorize another person to deflect a threat of serious bodily harm. Some moral personal dilemma proposed that the subject himself risk danger by inflicting harm to deflect a threat of serious bodily harm.

Researchers stated that these findings could have important consequences in organizations that rely on chronically sleep-deprived people when faced with a moral dilemma. Today's modern society's increases reliance on highly skilled professionals, such as the armed forces. They are expected to perform and excel in complex and demanding environments, with morally anchored rule-based decisions. These are important leadership responsibilities.

A study of the readiness of National Guard soldiers who were deployed to Iraq and Afghanistan found a striking prevalence of sleep apnea in 40% of the 265 soldiers. Some 40% of those with sleep apnea were smokers, they exercised less often, they ate fewer fruits and vegetables but more meat, and they had worse sleep and greater daytime sleepiness. Researchers concluded that soldiers with high stress, depression, poor sleep quality, and sleep apnea are at increased long-term risk for cardiovascular complications. They deserve focused interventions to encourage improved lifestyle changes.

Can Sleep-Deprived Troops Make Good Decisions?

According to a report released by the Navy and Marine Corps Public Health Center, nearly 30,000 sailors and marines suffer from sleep disorders. Researchers found that insomnia had nearly as strong an impact on mental health as did combat exposure, indicating the vital importance of sleep in protecting mental health.

A study of 21,499 military veterans from 2011-2013 and found that insomnia was part of post-traumatic stress disorder, so sleep assessments were recommended for PTSD patients.

A study on fleet readiness showed 70,000 sleep disorder medical appointments in a sample which included 85% men, 60% were aged 25-44, and 50% of enlisted ranks E5-E9. This displayed a major problem with fleet readiness and sleepy decision-making troops. Researchers concluded that key stakeholders across Navy Medicine should use programs, services, webinars, audio CD's on stress reduction, diet, exercise, and other strategies known to improve sleep hygiene.

More startling information was found when studying sleep disorders in active duty females. A study was done in 2016 of 101 women on active duty with an average age of 33.9 years. Research associates found that 49.6% of them were diagnosed with obstructive sleep apnea. Unbelievably, 96% were diagnosed with clinically significant sleep disorders. These figures were as high as on-duty military men. The authors recommended that more screening for sleep disorders in female military personnel was required. This demonstrated a major problem because so many men and women on active duty were found to have inadequate sleep.

A huge telephone survey was conducted from 2009 to 2011

wherein U.S. military personnel were asked about sleep in the past 30 days. They questioned 566,861 people eighteen to sixty-four years and 1,271,202 people sixty-five years or older. Among the younger group, daily insufficient sleep was 13.7% of those reporting recent duty. Those on active duty were 34% more likely to report daily insufficient sleep. Questions arose about what was needed to deal with sleep deprivation in the military?

Sleep Policy Recommendations for the Military

In 2015, the RAND National Defense Research Institute conducted a two-year study of sleep problems in the military, and it focused especially on force readiness. They also surveyed deployable service members across all four branches of the United States armed forces, forming a sample of 1,957. They chose and convened an amazing panel of 31 experts (clinician line leaders and researchers with expertise in sleep in the military). The study was called "Sleep in the Military: Promoting Healthy Sleep Among U.S. Service-members."

By pouring time, money and expertise into sleep problems in the military, they detected several important problems and made recommendations for improvement which can be seen by visiting their web site on the Internet. They put forth 16 policy recommendations pertaining to all military branches in the areas of: preventing sleep problems, identification and diagnosis of sleep problems, clinical management of sleep disorders, promoting sleep health, and improving sleep in training and operational contexts. The results were too large to include here but are currently being enacted in the various branches of the military.

Military Family and Spousal Sleep Problems

The role of the spouse in sleep problems was explored. Military families face many stresses such as deployments, relocations, marital struggles, as well as balancing work and family demands. One study investigated how 236 couples collectively coped and addressed challenges as a united front, and how the spousal relationship could influence sleeping and eating behaviors. Researchers found that at least one member of the couple must seek out needed help to link families to services and resources.

Another study of military service members found numerous stressors that place them at high risk for sleep disturbances. Some 1,480 female spouses of men expecting, or on deployment, were studied for sleep, health, marital satisfaction and depression. About 44% of spouses reported sleeping six hours or less per night. About 54% had daytime impairment due to sleep problems and 62% reported daytime fatigue at least one or two times per week. Improving sleep in spouses not only benefits the individual but can promote resilience in the military family unit.

More research has verified the depth of the military sleep problems. The "National Veteran Sleep Disorder Study" conducted 2000 to 2010 was published in 2016. Of veterans seeking care in U.S. Veterans Health Administration facilities over an eleven-year span, a stunning 9,786,778 were assessed for sleep diagnoses and sleep problems. Sleep apnea was found in 47% and insomnia in 26% among those patients. There was a *six-fold* increase in sleep disorders over the 11 years and a *tripling* of post-traumatic stress disorder (associated with sleep disorders) during that same time frame. Researchers concluded that there is a growing need for sleep disorder management among U.S. veterans.

Of 21 million veterans living in the United States today, more than 9 million receive health care from the Veterans Health Administration. The Veterans' study noted that the large increase in diagnosed sleep disorders over the 11-year span could be treated to reduce their cardiovascular disease and hypertension, which are commonly diagnosed conditions in veterans. However, it would require 600 more workers (physicians, clinical psychologists, sleep technologists and respiratory therapists) which is a huge financial burden. It has been proposed that the treatment of sleep disorders is a worthwhile investment for the Veterans Heaolth Administration to improve the quality of life for those who have served our country.

Unfortunately, the latest research shows that treating post-traumatic stress disorder may not remove sleep problems. The University of Texas Health Science Center at San Antonio studied 100 active military troops and 92% acknowledged difficulty falling or staying asleep before treatment, and 69% of them also suffered from nightmares. After treatment, for those who no longer met criteria for PTSD diagnosis, more than half continued to report insomnia and 13% continued to have problems with nightmares. There are few—if any—complete 'cures' in psychology and psychiatry, but that doesn't mean people can't go on to lead a rewarding and fulfilling life. Cognitive-behavioral therapy for insomnia has been proven successful for nightmares and insomnia in many people and should at least be tried to help sufferers.

Crew Fatigue and Accidents

The Air Force studied air crew fatigue as a factor in Class A mishaps. They found that fatigue and sleep deprivation was a factor in 101 accidents from 1977 to 1997. U.S. Air Force Lt. Col. Christian G. Watt in a 2009 paper dealt with sleep and air crew fatigue management. He said that all controls for insomnia, except sleep, should be considered a Band-Aid. He believed that suitable scheduling practices have not been adequately incorporated in field fatigue management strategies, and too much emphasis has been placed on drugs as a solution. He recommended drinking plenty of fluids, especially water, eating high protein meals, and having a carbohydrate in the evening, particularly when combined with a food high in tryptophan. He advised troops to avoid alcohol, nicotine, and caffeine prior to sleep.

Watt cited reports from military psychologists and others stating that during Operation Desert Storm (Gulf War), there were many friendly fire losses, and some of those were due to sleep deprivation. He commented that during Operation Enduring Freedom, 2001 to now, the increased length of fighter and bomber missions have extended to 44 hour flights. Pilots used drugs to counter the continuous hours awake. He believed that pharmacological methods masked a problem of poor scheduling practices. He proposed special and unique scheduling that allowed aircrews more rest.

Some Friendly Fire Incidents Stem from Sleep Deprivation

A compelling illustration of the possible safety consequence of fatigue-related impairment comes from debriefing after friendly fire incidents during Operation Desert Storm. Sleep deprivation was identified as contributing to Bradley fighting vehicle and M1 tank crews becoming disoriented and mistook friend for foe. They were, however, able to shoot straight while firing upon and destroying friendly vehicles.

Col. Gregory Belenky, the Army's leading expert on sleep management and Director of Neuropsychiatry at Walter Reed Army Institute of Research, was one of those who debriefed troops after friendly fire incidents. He concluded that no act of will or degree of training will preserve the ability to discriminate friend from foe after 96 hours of sleep deprivation. Research warns that danger lurks in drowsy eyes.

George Fink edited *Stress of War, Conflict, and Disaster* published in 2010 about the Gulf War. The authors stated that seeing an American wounded by their own friendly fire had great emotional impact. His book included estimates that 24% of our 148 dead and 15% of our wounded were caused by friendly fire in Operation Desert Storm.

The U.S. invasion of Afghanistan which began in 2001 ended in 2014. It resulted in killing our own U.S. Special Forces troops in some instances. Beyond the death and devastation caused by friendly fire, such incidents ripple through the ranks, making those left behind less aggressive, more likely to forfeit the initiative, leery of fighting at night or bad weather, and raising doubt in the minds of the commanders involved.

The 1980 movie *Breaker Morant* warned soldiers in the Boer War:

"Live every day as if it were to be your last. One day you're sure to be right."

Sleep deprivation was a known cause of friendly fire deaths of Canadian soldiers on April 18, 2002, when U.S. Air National Guard Major Harry Schmidt dropped a bomb from his F-16 jet fighter in a night firing exercise near Kandahar. Schmidt was charged with negligent manslaughter, aggravated assault, and dereliction of duty. During testimony Schmidt blamed the incident on his use of "go pills" (authorized mild stimulants), combined with the 'fog of war'. The four dead and eight wounded received United States medals for bravery, and an apology.

Exhaustion is a constant concern on lengthy missions. But this was the first time that the USAF tried pilots for criminal charges. Both pilots were each charged with four counts of manslaughter and eight counts of assault. The reprimand of Major Schmidt from General Bruce Carlson was not kind, and was made public:

> You acted shamefully on 17 April 2002 over Tarnak Farms, Afghanistan, exhibiting arrogance and a lack of flight discipline. When your flight lead warned you to 'make sure it's not friendlies' and the Airborne Warning and Control System aircraft controller directed you to 'stand by' and later to 'hold fire,' you should have marked the location with your targeting pod. ...You used the inherent right of self-defense as an excuse to wage your own war.

General Carlson made a powerful point and one likely to be felt by all pilots so that such accidents are now less likely to happen. Throughout time, military leaders and generals have had to make important points, whether they were on and off the battlefield themselves. They've had to set the level of operation for their troops and set the manner in which the troops would handle themselves and others. Leadership starts from the top!

Troop Suicides in Recent Military Operations

Suicide, not combat, kills more United States troops deployed to fight Islamic State militants in Iraq and Syria, according to Pentagon statistics released in January 2017. This program against ISIL, Inherent Resolve, began in 2014. Of the 31 troops who have died from August 8, 2014, to December 27, 2016, eleven took their own lives. Eight died in combat, seven in accidents and four died from illness or injuries. The causes of these suicides include post-traumatic stress, multiple combat deployments, and heightened anxiety in a military at war for so many years. So far, 2016 has been the most dangerous for United States forces since the war on ISIS began. The Inherent Resolve partner nations include Austria, Bahrain, Belgium, Canada, France, Jordan, Netherlands, Saudi Arabia, Turkey, and the U.K.

From 2001 to 2010, the rate of suicide in the military doubled, according to the Pentagon. The chief spike occurred around 2005 when fighting and combat deaths soared in Iraq and Afghanistan. The Army was responsible for most of the war's burden at that time, and the Army had the highest number of suicides among the service branches.

Of the 269 active-duty troops who took their own lives in 2014, 122 were soldiers. As a whole, the military's rate of suicide is about 20 per 100,000 troops.

Retired general Peter Chiarelli made suicide prevention a top priority when he was the Army's No. 2 officer as vice chief of staff from 2008 to 2012. He expressed frustration with the failure to drive down the rate of military and civilian suicides. He called for a research effort similar to the comprehensive initiative to attack HIV/AIDS.

Long Bomb Sorties Used on ISIS

At this time and for the future, America is at war with ISIS. Days before Barack Obama left office, two bomb strikes by the U.S. B-2 Spirit crews flew 32-hour sorties. Pilots flew to Libyan ISIS camps

5,700 miles away from Whiteman Air Force Base in Missouri and back. Each stealth bomber had a two-man cockpit and the planes refueled twice each way in route. Pilots had a crude toilet and a six-foot cot sleeping area behind their heads. The level of attention required for these 32-hour missions was extraordinary as they flew to the site, dropped 80 bombs, loitered to assess damage, and returned undetected by radar.

They prepared for this sortie with special diets so they would not need to relieve themselves as much. These long flights played hell with the pilots sleep and waking cycles. There are issues—dehydration, deep vein thrombosis, and fatigue. They sometimes used "go pills" like Dexedrine, as well as "no go pills" like Ambien to enforce the rest cycle.

Islamic troops challenge United States bombing strategists but Air Force pilots line up for these missions. Concerned crew chiefs scrutinize the bombers to maintain them and ensure that stealth coatings are on the surface. But sooner or later, the next planning order will come and the B-2s and crew will be called upon again.

Nuclear Regulatory Commission Time Limits on Duty

In May 2014, the United States Nuclear Regulatory Commission clarified that the Department of Energy has a limit of no more than 12 hours per day and no more than 60 hours per week for their protective force except in emergencies. But where is the enforcement arm of this program?

The document "Rulemaking for Enhanced Security at Fuel Cycle Facilities; Special Nuclear Material Transportations; Security Force Fatigue at Nuclear Facilities" stated: "The goal of safety is to prevent and mitigate accidents: the goal of physical protection is to prevent intentional acts that might negatively impact the facility or result in the theft or sabotage of nuclear weapons."

Certainly, these policies must be revisited and improved if their goal is to be satisfied and if we are to be kept safe from those with sleep problems.

General George Washington and Sleep

President George Washington was originally a General of the first Army of what became the United States during the American Revolution. He was a remarkable man who was limited only by the lack of money and sometimes manpower to defeat the English. In 1776, the British and their mercenaries, the German Hessians, had won almost every battle. But Washington planned a surprise attack on the morning after Christmas, assuming that the Hessians would be sleeping off their celebrations. The attack worked and morale was lifted.

However, by the following Christmas of 1777, General Washington's troops at Valley Forge were ill-equipped. Some went barefoot. Many did not have blankets. Food was scarce. Hundreds died after suffering from diseases such as flu, typhus, and dysentery in addition to wounds. Finally, the end of the war came and he returned to Mount Vernon.

After being elected president, since there was no White House most entertaining was done at his home. He had one of the largest distilleries of whiskey in the New World on his Mount Vernon plantation. He was proud to serve his visitors homemade drinks and those included a powerful eggnog.

This recipe contains enough protein and carbohydrates to ensure that people might get a good night's sleep, even if they cut down on much of the alcohol ingredients. Mount Vernon records (available on the Internet) were cut in half for this recipe, but a New Year's Eve celebration apparently offered this rich drink.

General George Washington Eggnog

½ cup rye whiskey
1 cup brandy
¼ cup Jamaican rum
¼ cup sherry
6 tablespoons sugar

2 cups cream
2 cups milk
6 egg yolks

Mix liquors together. Separate egg yolks from whites. Add sugar to beaten egg yolks. Mix well. Add milk and cream, slowly beating. Discard egg whites or use elsewhere.

General Dwight Eisenhower and Sleep

After his tremendous career in World War II, General Dwight Eisenhower was elected president. The peace and quiet of his time in office made some consider things as dull and uneventful. That's the way he wanted it because he knew the terrible cost of war on mankind.

By age 70 in January 1961, he had suffered a heart attack, a stroke, and was not in good health. He was taking too many sleeping pills and still not sleeping. He wanted to educate the callow young President-Elect John Kennedy about war and world conditions but he simply wasn't up to it.

Perhaps President Kennedy's best advice was "Ask not what your country can do for you, ask what you can do for your country!"

As we wind up the discussion of sleep in the military, we will offer one of General Eisenhower's favorite soups and a dessert prepared by his wife, Mamie, both of which are available on the Internet.

General Dwight Eisenhower Vegetable or Beef Soup

2 pounds stewing meat (optional, but cook longer if using meat)
If doing only vegetables, add barley or rice. Ike liked barley best.
1 pound small Irish potatoes
1 bunch small carrots

¾ pound small onions
2 fresh tomatoes
Spices (celery salt, thyme, bay leaves, garlic salt, Worcestershire sauce)
2 ½ pints beef stock
Salt and pepper

Stew the meat until tender. Add the vegetables and spices. When vegetables are done, add ½ cup of any canned vegetables desired such as peas and/or corn.

Mamie's dessert below contains fruits and cream with tryptophan and melatonin ingredients.

Mamie Eisenhower Frosted Mint Delight

Two one-pound cans crushed pineapple
¾ cup pure mint flavored apple jelly
1 pint of whipping cream
2 teaspoons of confectionary sugar
1 package of gelatin

Have all ingredients chilled. Melt the jelly and mix in the crushed pineapple. Dissolve the package of gelatin in one cup of the juice from the pineapple. Mix the gelatin mixture into the jelly mixture. Whip the cream, sweeten it with the sugar, and fold it into the mixture. Put in the freezer until firm but don't freeze solid. Makes enough for ten or twelve servings.

General Colin Powell and Sleep

After four-star General Colin Powell ended his Army career he became Secretary of State. When he retired, he wrote an autobiography called *It Worked for Me: In Life and Leadership.* He described a night during his career that very much interfered with his sleep and the sleep of all those with him. They were walking down a forested trail when they were hit by small arms fire from an enemy ambush. We returned fire but that night, as they tried to sleep on the forest floor, they were filled with the realization that the next morning they would probably be ambushed again.

Sleep was nearly impossible because they had to control fear and move on, just like every soldier since ancient times.

Colin Powell could have said, as in the movie *Scarface,* "Every day above ground is a good day." Colin Powell had his own recipe for a treat with tryptophan which can be used as a nighttime snack. He shared this recipe with Highland Foods and it can be found on their site on the Internet. Here is his main idea but you can use your own ideas for a good evening snack.

General Colin Powell Crispy Squash Seeds

Use squash seeds saved from pumpkin, acorn, butternut, blue hubbard, or butternut squashes. Use just enough olive oil to lightly coat the seeds. Then coat oiled seeds with a maple syrup and pepper seasoning. Add a dash of sea salt if you like. Scatter seeds on a lightly oiled cookie sheet. Place the sheet in a pre-heated 325-degree oven and roast for 15-20 minutes. Turn seeds at least once during roasting. Remove when lightly browned and crispy. When cooled put in a bowl to share with company.

The Institute of Medicine, Food and Nutrition Board published a 1994 book: *Food Components to Enhance Performance: An Evaluation of Potential Performance-Enhancing Food Components.* They looked at enhancing military performance by food components and sleep. They discussed the effects of sleep on performance and concluded that soldiers can fight for a long time with only fragmented sleep. However, they become less productive as days pass and are more likely to make abrupt and serious bad decisions. Commanders at all levels should encourage sleep, they concluded. Restricting sleep in the hope of getting more out of soldiers is unproductive. To paraphrase General George Patton, the idea is not to give up sleep for your country but to make the other "poor bastard" give up sleep for his.

Patton felt and talked about taking the life of the enemy. Many soldiers become sleepless thinking about the process of taking a man's life. It's like Clint Eastwood said in *The Unforgiven:* "It's a hell of a thing, killin' a man. You take away all he has, and all he's ever gonna have." As General Curtis LeMay said, "Every soldier thinks something of the moral aspects of what he is doing. But all war is immoral and if you let that bother you, you're not a good soldier."

Moving on, now that you have learned the importance of sleep deprivation, you want to get a good night's sleep. Like Kris Kristofferson said in his song, you're looking for something to "help me make it through the night". Here are some ideas about preparing for bed.

Chapter Fifteen

THIRTY MINUTES BEFORE BEDTIME

Consider your evening and try some sleep-inducing food, drink, and activities before bedtime. Begin some bedtime routines that add a pleasant serenity to your mind. But absolutely do not go to bed until you feel sleepy.

You must become your own sleep detective. You can try things and if they don't work, forget them. Be an experimenter and keep the solutions that work. Be a baloney detector. Don't do something just because people tell you it works for them. See if it works for you.

Remember what Benjamin Franklin said in 1784, "Living long has given me frequent opportunities of seeing certain remedies cried up as curing everything, and yet are soon after laid aside as useless."

Herbal Teas

The most acclaimed results for sleepiness brought on by herbal teas usually include chamomile, valerian, passion fruit, or special blends made by companies such as Celestial Seasonings. Decaffeinated green tea is also a stress reducer but doesn't contribute to sleepiness. Some people use a tea with hops (a beer ingredient) which can be purchased at health food stores. There is no scientific evidence of the effectiveness of herbal teas, but these teas have been used since prehistoric times for their relaxing qualities. The tea can include a little sugar or honey, and milk is optional. Mint leaves add another sleep-inducing ingredient to teas. Sipped slowly while sitting, the warmth invites one to relax.

Some people take a pill before bedtime and one such is aspirin. We already know the value of aspirin to prevent heart attacks, reduce blood clotting, lower fever temperatures, and ameliorate pain. It has some other uses such as preventing acne, protecting skin, and helping some people stay asleep. Some of its ingredients have a delayed effect of three to four hours. So, it may assist in keeping one asleep and more comfortable during the second half of the night. See Dr. Michael Roizen's article "Take Aspirin at Night to Reap its Health and Beauty Benefits."

Dr. Peter Hauri, sleep expert at Mayo, recommended an occasional dose of two aspirins of 325 mg. each with plenty of water before bedtime. The ancient Egyptians used willow bark (aspirin origins) as a remedy for aches and pains. They didn't know that what was reducing body temperature and inflammation was the salicylic acid. However, that acid can have a detrimental effect on the stomach with prolonged use.

Some people claim that Vitamin B6 in the evening is a good pill to take, but there is no particular supporting evidence. The *Journal of the American Geriatric Society* published in January 2011 that long-term care facilities for seniors offer melatonin, magnesium, and zinc for sleep and improved quality of life.

Three herbs noted for their hypnotic qualities are basil, mint and sage. A tea steeped with any of these herbs for 20 minutes is the easiest preparation. Sipping the tea can be a comforting drink in the evening. The herbs are also good when served with the evening meal as seasonings.

Some pills may be prescribed by a physician for sleep. It may be a pill the physician prescribes for another problem such as depression, but it has a side effect of sleepiness. It may be an actual sleeping pill. You may also choose to take a pill such as melatonin since it can be purchased without a prescription. There is no scientific evidence that melatonin pills aid sleep but they may not harm adults. However, there is some evidence of testosterone effects so they should not be given to children. Of course, any non-prescription pill may interact with other medicines so you must check out such pills with your physician to be sure they are safe.

What do sleep specialists say about these pills or "natural sleep aids?" Lisa Shives, a spokesperson for the American Academy of Sleep Medicine said, "The research has not been robust...but people like to feel they are taking something." She commonly refers people with sleep problems to a psychologist who specializes in cognitive behavioral therapy and may give them a short prescription for sleeping pills. She added: "Many of my patients have a desperate look in their eye by the time they come to see us. I know if they don't go away with a slip of paper in their hands it will be a dark day indeed.".

This advice reminds us that pseudoscience speaks to powerful emotional needs that science often leaves unfulfilled. Pseudoscience offers satisfaction of spiritual hungers, cures for disease, promises that death is not going to happen with a new product. It reassures us of our importance. At the heart of pseudoscience is the idea that wishing makes things happen. The genie from the lamp can give us three wishes just by rubbing the lamp or rubbing on the oil or the supposedly medical curative. Caveat emptor! Buyer beware, as the Romans said.

Cognitive behavioral therapy (CBT) for insomnia, according to Dr. Alan Ruth, is considered the ideal treatment for chronic insomnia. But unlike a pill, it takes some time and some effort.

In a nutshell, the main gain is that the therapist helps patients replace negative thoughts about sleep with positive ones. Dysfunctional thoughts about sleep are "I will have an awful day if I don't sleep well" or "I should fall asleep quickly." Changes in thinking help a patient shift from trying hard to sleep to allowing sleep to just happen. This is often accomplished in 4 to 6-weeks through regular appointments. You can attempt to make such a change in your thinking, and promise yourself that if it doesn't work after a short trial, you will invest in CBT to help your insomnia. Just the commitment to do something to help yourself may relax your vigilance.

Other Drinks

Although warm milk drinks with honey, cinnamon, nutmeg or black pepper have been labeled sleep-inducing, they are not as good as other ingredients. You benefit more by its warm relaxing quality, but sleep is not likely to come from the milk. Its placebo effect probably comes from years of hearing it is a good evening drink, so it's as comfortable as any old favorite. Hot chocolate is surely not good for sleep since chocolate has caffeine.

Anahad O'Connor wrote "The Claim: A Glass of Warm Milk Will Help You Get to Sleep at Night" in 2007. He contended that because milk has tryptophan, a sleep-inducing amino acid, it was thought by some to have sedative effects. The same is sometimes said about turkey. But if either of them have any soporific effect, it is not because of the tryptophan. We receive as friendly, those ideas which agree with us and our habits. However, the hard rule of science is that if ideas don't work, we must throw them out.

In fact, just the opposite was proven in a 2003 study published in the *American Journal of Clinical Nutrition*. Milk decreased the ability of tryptophan to enter the brain. But if carbohydrates are eaten, they stimulate the release of insulin which makes it easier for tryptophan to enter the brain. The routine of a glass of milk before bed may have more to do with psychology than sleep. However, it could counteract stomach acid that deters sleep.

Lettuce has a sedative-like ingredient which is akin to opiates. In ancient Greece, guests were served lettuce soup at the end of a meal to usher them into dreamland. It can be eaten in a salad as the last course, which is regularly done in France. It may be cooked with peas as a warm dinner vegetable, often accented with green onions, butter, salt, sugar, and chopped mint.

However, some prefer to just have lettuce in an evening tea. Place 3-4 leaves of any kind of lettuce in a cup of water and simmer for 15 minutes. Remove from heat, and add sprigs of mint and sip before bedtime. Or purchase Wild Lettuce extract and put several drops in a glass of warm water before bedtime. It works for me thanks to a recommendation by a vitamin therapist, Diane Patrick.

The wry author, James Thurber, best known for *The Secret Life of Walter Mitty*, wrote about lettuce in a 1931 book called *The Owl in the Attic*. He described an old female cat saying that she never seemed sleepy, or particularly happy. "Is there anything I could give her?" he asked someone. "There are no medicines which can safely be given to induce felicity in a cat, but you might try lettuce, which is a soporific." He found that it worked for his cat.

Beatrix Potter wrote a children's book called *The Tale of the Flopsy Bunnies* in 1909. Bunnies went across the field to a rubbish heap in the ditch outside Mr. McGregor's garden. One day—oh joy! There were many overgrown lettuces, which had "shot" into flower. The Flopsy Bunnies simply stuffed themselves with lettuces. By degrees, one after another, they were overcome with slumber, and lay down in the new-mown grass to sleep.

Melatonin is found in many common fruits and vegetables including tomatoes, grape skins, tart cherries and walnuts. It can also be found in olive oil, wine, and even beer. The *Journal of Pineal Research* cites studies that show significant increases in melatonin levels in the blood of people who consumed melatonin-rich foods. These findings have caused researchers to explore one of the largest sources of melatonin—tart cherries. However, the number of people in these trials were small.

In 2010, the *Journal of Medicine Food* published a study called "Effects of a Tart Cherry Juice Beverage on the Sleep of Older Adults with Insomnia." Fifteen participants 71 years or older who complained of insomnia, but were otherwise healthy, were tested. They were given morning and evening doses of 8 ounces of Montmorency tart cherries, or a placebo of black cherry Kool-Aid, for two weeks. Researchers found that the cherry juice modestly improved sleep. The cherry juice did not improve sleep as much as medically-prescribed sleeping pills, but did better than the teas, and about as well as store-bought melatonin.

The *European Journal of Nutrition* published a 2012 article "Effect of Cherry Juice on Melatonin Levels and Enhanced Sleep Quality." Twenty volunteers took Montmorency cherry juice or a placebo for seven days. Melatonin was significantly elevated in the bloodstream of the cherry juice group and increased their time in bed, total sleep time, and sleep efficiency.

A *Neutraceuticals World* article on May 1, 2014, was entitled "Tart Cherry Juice May Help Treat Insomnia." The researchers found that those who drank the tart cherry juice in the morning and at night slept an average of 84 more minutes per night compared to the placebo, and their sleep tended to be more efficient.

A drink which might promote sleep is a banana smoothie, made with ½ ripe banana and ½ cup of soy or almond milk. Some people prefer coconut water before retiring, and adding a half banana could be helpful as well.

Snacks

One of the best snacks before bedtime is a banana. If you want to improve on that, have a very small bowl of your favorite cereal with milk and cut-up banana. That dish has tryptophan, calcium, protein and fiber. These are the ideal ingredients for sleep.

A handful of almonds and walnuts bring sleep-inducing carbohydrates to the tummy if chewed well and followed with some liquid.

Cheese, peanut butter, or hummus on crackers provide excellent snacks before bedtime.

Have some jelly beans in honor of Ronald Reagan and remember his hilarious line to his younger presidential opponent: "I am not going to exploit my opponent's youth and inexperience."

Try a little *Jell-O*, applesauce, or pudding if desired.

Have two kiwis an hour before bedtime. In a 2011 study called "Effect of Kiwifruit Consumption on Sleep Quality in Adults with Sleep Problems" found that subjects who consumed two kiwis per night for four weeks were found to fall asleep sooner, and sleep one hour longer, than before the study.

Final Activities

Bathe and brush teeth. If a bath or shower does not suit you in the evening, you might want to soak your feet for ten minutes in a pail of hot water. Let the water cool a little before taking them out. This advice was prescribed for sleepless women by Dr. R. T. Trall in *Health and Diseases* of Women in 1872. Sleeplessness in women has been around a long time!

Handle pets and loved ones with loving care so they can sleep well but put them away from your bed. As Rod McKuen said: "Cats have it all—admiration, an endless sleep, and company only when they want it."

Wind up serious work, heavy reading, and disturbing television shows. Replace them with happier, funnier, or romantic past-times just before bed.

Review the list of recommendations for sleep at the beginning of the book and make the preparations listed in your bedroom.

Set your temperature for the right coolness. Turn on your side of an electric blanket to warm your bed, if it's a cold night.

In Your Bedroom.

When you are sleepy, go into your bedroom.

If you or your loved ones pray before getting in bed, consider an old familiar prayer with a change or two.

Old version:
Now I lay me down to sleep,
I pray the Lord my soul to keep.
If I should die before I wake
I pray the Lord my soul to take.

New version:
Now I lay me down to sleep,
I pray the Lord my soul to keep.

Sweetest dreams all through the night
And wake me with the morning light.

Sit on your bed. Gently rub your temples with your hands. Have flowers or flower oil, described earlier, by your bed to breathe and smell. Rub a drop or two of your chosen oil on your forehead (rose or lavender).

Spread rose petals on your bed if desired. Damask roses would be best, but others will do.

Rub or have your mate rub the spine from top to bottom and legs from hip to foot.

Dr. Mehmet Oz suggested that massaging the forehead could relax one and stimulate the "feel good" hormones. He said to massage between the eyebrows, an area that is connected to the pineal gland, where melatonin is released. He said to begin by placing gentle pressure right between the eyebrows, then move toward the middle the brow. You can move back and forth or pull your fingers along your eyebrow. All of this plus gentle massage of the temples can be done in less than five minutes. He added that there's no harm in doing these massages more than once a day.

Cuddle up to your loved one and chat or fool around. Then just lie quietly together with mild caresses. After a final nice kiss, get into your desired position (together or apart) and let yourself go. You are safe and don't need to maintain your vigilance. You can write down any problems to take up the next day on a pad by your bed in the dark.

Don't *decide* to go to sleep. Just let things float around in your mind and allow all parts of your body to relax and fall where they may. Don't fret if your mind wanders all over the place because that is what it needs to do.

Good night, my dears!

APPENDIX I
CARBOHYDRATES THAT HELP PROTEIN PRODUCE MELATONIN

This appendix shows the *main* carbohydrates that are likely to help foods with tryptophan pass into the brain and help to produce serotonin, which in turn leads to the production of melatonin to make one sleepy. Enjoy these with or after your evening meal of some protein.

Almonds
Apples
Bananas
Barley
Beer
Cherries
Cherry (tart) juice
Fennel seeds
Ginger
Grapes
Grape juice
Kiwi
Oats
Oranges
Peppers

Pineapple
Radishes
Rice (especially Jasmine)
Spinach
Sunflower seeds
Strawberries
Sweet corn
Tomatoes
Wine

APPENDIX II

FOODS WITH MELATONIN (NG/100G)

Enjoy these with your evening meal or as evening snacks

Melatonin, ng/100 g.	Foods (A nanogram—ng-- is one billionth of a gram)
17,535	Tart (sour) cherry juice concentrate
1,350	Tart (sour) cherries
270	Walnuts
191.33	Mustard seed
187.80	Corn
149.80	Rice
142.30	Ginger root
116.70	Peanuts
87.30	Barley grains
79.13	Rolled oats
76.62	Asparagus
75.8	Radish
58.7	Garlic
53.95	Tomatoes

49.66	Fresh mint
49.4	Carrot
40.50	Black tea
31.40	Under ripe banana
30.9	Cabbage
29.9	Onion
27.8	Pineapple
26.67	Broccoli
21	Pomegranate
21	Strawberries
18.50	Ripe banana
16.88	Brussels sprouts
16.1	Apple
9.20	Green tea
8.94	Black olives
8.36	Green olives
5.93	Cucumber
4.26	Sunflower seeds
1.94	Red grapes (whole)
1.71	Concord grapes (whole)
1	Red wine

APPENDIX III

FOODS WITH TRYPTOPHAN
(BASED ON 200 MG. PORTIONS)

Enjoy these foods in a light evening meal accompanied by carbohydrates

Trytophan mg.	Food
746	Game meat, elk, cooked, roasted
690	Spinach, frozen, chopped or leaf
660	Soy protein isolate
659	Seeds, sesame
641	Seaweed, spirulina, dried
603	Soy sauce made from soy (tamari)
588	Crustaceans, shrimp, cooked
582	Crustaceans, lobster, cooked
578	Crustaceans, crab, canned
571	Crustaceans, crayfish, cooked
545	Watercress, raw
543	Duck, boneless, cooked

518	Cheese, parmesan
515	Egg white
513	Tofu, silken, lite firm
493	Fish, tuna, light, canned in water
490	Turkey, light meat, cooked
489	Pumpkin seed, cooked
486	Fish, haddock, cooked
484	Fish, tuna, cooked
475	Fish, perch, cooked
474	Chicken, fryer, breast
462	Fish, walleye pike, cooked
438	Fish, orange roughy, cooked
435	Fish, salmon, canned, bones removed
434	Ham, sliced, cooked
429	Cheese, Romano
418	Turkey, leg meat, cooked
415	Mushrooms, brown, raw
414	Fish, tilapia, cooked
413	Pork, loin, cooked
410	Fish, roe, raw
406	Chicken, Cornish game hen, cooked
405	Chicken, dark meat, cooked
400	Turnip greens, cooked
400	Chicken, canned with water
399	Cheese, mozzarella
394	Fish, catfish, cooked

392	Pork chops, cooked
391	Broccoli, raw
389	Lamb, cooked
385	Ham, cured, boneless, cooked
384	Fish, pink salmon, cooked
381	Parsley
381	Cheese, cottage, non-fat
379	Chicken salad without dressing
377	Veal, cubed for stew, cooked
373	Shrimp salad without dressing
372	Crustaceans, canned shrimp
370	Sesame seeds
366	Fish, swordfish, cooked
364	Fish, tuna, cooked
363	Cheese, cottage 2% milkfat
361	Chicken, giblets, neck, skin cooked
360	Cashew nuts
353	Lamb, cubed for stew, kabob, cooked
352	Turnip greens and turnip
351	Chicken, wing meat, cooked
350	Fish, smoked salmon
350	Chicken broth 99% fat free
348	Fish, anchovies raw
348	Spinach, cooked
347	Cheese, cream fat-free
345	Cheese, provolone

343	Fish, trout, cooked
339	Tofu, raw, firm
339	Basil, fresh
339	Spinach, raw
333	Mustard greens, cooked
333	Pumpkin leaves, cooked
331	Cheese, cheddar or Colby
331	Pastrami beef, 98% fat-free
322	Asparagus, cooked
320	Turkey, canned, with broth
318	Beet greens, raw
318	Mushrooms, white, raw
317	Beans, cooked
303	Beans, kidney, cooked
296	Beet greens, cooked
295	String beans, cooked
295	Spinach, canned
295	Chicken, canned with broth
294	Chia seeds, dried
286	Mushrooms, portabella, cooked
285	Oat bran, cooked
280	Soy beans, cooked
275	Lettuce, red leaf, raw
275	Split peas, cooked
274	Milk
272	Peanuts

270	Pistachio nuts
270	Asparagus, raw
270	Parmesan cheese, shredded
267	Bamboo shoots, cooked
265	Fish, sardines
264	Peanut butter
250	Cauliflower, cooked or raw
250	Cabbage, cooked
248	Corn salad
247	Chives, raw
229	Broccoli, cooked
229	Squash, zucchini
227	Mint leaves
210	Eggs, cooked
200	Walnuts
200	Almonds
200	Oats
190	Brussels sprouts, cooked
190	Pinto beans, cooked
166	Lima beans, cooked
164	Hearts of palm, canned
164	Navy beans, cooked
160	Green peas, cooked
146	Sweet pepper, cooked or raw
145	Okra, cooked
140	Ground beef

140	Macaroni/spaghetti
134	Whole wheat bread
126	Onions, raw or cooked
122	Celery, raw
112	Beef, ground, cooked
110	Crackers
102	Noodles, made with egg
100	Tomatoes, raw
98	Potato, white, with skin, cooked
94	Bread, white
89	Potato, sweet, cooked
89	Tomatoes, cooked
80	Egg, whole, uncooked
83	Rice, brown, cooked
76	Pineapple, canned
75	Potato, white, no skin, cooked
73	Rice, white, cooked
61	Corn, cooked
61	Carrots, cooked
57	Potato chips
53	Soy milk
49	Milk, 2% low fat
49	Red potatoes
47	Yogurt
44	Coleslaw
44	Apple pie

42	Cherries, sweet
41	Sour cream
33	Avocado
14	Kiwi
13	Strawberries
12	Butter
11	Banana
7.4	Melon
6.8	Pineapple
4	Raspberries

REFERENCES

Chapter One: Common Sense about Sleep

Arendt, J. "Importance and relevance of melatonin to human biological rhythms." *Journal of Neuroendocrinology.* 15:427-431, 2003.

"Blue Light Has a Dark Side." *Harvard Health Publications.* Retrieved from: www.health.harvard.edu/staying-healthy/blue-light-has-a-dark-side. 2015.

Brzezinski, A., Vaugel, M.G., Wurtman, R.J., Norrie. G., Zhdanoru, I., Ben-Shushan, A. and Ford, I. "Effects of exogenous melatonin on sleep: A meta-analysis." *Sleep Medicine Reviews.* 9:41-50, 2003.

Cardinali, D.P., Brusco, L.I., Llorett, S.P. and Furio, A.M. "Melatonin in sleep disorders and jet lag." *Neuroendocrinology Letters,* 1:9-13, 2002.

Cartwright, R. *The 24-Hour Mind: The Role of Sleep and Dreaming in Our Emotional Lives.* New York: Oxford University Press, 2010.

Ekirch, A. Roger. *At Day's Close: Night in Times Past.* New York: W.W. Norton, 2005.

Lipman, D. S. *Snoring from A to ZZZZ.* Portland, OR: Spencer Press, 1996.

Ng, W.L., Stevenson, C.E., Wong, E., Tanamas, S., Boelsen-Robinson, T., Shaw, J.E., Naughton, M.T., Dixon, J., and Peeters, A. "Does intentional weight loss improve daytime sleepiness? A systematic review and meta-analysis." *Obesity Reviews*. January 24, 2017. doi: 10.1111/obr.12498. 2017.

Schmerler, J. "Why is blue light before bedtime bad for sleep?" *Scientific American Mind*, 2015.

Winters, C. "How to stop snoring." *Consumer Reports*. Retrieved from: www.consumerreports.org/sleeping/how-to-stop-snoring/ 2016.

Chapter Two: Sleep Through the Ages

The Holy Bible. American Standard Version. New York: Thomas Nelson and Sons, 1929.

Aries, P, Duby, G., and Veyne, Paul. *A History of Private Life: From Pagan Rome to Byzantium*. Cambridge: Harvard University Press, 1992.

Badawy, A.A. and Dougherty, D.M. "Standardization of formulations for the acute amino acid depletion and loading tests." *Journal of Psychopharmacology*; 29: 363-371, 2015.

Bondy, S.C. and Sharmar, E.H. "Melatonin and the aging brain." *Neurochemistry International*, 50:571-80, 2007.

Borsay, P. *The English Urban Renaissance: Culture and Society in the Provincial Town*. Oxford: Oxford University Press, 1989.

Boynton, L.O.J. "The bed-bug and the age of elegance." *Furniture History* 1:15-31, 1965.

Brotto, L.A. and Gorzalka, B.B. "Melatonin enhances sexual behavior in the male rat." *Physiology and Behavior*, 68: 483-486, 2000.

Burgess, A. *On Going to Bed*. New York: Abbeville Press, 1982.

Burton, N. "Ten reasons you should be having a lot more morning sex." Retrieved from: www.cosmopolitan.com/sex-love/advice/a4803/why-morning-sex/ 2013.

Casanova, Giovanni. *The Complete Memoirs of Casanova: The Story of My Life*. Oxford: Benedictine Classics, 2015.

Cervantes, Miguel. *Don Quixote de la Mancha*. New York: Harper Perennial, 2005.

Chaucer, Geoffrey. *Canterbury Tales*. London: Penguin Classics, 2003.

Columbus, Christopher. *Letters of Christopher Columbus*. Rare books and special collections div. Library of Congress (048.00) 1493.

Crayton, J.W. "Focus on tryptophan." *Nutrition Digest* 38(1) American Nutrition Association. Retrieved from: www.superiorsites3.com/NNW01Trypt.html. 2001.

Davidoff, H. *A World Treasury of Proverbs from Twenty-Five Languages*. New York: Random House, 1946.

Davidson, P. (ed.) *Russian Literature and Its Demons*. Oxford, New York: Berghahn Books, 2000.

Dold, C. American cannibal. Retrieved from: discovermagazine.com/1998/ref/americancannibal1407. 1998.

Ekirch, A. Roger. *At Day's Close: Night in Times Past*. New York: W. W. Norton, 2005.

Ekirch, A. R. *Bound for America: The Transportation of British Convicts to the Colonies, 1718-1775*. Oxford: Clarendon Press, 1990.

Ferrari, C.K. "Functional foods, herbs, and nutraceuticals: Toward biochemical mechanisms of health aging." *Biogerontology*, 5:275-89, 2004.

Field, Eugene. *The Prose and Verse of Eugene Field*. New York: Charles Scribner's Sons, 1889.

Grape Dumplings (Tsalagi) recipe retrieved from: www.snowwowl. com/recipes/recsweets.html

Harrison, M. and Royston, O.M. *How They Lived: An Anthology of Original Accounts Written between 1485 and 1700*. Oxford: Basil Blackwell, 165:122-25, 1962.

Hotchner, A. E. *Papa Hemingway*. New York: Random House, 1966.

Jones, G. *Oxford Book of Welsh Verse in English*. Oxford: Oxford University Press, 1977.

Kiel, G. and Wolfegg, C.W. (Eds.) *The Medieval Housebook*. Munich: Prestel Publications, 1997.

Killigrew, W. *The Artless Midnight Thoughts of a Gentleman at Court Who for Many Years Built on Sand, Which Every Blast of Cross Fortune Has Defaced, But Now He Has*. Proquest, Eebo Editions, 2011.

Kipling, Rudyard. *The Day's Work*. London: Macmillan, 1898.

Lohmann, R. "Sleeping among the Asabano: Surprises in Intimacy and Society at the Margins of Consciousness." *Sleep Around the World*. Edited by Glaskin, K. and Chenhall, R. New York: Polgrave Macmillan, 2013.

McKeon, M. *The Secret History of Domesticity*. Cambridge: John Hopkins University Press, 2005.

McNamara, P. "The mystery of REM-related penile erections." *Psychology Today*, June 18, 2914.

Musharbash, Y. "Night, sight, and feeling safe: An exploration of aspects of Warlpiri and Western sleep." *Australian Journal of Anthropology*, 24:48-63. doi: 10.1111/taja.12021. 2013.

Paredes, S.D.; Barriga, C.; Reiter, R.J. and Rodriguez, A.B. "Assessment of the potential role of tryptophan as the precursor of serotonin and melatonin for the aged sleep-wake cycle and immune function." *International Journal of Tryptophan Research*, 2:23-36, 2009.

Pinker, Steven C. *The Better Angels of Our Nature: Why Violence Has Declined.* New York: Viking, 2011.

Polo, Marco. *The Travels of Marco Polo.* London: Penguin Books, 1958.

"L-Tryptophan manipulation." *Neurobehavioral Research Laboratory and Clinic.* 2016. Retrieved from: http://www.nrlc-group. net/proceduresAndFacilities/Tryptophan.php. 2016.

"Sleep Positions." *Better Sleep Council.* Retrieved from: www. bettersleep.org/better-sleep/sleep-positions. n.d.

Stevenson, Robert Louis. *A Child's Garden of Verses.* New York: Simon and Schuster, 1885.

Stoleru, S., Fonteille, V., Cornelis, C., Joyal, C. and Moulier, V. "Functional neuroimaging studies of sexual arousal and orgasm in health men and women: a review and meta-analysis." *Neuroscience Biobehavioral Review*, 36(6):1481-1509, 2012.

Van Driel, M. F. "Sleep related erections throughout the ages." *Journal of Sexual Medicine*, 11:(7), 2014.

Willett, C. and Cunnington, P. *The History of Underclothes.* London: Dover Publications, 41-61, 1951.

Chapter Three: Sleep in Songs and Fairy Tales

Arendt, J. "Importance and relevance of melatonin to human biological rhythms." *Journal of Neuroendocrinology.* 15:427-431, 2003.

Beauvillier, Antoine. *The Art of French Cookery.* Memphis, TN: General Books, 2012.

Bettelheim, Bruno. *The Uses of Enchantment.* New York: Vintage Books, 2010.

Brown, M.W. and Hurd, C. *Goodnight Moon.* New York: Harper and Row, 1947.

Brzezinski, A., Vaugel, M.G., Wurtman, R.J., Norrie, G., Zhdanoru, I., Ben-Shusahn. A. and Ford, I. "Effects of exogenous melatonin on sleep: A meta-analysis." *Sleep Medicine Review.* 9:41-50, 2003.

Cardinali, D.P., Brusco, L.I., Llorett, S.P. and Furio, A.M. "Melatonin in sleep disorders and jet lag." *Neuroendocrinology Letters,* I:9-13, 2002.

Cartwwright, R. *The 24-Hour Mind: The Role of Sleep and Dreaming in Our Emotional Lives.* New York: Oxford University Press, 2010.

Chandler, S.B. "Shakespeare and sleep." *Bulletin of the History of Medicine* 29: 255-260, 1955.

Fernando, S. and Rombauts, L. "Melatonin: Shedding light on infertility? A review of the recent literature." *Journal of Ovarian Research.* 7:98, 2014.

Fortescue, A. *The Seven Sleepers of Ephesus.* The Catholic Encyclopedia. New York: Robert Appleton Company, 1909.

Heffron, T.M. *I See the Animals Sleeping: A Bedtime Story.* Darien, IL: American Academy of Sleep Medicine, 2011.

Holloway, Diane. *Authors' Famous Recipes and Reflections on Food.* Lincoln, NE: Writers Club Press, 2002.

Irving, Washington. *Rip Van Winkle.* Philadelphia: David McKay Company Publishers, 1921.

Moreno, M.A. "Sleep terrors and sleepwalking." *Journal of the American Medical Association of Pediatrics.* 169(7):704, 2015.

Owens, J. and Mohan, M. "Behavioral interventions for parasomnias." *Current Sleep Medicine Reports*, 2:81, 2016.

Petit, D., Penestri, M.H., Paquet, J., Desautels, A., Zadra, A., Vitaro, F. Tremblay, R.E., Boivin, M. and Montplasir, J. "Childhood sleepwalking and sleep terrors." *Journal of the American Medical Association of Pediatrics.* 169(7): 653-658, 2015.

Price, Vincent and Price, Mary. *Come into the Kitchen.* New York: Stravon Educational Press, 1969.

Shaw, P., Tafti, M. and Thorpy, M. (Eds.) *The Genetic Basis of Sleep and Sleep Disorders.* Cambridge: Cambridge University Press, 2013.

Stevenson, Robert Louis. *A Child's Garden of Verses.* New York: Simon and Schuster, 1885.

Wright, L. *Warm and Snug: The History of the Bed.* Charleston, SC.: The History Press, 2004.

Chapter Four: "I Have a Dream!"

Ball, P. "Electric dreams." *The Lancet.* 389 (10073): 999-1000, 2017.

Baudelaire, Charles. *Les Paradis Artificiels (The Artificial Paradise)* New York: Citadel Press, 1996.

Benfry, O. T. "August Kekule and the birth of the structural theory of organic chemistry in 1858." *Journal of Chemical Education,* 35 (1):21-23, 1958.

Bolton, S.K. *The Story of Elias Howe and the Sewing Machine.* Bayside, NY: A. J. Cornell Publications, 2012.

Brian, D. *Einstein: A Life.* New York: John Wiley and Sons, 1996.

Carroll, Lewis. *Alice in Wonderland.* Kingspoint, TN: Grosset and Dunlap, 1946.

Davidson, Alan and Davidson, Jane. *Dumas on Food.* Oxford: Oxford University Press, 1978.

DeQuincy, Thomas. *Confessions of an Opium Eater.* New York: Penguin Classics, 2003.

Dickens, Charles. *Lying Awake.* NY, NY: The Literature Network, 1852.

Dostoyevsky, Fyodor. *The Brothers Karamazov.* New York: Farrar, Straus, and Giroux, 1990.

Dostoyevsky, Fyodor. *The Dream of a Ridiculous Man.* West Valley City, UT: Waking Lion Press, 2006.

Dumas, Alexander. *The Count of Monte Cristo.* New York: Wordsworth Editions, 1998.

Durant, Will and Durant, Ariel. *The Lessons of History.* New York: Simon and Schuster Paperbacks, 1968.

Fogg, A. *The Secrets of Hypnotic Golf: Play Better Golf in Your Unconscious Mind with Hypnosis and NLP.* Andrew Fogg Publications, 2010.

French, A. P. and Kennedy, P.J. *Niels Bohr: A Centenary Volume*. New York: Harvard University Press, 1987.

Freud, Sigmund. *The Interpretation of Dreams*. New York, NY: Basic Books, 2010.

Hall, A. "Six Ways smoking affects your sleep." Retrieved from: www. huffingtonpost.com/2015/03/05/how-smoking-affects-sleep_n_679 2954.html.

Haney, L. *Gregory Peck: A Charmed Life*. Cambridge: DeCapo Press, 2009.

Hitler, Adolf. *Mein Kampf.* New York: Houghton Mifflin Company, 1998.

Hopkin, M. "Sleep Boosts Lateral Thinking." *Nature*, 2004.

"Smoking affects Circadian Rhythm, study finds." Retrieved from: www.huffingtonpost.com/2014/01/06/smoking-circadian-rhythm-lungs_n_4532049.html.

Jouvet, Michel. "Behavioral and EEG Effects of Paradoxical Sleep Deprivation in the Cat." *Excerpta Medica International Congress* Series No. 87, 1965.

Kimball, M. *Thomas Jefferson's Cookbook*. Hartsville, OH: James Direct, Inc., 2007.

Komaroff, A.L. *Ask Dr. K*. Hookahs are not harmless, despite what teens may think. Retrieved from: www.uexpress.com/ask-dr-k/2016/11/21/ hookahs-are-not-harmless-in-spite. 2014.

Kyle, R.A. and Shamp, M.A. "Otto Loewi (1873-1961)". *Journal of the American Medical Association*. 241:463, 1979.

Mann, Thomas. *The Magic Mountain.* New York: Everyman's Library, 1924.

Mednick, S. "Remote Associates Test (RAT)." *The Science of Sin: The Seven Deadlies (and Why They Are So Good For You.* New York: Three Rivers Press, 2012.

Moreau, J.J. *Hashish and Mental Illness.* New York: Raven Press, 1973.

Rocke, A.J. *Image and Reality: Kekule, Kopp, and he Scientific Imagination.* Chicago: Chicago Press, 2010.

Rosa, J.A. "Why you should think twice about smoking hookah." *Cosmopolitan,* 2013.

Stevenson, Robert Louis. *The Strange Case of Dr. Jekyll and Mr. Hyde.* New York: Charles Scribner's Sons, 1886.

Stevenson, Robert Louis. *Across the Plains.* New York: Charles Scribner's Sons, 1892.

Spiers, H.J. and Caswell, B. "Neural systems supporting navigation." *Current Opinion in Behavioral Sciences.*1:47-55, 2015.

Thapoung, K. "The surprising damage of one night at a Hookah Bar." *Womens Health Magazine,* 2014.

Tolstoy, Leo. *Anna Karenina.* New York: Penguin Books, 2000.

Valenstein, E. The discovery of chemical neurotransmitters. *Brain and Cognition,* 49(1): 73-95, 2002.

Wilson, M.A. and Louie, K. "Temporally structure replay of awake hippocampal ensemble activity during rapid eye movement sleep." *Neuron,* 29(1): 145-56, 2002.

Chapter Five: Is the Universe on Circadian Rhythm?

Abbassi, J. "Do Apollo astronaut deaths shine a light on deep space radiation and cardiovascular disease?" *Journal of the American Medical Association.* 316(23):2469-70, 2016.

Annas, G.J. and Crosby, S.S. "Post-9/11 Torture at CIA 'Black Sites'— Physicians and Lawyers Working Together". *New England Journal of Medicine.* 372:2279-2281, 2015.

Barger, L.K., Flynn-Evans, E.E., Kubey, A., Walsh, L., Ronda, J.M., Wang, W., Wright, K.P., Jr. and Czeisler, C.A. "Prevalence of sleep deficiency and use of hypnotic drugs in astronauts before, during, and after spaceflight: An observational study." *Lancet Neurology*, (9):904-12, 2014.

Borchelt, G. and Pross, C. "Systematic use of psychological torture by U.S. forces." *Torture*, 3(1), 2005.

Burroughs, J. *Our Vacation Days of 1918*. The Adventures of the Four Vagabonds. The Harvard Library Shelf, 2013.

Drake, N. "Potentially habitable planet found orbiting star closes to sun." *National Geographic*, 2016.

Flynn-Evans, E., Gregory, K., Arsintescu, L. & Whitmire, A. "Risk of performance decrements and adverse health outcomes results from sleep loss, circadian desynchronization and work overload." Houston, TX: NASA Technical Reports Services, 2016.

Glaberson, W. "Detainee's lawyers make a claim on sleep deprivation". *New York Times*, 2008.

Gordon, R.V. "New food for third Skylab mission." Houston, TX: *NASA*, 1979.

Gottlieb, D.J., Punjabi, N.M. Newman, A.B., Resnick, H.E., Redline, S. and Baldwin, C.L. "Association of sleep time with diabetes mellitus and impaired glucose tolerance." *Journal of the American Medical Association Internal Medicine.* 165(8), 2005.

Grandner, M.A., Jackson, N.J., Pigeon, W.R., Gooneratne, N.S. and Patel, N.P. "State and Regional Prevalence of Sleep Disturbance and Daytime Fatigue." *Journal of Clinical Sleep Medicine.* 9(1):77-86, 2012.

Hlavaty, C. "Early NASA Diapers Forced Astronauts to Disclose the Size of Their Manhood." *Chron,* 2014.

Howell, E. "The Six Earth-like Alien Planets." *Space.com.* 2015.

"Inquiry into the Treatment of Detainees in U.S. Custody." *Report of the Committee on Armed Services, United States Senate,* 2008.

Klein, C. "Ford and Edison's Excellent Camping Adventures." *History Channel.* July 30, 2013.

Nilssen, O, Lipton, R., Brenn, T., Hoyer, G. Boiko, E. and Tkatchev, A. "Sleeping Problems at 78 Degrees North: The Svalbard Study." *Acta Psychiatric Scandinavia.* 95(1):44-48, 1997.

Siems, Larry. *The Torture Report.* Amazon Nook Edition, 2012.

Sommerer, J.C. "Charting a Course: Expert Perspectives on NASA's Human Exploration Proposals." *U.S. House of Representatives Committee on Science, Space, and Technology,* 2016.

Stirling, A. "Borscht by Tube? Space Menu Served Up to Mark Soviet Achievements." *The Guardian,* U.S. edition, 2015.

Willemse, Jan. *Cooking for Henry.* Virginia Beach, VA: The Donning Company, 1993.

Woollaston, V. "How to Throw Up in Space." *Daily Mail,* UK edition, 2013.

Chapter Six: People Sleeping Together

Aligheri, Dante. *The Divine Comedy.* New York: Penguin Books, 2003.

Bacall, Lauren. *Lauren Bacall by Myself.* New York: Knopf, 1978.

Baggaley, K. "Why We Like to Touch Soft, Fluffy Things." Retrieved from: https://braindecoder.com/post/why-we-like-touching-soft-fluffy-things-1262780083. n.d.

Borreli, L. "Sleep positions to stay healthy: The best and worst ways to sleep during the night." Healthy Living. Retrieved from www.medicaldaily.com. August 5, 2014.

Boskabady, M. H., Shafei, M.N., Saberi, Z. and Amini, S. "Pharmacological effects of Rosa Damascena." *Iran Journal of Basic Medical Science.* 14(4):295-307, 2011.

Brech, A. "Couples who sleep naked together have a happier relationship, study reveals." *Stylist(UK),* 2016.

Breus, M. J. "Coping with couples' different sleep needs." Retrieved from: www.webmd.com/sleep-disorders/feature/coping-with-couples-difference-sleep-needs#1. 2004.

Bulkeley, K. *Big Dreams: The Science of Dreaming and Origins of Religion.* New York: Oxford University Press, 2016.

Burdick, A. "Present tense: How time became psychological." *The New Yorker,* 2016.

Cerwin, H. (Ed). *Famous Recipes by Famous People*. San Francisco: Lane Publishing Company, 1940.

Cervantes, Miguel. *Don Quixote*. Ware, England: Wordsworth Editions, Ltd., 1997.

Coffey, L. "Relationships and Sleep." *Better Sleep Council,* Retrieved from: http://bettersleep.org/better-sleep/healthy-sleep/relationships-sleep. Dec. 31, 2016

Coren, Stanley. *Sleep Thieves*. New York: Simon and Schuster, 1991.

DeMunck, V.C. (Ed.) *Romantic Love and Sexual Behavior: Perspectives from the Social Sciences*. Connecticut: Praeger Publishers, 1998.

Dietrich, Marlene *ABC: Wit, Wisdom & Recipes*. New York: Open Road, 1984.

Edwards, S. "Love and the brain." *Harvard Medical School: On the Brain*, 2015.

Ekirch, A.Roger. *At Day's Close: Night in Times Past*. New York: W. W. Norton, 2005.

Feiler, B. The lark-owl scale: When couples' sleep patterns diverge." *The New York Times*, 2016.

Field, T., Field, T., Cullen, C., Largie, S., Diego, M., Schanberg, S. and Kuln, C. "Lavender bath oil reduces stress and crying and enhances sleep in very young infants." *Early Human Development*. 84(6) 399-401, 2008.

Fisher, Helen. *Anatomy of Love: A Natural History of Mating, Marriage, and Why We Stray*. Washington, D.C.: Ballantine Books, 1994.

Fleming, J. "Psychiatric disorders and insomnia: Managing the vicious cycle." *Insomnia Rounds*. 2(1):1-5, 2013.

Frankel, V. "Exploring the love drug, joy and sex." *CNN: Oprah.com.* 2010.

Fromm, Erich. *The Art of Loving.* NY: Perennial Classics. 2000.

Gandhi, Mohatmas K. *Diet and Diet Reform.* Ahmedabad, India: Navajivan Publishing House. 1949.

Gandhi, Mohatmas K. *Autobiography: My Experiments with Truth.* Washington, D.C.: Dover Publications. 1983.

Gavrilets, S. "Human origins and the transition from promiscuity to pair bonding." *Proceedings of the National Academy of Sciences 109* (25):9923-9928. 2012.

Goldsmith, B. "The importance of sharing a bed with your lover." *Psychology Today,* 2013.

Graczyk, M. "Prison plays hide-and-seek with FLDS leader Warren Jeffs." Retrieved from: www.deseretnews.com/article/865650018/prison-plays-hide-and-seek-with-flds-leader-warren-jeffs.html. 2016.

Gray, P. "How hunter gatherers maintained their egalitarian ways." *Psychology Today,* 2011.

Gray, P. "Play as a foundation for hunter-gatherer social existence." *American Journal of Play.*1(4):476-522, 2009.

Griffith, L.L. "Sleeping apart may mean trouble for couples." *San Luis Obispo Tribune,* 2015.

Hammett, Dashiell. *Dashiell Hammett Five Complete Novels.* Avenel, NJ: Avenel Publishing, 1980.

Hellmann, Lillian and Feibleman, P. *Eating Together: Recollections and Recipes.* Boston: Little, Brown and Company, 1984.

Hinohara, S. and Niki, H. *Osler's "A Way of Life" and Other Addresses with Commentary and Annotations*. Durham: Duke University Press, 2001.

Holloway, Diane and Cheney, Bob. *American History in Song*. Lincoln, NE: Authors Choices Press, 2001.

Ju, Y.E., McLeland, J.S., Todedbusch, C.D., Xiong, C., Fagan, A.M., Duntley, S.P., Morris, J.C. and Holtzman, D.M. "Sleep quality and preclinical Alzheimer disease." *Journal of the American Medical Association Neurology*. 79(5):587-93, 2013.

Kalmbach, D.A., Amedt, J.T., Pillai, V., and Ciesla, J.A. "The impact of sleep on female sexual response and behavior: A pilot study." *Journal of Sexual Medicine*. 12:1221-1232, 2015.

Komori, T., Matsumoto, T., Motomura, E. and Shiroyama, T. "The sleep-enhancing effect of valerian inhalation and sleep-shortening effect of lemon inhalation." *Chemical Senses*. 31(8):731-7, 2006.

Kipling, Rudyard. *The Collected Poems of Rudyard Kipling*. London: Wordsworth Editions, 2001.

Kottak, C.P. *Cultural Anthropology*. New York: McGraw-Hill, 2006.

Lewis, J.G. "Alcohol, sleep and why you might rethink that nightcap." *Psychology Today*. October 28, 2013.

Lott, T. "Are separate beds the key to a good night's sleep?" *The Guardian*, 2013.

Mahboubi, M. "Rosa damascena as holy ancient herb with novel applications." *Journal of Traditional Complementary Medicine*. 6(1):10-16, 2016.

Methven, J. "Why we sleep together." *The Atlantic*, 2014.

Morley, C. *Modern American Literature: The Lost Generation.* Edinburgh: Edinburgh University Press, 157, 2012.

Musherbash, Y. "Night, sight, and feeling safe: An exploration of aspects of Warlpiri and Western sleep." *The Australian Journal of Anthropology.* Doi: 10.1111/4aja.12021. 2013.

Olds, J. "Hypothalamic substrates of reward." *Physiological Reviews* 45:554-604, 1962.

Park, Shin-Jung. "Effects of softness of bedding materials upon overnight excretion of urinary catecholamines and sleep quality in warm environmental conditions." *Journal of Biological Rhythm Research.* 46(1) 91-101. doi.org/10.1080/09291016.2014.950090. 2015.

Revenson, T.A., Marin-Chollom, A.M., Rundle, A.G., Wisnivesty, J.and Neugut, A.I. "Hey Mr. Sandman: Dyadic effects of anxiety, depressive symptoms and sleep among married couples." *Journal of Behavioral Medicine* 39(2):225-232, 2016.

Rosenblum, Gail. "Suite idea: Dual master bedrooms." *Star Tribune,* 2015.

Shore, Dinah. *Someone's in the Kitchen with Dinah.* New York: Doubleday and Company, 1971.

Slater, L. "True love." *National Geographic Magazine,* 1-7, 2006.

Toklas, Alice B. *The Alice B. Toklas Cook Book.* New York: Harper Perennial, 1954.

Troxel, Wendy M., Robles, T.F., Hal, M. and Buysse, D.J. "Marital quality and the marital bed: Examining the covariation between relationship quality and sleep." *Sleep Medicine Review.* 11(5):389-404, 2007.

Troxel, Wendy M. "Exploring the dyadic nature of sleep and implications for health." *Psychosomatic Medicine* 72(6):578-586, 2010.

Wehr, Thomas A. "In short photoperiods, human sleep is biphasic." *Journal of Sleep Research.* 1(2):103-107, 1992.

"WJU professor and students find Jasmine odor leads to more restful sleep, decreased anxiety and greater mental performance. Wheeling Jesuit University in Wheeling, West Virginia." Retrieved from: www. wju.edu/about/adm_new_story.asp?iNewsID=5398strBack=/about/ adm_news_archive.asp. n.d.

Wilding, R. "Romantic love and 'getting married': narratives of the wedding in and out of cinema texts." *Journal of Sociology.* 39.4 (2003): 373-390, 2003.

Zuffoletti, A.R. *Arranged Marriages.* Retrieved from: http://iml.jou.ufl. edu/projects/spring07/Zuffoletti/love.html. 2007.

Chapter Seven: Sleep Loss in Leaders! Are We Safe?

Blair, Cherie. *My Speaking for Myself: My Life from Liverpool to Downing Street.* London: Little Brown Company, 2008.

Braebner, W. *My Dear Mister Churchill.* New York: Simon and Schuster, 1965.

Buchanan, Patrick J. *The Greatest Comeback: How Richard Nixon Rose from Defeat to Create the New Majority.* New York: Crown Forum, 2014.

Bush, George H.W. *All the Best, George Bush.* New York: Scribner, 2013.

Caldwell, D and Hocking, W.G. "How jet lag hurts diplomats without them even knowing it." *The Washington Post,* 2015.

Cummings, D. "American time zones established by railways." *On This Day* web site produced by Dulcinea Media, 2011.

Diliberto, G. "Biologist Charles Ehret says jet lag is avoidable even on a fast plane to China." *People,* 21 (17), 1984.

Ecker, W.B. and Kenneth, V.J. *Blue Moon over Cuba: Aerial Reconnaissance during the Cuban Missile Crisis.* Oxford, England: Osprey Publications, 2012.

"Fatal Familial Insomnia." U.S. Department of Health and Human Services: National Institute of Health (NIH) web site.

Foster, P. "Nixon tapes reveal secret of time-delay lock on Soviet leader's cigarette box." *The Telegraph,* 2013.

"Neville Chamberlain and appeasement." *The Guardian,* 2009.

Gupta, S. and Cohen, E. "Get some sleep: Jet lag?" *CNN* on line, 2010.

Ho, E. "How presidents beat jet lag." *Business Insider,* 2014.

Holloway, Diane and Cheney, Bob. *Analyzing Leaders, Presidents and Terrorists.* Lincoln, NE: Writers Club Press, 2002.

Kennedy, John F. *Why England Slept.* Melbourne: London, 1940.

Kreitzman, L. "Who put the lag in jet lag?" *New York Times—The Opinionator,* 2009.

Kristen, A.L. "Soon-to-be secretary of state John Kerry, with tongue in check, shares his tips for fighting jet lag." *New York Daily News,* 2013.

Maas, J.B., Wherry, M.L., Axelrod, D.J., Hogan, B.R. and Blumin, J.A. "Review of power sleep." *New York Times on the Web,* 1988.

Mikoyan, Anastas. *Book of Tasty and Healthy Food.* Moscow: USSR Institute of Nutrition of the Academy of Medical Sciences, 1939.

Valkeinen, J. "No time for jet lag." *GB Times Oy Limited,* 2010.

Weisberg, J. *W's Greatest Hits.* Retrieved from: www.slate.com/ articles/news_and_politics/bushisms/2009/01/wc_greatest_hits. html. 2009.

Wills, G. *The Kennedy Imprisonment: A Meditation on Power.* Boston: Mariner, 2002.

Wines, M. "Bush in Japan: Bush collapses at state dinner with the Japanese." *The New York Times,* 1992.

Chapter Eight: Sleep and Various Cultures: Who Sleeps with Who?

Abbott, S. "Holding on and pushing away: comparative perspectives on an eastern Kentucky child-rearing practice." *Ethos 20*(1):33-65, 1992.

Bixler, E.O., Papaliaga, M.N., Vgontzas, A.N., Lin, H.M., Pejovic, S., Karataraki, M., Vila-Bueno, A. and Chrousos, G.P. "Women sleep objectively better than men and the sleep of young women is more resilient to external stressors: Effects of age and menopause." *Journal of Sleep Research 18*(2): 221-228, 2009.

Brooks, Megan. "On-line sleep education tool promising in college students." *Medscape,* 2016.

Bursztyn, M. "Mortality and the siesta, fact and fiction." *Sleep Medicine.* http://dx.doi.org/10.1016/j.sleep.2012.09.010. 2012.

"1 in 3 adults don't get enough sleep." *Centers for Disease Control and Prevention* web site, 2016.

Caudill, W. and Plath, D.W. "Who sleeps by whom? Parent-child involvement in urban Japanese families." *Psychiatry 29*:344-366, 1966.

Caudill, W. & Weinstein, H. (1969) Maternal care and infant behavior in Japan and America. *Psychiatry 32*:12-43.

Chekov, A. Sleepy. (1906) *Cosmopolitan Magazine*, 41:151.

Chu, C., Hom, M.A., Rogers, M.L., Ringer, F.B., Hames, J.L., Suh, S. & Joiner, T.E. (2016) Is insomnia lonely? Exploring thwarted belongingness as an explanatory link between insomnia and suicidal ideation in a sample of South Korean university students. *Journal of Clinical Sleep Medicine 12*(5):647-652.

Cortesi, F., Giannotti, F., Sebastiani, T. & Vagnoni, C. (2004) Co-sleeping and sleep behavior in Italian school-aged children. *Journal of Developmental Behavioral Pediatrics 25*:28-33.

Dickens, C. (1875) *The Pickwick Papers*. New York: Hurd and Houghton.

Dinges, D.F. & Broughton, R.J. (1989) The significance of napping: a synthesis. In: Dinges DF, Broughton RJ, eds. *Sleep and Alertness: Chronobiological, Behavioral, and Medical Aspects of Napping*. New York, NY: Raven Press.

Donovan, L.M. & Kapur, V.K. (2016) Prevalence and characteristics of central compared to obstructive sleep apnea: Analyses from the sleep heart health study cohort. *Sleep 39*(7):1353-9.

Feder, M. & Feder, K. (2007) *Joy of Liberace*. Santa Monica, CA: Angel City Press.

Ferber, R. (1985) *Solve Your Child's Sleep Problems*. New York: Simon and Schuster.

Forbes, J.F., Weiss, D.S. & Folen, R.A. (1992) The co-sleeping habits of military children. *Military Medicine 157*:196-200.

Gannon, L. (2007) Grand Slam: Maria Sharapova. *MailOnline*.

Hafner, M. & Troxel, W.M. (2016) Americans don't sleep enough, and it's costing us $411 billion. *The Washington Post.*

Hershner, S.D. & Chervin, R.D. (2014) Causes and consequences of sleepiness among college students. *National Science of Sleep* 6:73-84.

Kawakami, K. (1987) Comparison of mother-infant relationships in Japanese and American families. Paper presented at the meetings of the International Society Study of Behavioral Development in Tokyo, Japan.

Kellum, B.A. (1974) Infanticide in England in the later middle ages. *History of Childhood Quarterly* 1(3):367-388.

Klonoff-Cohen, H.S. & Edelstein, S.L. (1995) Bed sharing and the sudden infant death syndrome. *British Medical Journal* 311:1269-1272.

Koyanagi, A., Garin, N., Olaya, B., Aguyso-Mateos, J.L., Chatterji, S.,Leonardi, M., Koskinen, S., Tobiasz-Adamczyk, B. & Haro, J.M. (2014) Chronic conditions and sleep problems among adults aged 50 years or over in nine countries *PLoS ONE* 9(12): e114742.

Kripke, D.F., Garfield, L., Wingard, D.L., Klauber, R. & Marlar, M.R. (2002) Mortality associated with sleep duration and insomnia. *Archive of General Psychiatry* 59(2):131-36.

Leng, Y., Wainwright, N.W.J., Cappuccio, F.P., Surtees, P.G., Hayat, S., Luben, R., Brayne, C. & Khaw, K. T. (2014) Daytime napping and the risk of all-cause and cause-specific mortality: A 13-Year follow-up of a British population. *American Journal of Epidemiology* 179(9):1115-1124.-

Levy, D.J., Heissel, J.A., Richeson, J.A. & Adam, E.K. (2016) Psychological and biological responses to race-based social stress as pathways to disparities in educational outcomes. *American* Psychologist 71(6):455-473.

Liu, X., Zhao, Z., Jia, C. & Buysse, D.J. (2008) Sleep patterns and problems among Chinese adolescents. *Pediatrics 121*(6):1165-73.

Loren, S. (1998) *Recipes and Memories.* New York: GT Publishing.

Marriott, B. (1994) Food components to enhance performance: An evaluation of potential performance-enhancing food components. Washington, DC: *Institute of Medicine, Food and Nutrition Board. National Academies Press.*

McKenna, J. (1998) Bedsharing promotes breast feeding and the AAP task force on infant positioning and SIDS. *Pediatrics 102* (3):663-664.

Mead M. (1970) Children and ritual in Bali. In: Belo, J. ed. *Traditional Balinese Culture.* New York, NY: Columbia University Press.

Medoff, D. & Schaefer, C.E. (1993) Children sharing the parental bed: a review of the advantages and disadvantages of co-sleeping. *Psychology Journal of Human Behavior 30*(1):1-9.

Morelli, G.A., Rogoff, B., Oppenheim, D., Goldsmith, D. (1992) Cultural variation in infants' sleep arrangements: questions of independence. *Developmental Psychology 28*:604-613.

Mosko, S., Richard, C. & McKenna, J. (1996) Maternal sleep and arousals during bedsharing with infants. *Sleep 20*(2):142-150.

Nashka, A., Oikonomou, E., Trichopoulou, A., Psaltopoulou, T. & Trichopoulos, D. (2007) Siesta in health adults and coronary mortality in the general population. *Archives of Internal Medicine 167*(3):296-301.

Ozturk, M. & Ozturk, O.M. (1977) Thumbsucking and falling asleep. *British Journal of Medical Psychology 50*:95-103.

Pinker, S. (2011) *The Better Angels of Our Nature: Why Violence Has Declined.* NY: Viking, 2011.

Preston, D. (1998) Cannibals of the canyon. *New Yorker.*

Schachter, F.F., Fuchs, M.L., Bijur, P.E. & Stone, R.K. (1989) Co-sleeping and sleep problems in Hispanic-American urban young children. *Pediatrics 84*:522-530.

Sleep in America, 2006. Washington, D.C.: National Sleep Foundation, Washington, DC.

Soldatos, C.R., Madianos, M.G. & Vlachonikolis, I.G. (1983) Early afternoon napping: a fading Greek habit. In: Koella, W.P. ed. *Sleep '82.* Basel, Switzerland: Karger Verlag.

Spitzer, K. (2016) Japanese are working themselves to death—literally. *USA Today.*

Spock, Benjamin. (1968) *Baby and Child Care.* New York: Pocket Books.

Steger, B. & Brunt, L. eds. (2003) *Night-time and Sleep in Asia and the West: Exploring the Dark Side of Life.* London, England: Routledge Curzon.

Stone, L. (1977) *The Family, Sex and Marriage in England, 1500-1800.* New York: Harper and Row.

Sullivan, K. (2015) Cowboy Wash: The mystery of the 7 cannibalized victims in an abandoned Anasazi village. *Ancient Origins.*

Tamaki, M., Bang, J.W., Watanabe, T. & Sasaki, Y. (2016) Night watch in one brain hemisphere during sleep associated with first-night effect in humans. *Current Biology* 26(9):1190-1194.

Thompson, S.A. (2014) Which cities get the most sleep? *The Wall Street Journal.*

Tynjala, J., Kannas, L. & Valimaa, R. (1993) How young Europeans sleep. *Health Education Research 8*:69-80.

White, S. (2016) Death by overwork on rise among Japan's vulnerable workers. *Business News.*

Who Gets Any Sleep These Days? Sleep Patterns of Canadians. (2005) Statistics of Canada: General Social Survey.

Wolf, A.W. & Ozoff, B. (1989) Object attachment, thumb sucking, and the passage to sleep. *Journal of the American Academy of Child & Adolescent Psychiatry 28*:287-292.

Yang, C.K. & Hahn, H.M. (2002) Co-sleeping in young Korean children. *Journal of Developmental and Behavioral Pediatrics 23*:151-157.

"Yoko Ono Off B'way Epic Hiroshima Hits". (1997) October 9.

Chapter Nine: Drowsy Drivers

Aldridge, J. (2005) Saint Paul *The Guardian*, New York City.

Algeo, M. (2009) *Harry Truman's Excellent Adventure: The True Story of a Great American Road Trip.* Chicago: Chicago Review Press.

Butel, J. (2008) *Chili Madness.* New York: Workman Publishing Company.

Carney, C., McGehee, D., Harland, K., Weiss, M. & Raby, R.M. (2016) Using Naturalistic Driving Data to Examine Teen Driver Behaviors Present in Motor Vehicle Crashes 2007-2015. AAA Foundation for Traffic Safety.

Flannigan, J., Talpins, S.K. & Moore, C. (2017) Oral fluid testing for impaired driving enforcement. *The Police Chief.*

History of electric cars: Retrieved from https://energy.cov/articles/history-electric-car.

Hotchner, U. & Newman, N. (1985) *Newman's Own Cookbook.* Chicago: Contemporary Books.

Huffington, A. (2016) *The Sleep Revolution: Transforming Your Life, One Night at a Time.* New York: Harmony Books.

Johnson, K.D., Patel, S.R., Baur, D.M., Edens, E., Sherry, P., Malhotra, A. & Kales, S.N. (2014) Association of sleep habits with accidents and near misses in U.S. transportation operators. *Journal of Occupation Environmental Medicine 56*(5):510-515.

Lancet editorial: The USA's Dangerous Driving Culture. (2016) Lancet 388(10041):212.

Lind, H. (2017) The History of the Electric Car and Self-Driving Cars. Address at: West Valley Engineers, Science and Technology Association" on March 3, 2017.

Nascar.com: Danica Patrick Breakfast Hash on AllRecipes.

Rousseau, B. (2016) Napping in public? In Japan, that's a sign of diligence. *NY Times.*

Santos, F. (2005) No light-speeding: Safe-driving message get 'Star Wars' twist. *New York Times,* December 21, 2005. Retrieved from: www.nytimes.com/2015/12/22/us/star-wars-arizona-drunk-driving.html?_r=3

Schwartz, C. (1979) *Cole Porter: A Biography.* Boston: DaCapo Press.

Seabaugh, C. (2012) The life of a legend through the years: Carroll Shelby 1923-2012. *Motortrend News.*

U.S. Nuclear Regulatory Commission: (2014) *Rulemaking for Enhanced Security at Fuel Cycle Facilities; Special Nuclear Material Transportations; Security Force Fatigue at Nuclear Facilities.*

Vartabedian, R. & Hennigan, W.J. (2017) This troubled, covert agency is responsible for trucking nuclear bombs across America each day. *Los Angeles Times.*

Chapter Ten: Catastrophes and Sleep Deprivation

1988 Presidential Commission on the Space Shuttle Challenger Accident (Volume 2, Appendix G—Human Factor Analyses).

Balsamo, M. & Klepper, D. (2016) Engineer in crash had undiagnosed sleep apnea. *APNewsBreak on MSN News.*

Boardman, B. (1942) *Sincerely Yours.* San Francisco: Grabhorn Press, 1942.

Findings of accidents caused by sleep deprivation were reported on June 9, 2016. Retrieved from: http://www.ncbi.nlm.nih.gov/pmc/articles/PMC2517096/

Harper, K. (2001) Chernobyl stories and anthropological shock in Hungary. *Anthropological Quarterly 74*(3):114-123.

Hatch, M.C., Wallenstein, S., Beyea, J., Nieves, J.W. & Susser, M. (1991) Cancer rates after the Three Mile Island nuclear accident and proximity of residences to the plant. *American Journal of Public Health 81*(6): 719-724.

McGeehan, P., Rosenburg, E. & Fitzsimmons, E. (2016) Hoboken train crash kills 1 and injures over 100. *The New York Times.*

Mittler, M.M., Carskadon, M.A., Czeisler, C.A., Dement, W.C., Dinges, D.F. & Graeber, R.C. (1988) Catastrophes, sleep and public policy. *Sleep 11*(1):100-109.

NTSB Press Release of 10/4/15: Fatigue, Drug Use Caused Multi-Vehicle Crash in Tennessee.

Refinery Explosion and Fire. (2007) *U.S. Chemical Safety and Hazard Investigation Board*. Report No. 2005-04-I-TX.

Shaer, M. (2016) The wreck of Amtrak 188. *New York Times Magazine*.

Sisak, M.R. (2016) Feds target sleep apnea, speeding after train crash. *The Arizona Republic*.

Smolensky, M., Halberg, F. & Sargent, F. (1972) Chronobiology of the life sequence in *Advances in Climatic Physiology*. Tokyo: Igaku Shoin; pp. 515-516.

Wing, S. (2003) Objectivity and ethics in environmental science. *Environmental. Health Perspectives 111*(14):1809-1818.

Chapter Eleven: Aviation and Sleep Deprivation

Ahlers, M.M. (2011) FAA reports another sleeping air traffic controller. *CNN News*.

Albuquerque, New Mexico, mourns loss of medical personnel after plane crash in California." *EMS World*, reported by Associated Press, October 25, 2004.

Badam, R.T. (2013) Three years on, memories of crash of Air India's Dubai flight still haunt, *The National/AE* Retrieved from: www.thenational.ae/news/uae-news/three-years-on -memories-of-crash-of air indias-dubai-flight-still-haunt.

Beck, K. & Clark, J. (1995) *The All-American Cowboy Cookbook*. Nashville, TN: Rutledge Hill Press.

Challenger with frost on wings enters uncontrolled roll on takeoff. (2005) Challenger 604 crash in Birmingham, England on January 4, 2002. *Flight Safety Foundation. Accident Prevention 62*(1).

Deangelis, T. (2016) Behavioral therapy works best for insomnia. *Monitor on Psychology 47*(9).

Eatherly, C. (2015) *Burning Conscience: The Case of the Hiroshima Pilot Claude Eatherly.* Cleveland, Ohio: Pickle Partners Publishing.

Eckert, B. (2002) The Long Good-by. *New York Magazine,*

Fatigue and Sleep Management: Personal Strategies for Decreasing the Effects of Fatigues and Traffic Control. Retrieved from: *Eurocontrol.* SKYbary.aero/bookshelf/books/220.pdf.

Ferran, L. (2009) Beverly Eckert, September 11 widow, died in fiery Buffalo flight 3407 crash. *ABC News*

Freedman, R. (1977) *Eleanor Roosevelt: Life of Discovery.* NY: Houghton-Mifflin.

George, F. (2015) Preventing crew fatigue from A to Azz. *Aviation Week* Retrieved from: http://aviationweek.com/business-aviation/preventing-crew-fatigue-zzz.

Gronner, C.J. (2004) *The Family of Ronald W. Reagan.* Baltimore, MD: Genealogical Publications. Also see: www.genealogical.com and insert Ronald W. Reagan.

Holloway, D. & Cheney, B.)2001) *American History in Song.* Lincoln, NE: Authors Choices Press.

Hunsicker, J. (2014) Emotional scars run deep for survivors of corporate airlines flight 5966. *Kirksville Daily Express.*

Kegley, J. (2012) Comair 5191 crash's surviving copilot speaks in documentary film. *Lexington Herald Leader.*

Kessler, L. (2000) *The Happy Bottom Riding Club: The Life and Times of Pancho Barnes.* NY: Random House.

Kessner, T. (2010) *The Flight of the Century.* New York: Oxford University Press.

Lacagnina, M. (2006) CFIT on a dark night departure. *Aviation Safety.*

Lawton, R. (1994) Steep turn by captain during approach results in stall and crash of DC-8 freighter. *Flight Safety Foundation. Accident Prevention 51*(10): 1-8.

Maxon, T, (2011) FAA wants to fire air traffic controller napping in Knoxville. *Dallas News.*

Mele, C. (2017) FAA investigates errant flight involving Harrison Ford. *New York Times.*

Memmott, M. (2014) Deborah Hersman stepping down as head of NTSB. Retrieved from: http://www.npr.org/sections/thetwo-way/2014/03/11/289056642/deborah-hersman-stepping-down-as-head-of-ntsb.

Morris, S.L. (2006) *What Archives Reveal: The Hidden Poems of Amelia Earhart,* West Lafayette, IND. *Purdue Univ. Lib.* West Lafayette, IND, 2006. Retrieved from: http://docs.lib.purdue.edu/lib_research/28

National Transportation Safety Board. (1993) Uncontrolled collision with terrain. Guantanamo Bay, Cuba.

National Transportation Safety Board. (1999) Runway overrun during landing. Little Rock, Arkansas.

National Transportation Safety Board. (2004) Collision with trees and crash short of the runway" Kirksville, Missouri.

National Transportation Safety Board. (2004) Controlled flight into terrain. Albuquerque, New Mexico.

National Transportation Safety Board. (2006) Attempted takeoff from wrong runway, Lexington, Kentucky.

National Transportation Safety Board. (2009) Loss of control on approach, Clarence Center, New York.

Pannel, E. (2009) Ouachita singers meet to remember plane crash. *Three Rivers Edition.*

Patel, P. (2010). DYFI joins crash victims' cause. *Times of India.*

Pilkington, E. (2011) US air traffic controller suspended for watching Samuel L. Jackson film, April 19, 2011. Retrieved from: www.theguardian.com/world/2011/apr/19/us.

Porter, D.. (2005) *Hell's Angel.* NY: Blood Moon Prod. Ltd.

Porter, D.J. (2013) *Howard Hughes Amazing Pioneering Helicopter Exploits.* Oxford, England: Fonthill Media.

Post, W. & Gatty, H. (1931) *Around the World in Eight Days.* NY, Rand McNally & Company.

Rentz, C. (2010) Regional airlines cut cost of flying, at what price? *Investigative Reporting Workshop.*

Review of Flightcrew-Involved Major Accidents 1978 through 1990. National Transportation Safety Board Washington, DC. January, 1994.

Ross, B. & Lieberman, D. (2016) Captain Sullenberger exclusive: Airline industry must take care of tired pilots. *ABC News.* Retrieved from: https://www.boxer.senate.gove/?p=release&id=3283.

Transcript of cockpit voice records in Buffalo crash. (2009) *Wall Street Journal.* Retrieved from: www.wsj.com/articlesISB124214197938010949.

Sonati, J. (2016) Quality of life, sleep and health of air traffic controllers with rapid counterclockwise shift rotation. Workplace Health and Safety. Retrieved from: Doi:10.1177/2165079916634710.

Song, J. (2008) FAA suspends pilots who fell asleep on Hawaii flights, overshooting airport. *The Seattle Times.*

Sole Survivor of Flight 5191, Lexington, KY on August 27, 2006. Retrieved from: www.WKYT.com/home/headlines/For_first_time_flight_5191_co-pilot_and_sole_survivor_talks_about_crash__150472865.html.

Turner Farms Living: See www.turnerfarmliving.com. (Put in: Mothers Day Desert Eleanor Roosevelt Pink Clouds on Angel Food cake.)

Yeager, C. & Janos, L. (1985) *Yeager: An Autobiography.* NY: Bantam, 1985.

Young, R. (2010) Frontline: Flying Cheap. First aired on February 9, 2010. One-hour *Frontline* show available at Amazon and Barnes and Noble.

Walker, P. (2010) Pilot was snoring before the Air India crash. *The Guardian.*

Wickiwand website for Harrison Ford: www.wickiwand.com/en/Harrison_Ford.

Chapter Twelve: Sleep in the Fittest: Athletes, Police and Firefighters

Ansell, Tom IAFF. Retrieved from: http://www.iaff.org/hs/fts/SuccessStories/ChoosingHealthyFoods1.asp.

Bair, D. & Czink, K. (2016) Firefighters' fights against PTSD: Before death, firefighter makes plea to others. *WGNTV.* Retrieved from: WGNTV.com/2016/11/15/firefighters-fight-against-ptsd-before-death-firefighter-makes-plea-to-others/

Bakalar, N. (2014) Firefighter accidents are linked to sleep problems, *The New York Times*, Nov. 13, 2014.

Berninger, A., Webber, M.P., Niles, J.K., Gustave, J., Lee, R., Cohen, H.W., Kelly, K., Corrigan, M. & Prezant, D.J. (2010) Longitudinal study of probable post-traumatic stress disorder in firefighters exposed to the World Trade Center disaster. *American Journal of Industrial Medicine 53*:117-1185.

Boivin, P. (2016) Cardinals are true believers in naps. *Arizona Republic.*

Carey, M.G., Al-Zaiti, S.S.; Dean, G.E., Sessanna, D.N.S. & Finnell, D.S. (2011) Sleep problems, depression, substance use, social bonding, and quality of life in professional firefighters. *Journal of Occupational Environmental Medicine 53*(8):928-933.

Chapman, B. (2016) Supporting officer wellness within a changing policing environment: What research tells. *Police Chief Magazine*, pp. 22-24.

Cox, T. (2017) Police union: Hire more cops instead of paying $93M in overtime. Retrieved from: (//www.dnainfo.com/Chicago/about-us/our-team/editorial-team/ted-cox)

Denison, K.J. (2012) The effect of fatigue and training status on firefighter performance. *Journal of Strength and Conditioning Research 26*(4):1101-1109.

Dougherty, J. (2015) After years of delay, the Granite Mountain Hotshot autopsy records are released. *Investigative Media.*

Elliott, D.L. &. Kuehl, K.S. (2007) The effects of sleep deprivation on fire fighters and EMS responders. *International Association of Fire Chiefs.*

Fatigue Science. (2013) Why athletes should make sleep a priority in their daily training.

Goldberg, J. (2016) Fairfax Fire Department plugs 5K in Fairfax. *WJLA,* Washington, D.C.

Haddock, C.K., Jahnke, S.A., Poston, W.S.C., Jitnarin, N., Kaipust, C.M., Tuley, B. & Hyder, M, L. (2012) Alcohol use among firefighters in the Central United States. *Occupational Medicine* (Lond) *62*(8):661-664.

Harven, S.B., Milligan-Saville, J.S., Paterson, H.M., Harkness, E.L., Marsh, A.M., Dobson, J., Kemp, R. & Bryant, R.A. (2016) The mental health of fire-fighters: An examination of the impact of repeated trauma exposure. *Australian New Zealand Journal of Psychiatry 50* (7):649-658.

Jahnke, S.A., Poston, W.S.C., Haddock, C.K., Jitnarin, N., Hyder, M.L. & Horvath, C. (2012) The health of women in the US Fire Service." *Biomed Central Womens' Health.* doi:10.1186/1472-6874-12-39.

Jitnarin, N., Haddock, C.K., Poston, W.S.C. & Jahnke, S.A. (2013) Smokeless tobacco and dual use among firefighters in the Central United States. *Journal of Environmental Public Health (35):* 675426.

Jitnarin, N., Haddock, C.K., Poston, W.S.C., Jahnke, S.A. & Day, R.S. (2015) Tobacco use pattern among a national firefighter cohort.

University of Texas. Retrieved from: www.uthealth.influuent.utsystem.edu/en/publications/tobacco-use-pattern-among-a-national-firefighter, p. 66-73.

Jones, C. (2016) Many companies force workers to use time off. *USA Today.*

Kerwood, S. (2016) Firefighter mental health—It's your responsibility. *On Scene--International Fire Chiefs Association Newsletter.*

Larraneta, I. (2014) Daughter of Groton City police lieutenant who committed suicide pushes for more mental health support for officers. *The Day.*

Mansourian, J. (2011) Fatal Fatigue: The consequence of sleep deprivation on officer safety. *COPS, U.S. Department of Justice Journal 4(6).*

Mayer, K. (2016) Is sleep the next frontier of workplace wellness? *Employee Benefit News* from Employee Benefit Association.

McLean, K. (2017) Taking care of your own: Sustaining a culture of crash prevention efforts in law enforcement. *The Police Chief Magazine.*

Mehrdad, R., Haghighi, K.S. & Esfahani, A.H.N. (2013) Sleep quality of professional firefighters. *International Journal of Preventive Medicine* 4(9):1095-1100.

Metz, D. (2016) Companies can't afford to ignore sleep in wellness offerings. *Employer Benefit News* from Employee Benefit Association.

Neylan, T.C., Metzler, T.J., Best, S.R., Weiss, D.S., Fagan, J.A., Liberman, A., Rogers, C., Vedantham, K., Brunet, A., Lipsey, T.L.& Marmar, C.R. (2002) Critical incident exposure and sleep quality in police officers. *Psychosomatic Medicine* 64:345-352.

Nintzel, J. (2015) A new twist in the death of Granite Mountain Hotshots. *Tucson Weekly,* Retrieved from: www.tucsonweekly.com/ TheRange/archives/2015/12/a-new-twist-in-the-death-of-the-granite-mountain-hotshots

Nova Southeastern University, Broward County Florida (2016) Sleep quality: A key component to overall mental and physical health among firefighters. Retrieved from: http://nsubso.nova.edu/ programs/research/abstract_firefighters_sleep.html

Nuwer, R. (2014) Lack of sleep seems to be more deadly for firefighters than fire. *Smithsonian Magazine.*

O'Brien, Chef Marshall. Minneapolis Fire District Guide to Improving Fire Fighter Energy, Performance and Safety. Retrieved from: www.minneapolismn.gov/www./groups/public/@communications/ documents/images/wcms1p-124030.pdf.

Piazza-Gardner, A.K., Barry, A.E. Chaney, E., Dodd, V., Wester, R. & Delisle, A. (2014) Covariates of alcohol consumption among career firefighters, *Occupational Medicine,* (Lond) *64*(8):580-2.

Poole, T.L. (2012) The 48/96 Work Schedule: A Viable Alternative? Retrieved from: http://www.fireengineering.com/articles/ print/volume-165/issue-2/features/the-48-96-work-schedule-a-viable-alternative.html

Rajaratnam, S.M.W., Barger, L.K. & Lockley, S.W. (2011) Sleep disorders, health and safety in police officers. *Journal of the American Medical Association 306*(23):2567-2578.

Rickman, K. (2013) 19: The true story of the Yarnell Hill Fire. *Outside.* Retrieved from: www.outsideonline.com/1926426/19-true-story-yarnell-hill-fire.

Roy, J. & Forest, G. (2016) A five-year retrospective study on the circadian disadvantage in three major sport leagues in North America. *SLEEP*, Vol. 39.

Sanders, L. (1981) *The Third Deadly Sin*. NY: Putnam.

Sports Injury Handbook, November 30, 2012. Retrieved from: www.sportsinjuryhandbook.com/features_archive/lack_of_sleep.html.

Stout, R. (1973) *The Nero Wolfe Cookbook*. Nashville, TN: Cumberland House Publisher.

Thomas, R.J. (2015) Sleepiness and driving: multidimensional legal, social, technological and biological challenges. *SLEEP*.

Vila, B. & Kenney, D.J. (2002) Tired cops: The prevalence and potential consequences of police fatigue. *National Institute of Justice Journal*, 16-21. Retrieved from: http://www.ncjrs.gov/app/publication/abstract.aspx?ID=190634.

Violanti, J.M. (2014) *Dying for the Job*. Springfield, IL: Charles C. Thomas Publications Ltd.

Wadsworth, J. (2016) San Jose grapples with police overtime, officer fatigue. *San Jose Inside*.

Whyman, A. (2015). The stressful lives of police officers: Mental health matters. *Sierra Sun*. Retrieved from http://www.sierrasun.com/news/opinion/the-stress-lives-of-police-%C2%AD-mental-health-matters/

Wickman, T. (2016) An ideal diet for improved heart health. *The Police Chief Magazine*, 12-13.

Weich, S. (2011) Change in schedule doubles firefighters' time on duty. *St. Louis Dispatch*, June 19th.

Willing, L. (2014, December 1) Firefighter sleep: 7 ways to improve your crews' sleep and safety. Retrieved from https://www.firerescue1. com/fire-chief/articles/20311999-Firefighter-sleep-7-ways-to-improve-your-crews-sleep-and-safety/

Wolski, C.A. (2015). Helping athletes find their (circadian) rhythm. *Sleep Review*. Retrieved from http://www.sleepreviewmag.com/2015.03/ helping-athletes-find-circadian-drhythm/.

Wyllie, D. (2014) How lack of sleep may cause deadly police errors. *PoliceOne.com*

Chapter Thirteen: Sleep in the Medical Professions

Barnard, C.N. (1967). A human cardiac transplant. *South African Medical Journal, 41*, 1257-1278.

Bates, D.W; Spell, N., & Cullen, D.J. (1997) The costs of adverse drug events in hospitalized patients. *JAMA, 277*(4), 307-311. doi:10.1001/ jama.1997.03540280045032

Bennett, C.L., Finch, A., Vuong, K., McDonald, D., & Rennie, S. (2016) Surgical resident duty hours. *New England Journal of Medicine 374*(24), 2399-2401. doi:10.1056/NEJMc160 2016; 374(24)2399-2401.

Berwick, D.M. & Leape, L.L. (1999) Reducing errors in medicine, Quality & Safety in Health Care, 8(3), 145-146. doi:10.1136/qshc.8.3.145.

Birkmeyer, J.D. (2016). Surgical resident duty-hour rules: Weighing the new evidence. *New England Journal of Medicine, 374*,783-784. doi:10.1056/NEJMe1516572.

Blum, A.B., Raiszadeh, F., Shea, S., Mermin, D., Lurie, P., Landrigan, C.P., & Czeisler, C.A. (2010). U.S. public opinion regarding proposed limits on resident physician work hours. *BMC Medicine, 1*(8), 33. doi: 10.1186/1741-7015-8-33.

Brennan, T.A. et al. (1991). Incidence of adverse events and negligence in hospitalized patients. *New England Journal of Medicine, 324*, 370-376. doi:10.1056/NEJM199102073240604

Carson, B. & C.(2016). Cooking with 'Friends': Dr. Ben and Candy Carson's coconut spinach. [web log]/ Retrieved from http://www. foxnews.com/on-air/fox-and-friends/blog/2016/07/19/cooking-friends-dr-ben-and-candy-carsons-coconut -spinach

Carson, B. (1992) *Gifted hands: The Ben Carson story.* Grand Rapids, MI: Zondervan.

Centor, R.M., Morrow, R.W., Poses, R.M., & Vega, C.P. (2012) Doc burnout: Worse than other workers. Retrieved from http://www. medscape.com/viewarticle/774013

Cohen, M.R., Jenkins, R.H., Vaida, A, & Litman, R.S. (2016) The effects of residents' work-hour restrictions on the occurrence of medication errors. *Institute for Safe Medication Practices.* Retrieved from:

https://www.acgme.org/Portals/0/PDFs/Position%20Papers/ Institute%20for%20Safe%20 Medication%20Practices.pdf

DePietro, R.H. Knutson, K.L. Spampinato, L., Anderson, S.L., Meltzer, D.O., Van Cauter, E. & Arora, V.M. (2016) Association between sleep loss and hyperglycemia of hospitalization. *Diabetes Care.* doi. org/10.2337/dc16-1683

Ellenbogen, J.M. (April 2005) Cognitive benefits of sleep and their loss due to sleep deprivation. *Neurology 64*, E25-E27.

Frampton, S.B., Guastello, S., Hoy, L., Naylor, M., Sheridan, S. & Johnston-Fleece, M. (2017) Harnessing evidence and experience to change culture: A guiding framework for patient and family engaged care. *National Academy of Medicine.* Retrieved from: https://nam.edu/perspectives

Gefell, A.W. (July 2003) Dying to sleep: Using federal legislation and tort law to cure the effects of fatigue in medical residency programs. 1 Journal of Law and Policy 645. *Committee of Interns and Residents Service Employees International Union Journal.*

Gold, D. Rogacz, S. & Bock, N. (1992) Rotating shift work, sleep, and accidents related to sleepiness in hospital nurses. *American Journal of Public Health. 82*(7):1011-1014.

Graeme, D. (2013) *The Accidental Scientist. The Role of Chance and Luck in Scientific Discovery.* London: Michael O'Mara Books, 2013.

Gyorffy, A., Dweik, D., & Girasek, E. (2016) Workload, mental health and burnout indicators among female physicians. *Human Resources for Health 14* (12):1-10.

Hill, A.B. (2017) Breaking the stigma—A physician's perspective on self-care and recovery. *New England Journal of Medicine. 376* (12): 1005-1007.

Hinohara, C & Niki, H. (2001) *Osler's "A Way of Life" & Other Addresses with Commentary and Annotations.* Durham: Duke University Press.

Hoffenberg, Raymond. (December 2001) Christiaan Barnard: His first transplants and their impact on concepts of death. *British Medical Journal.* 323(7327):1478-1480.

Klass, P. (2013) Getting through the night. *New England Journal of Medicine 369*:2279-2281.

Kohn, L.T., Corrigan, J.M., & Donaldson, M.S. editors. (2000) To err is human: Building a safer health system. *Institute of Medicine,* Washington (DC), National Academies Press (US).

Krumholz, H. M. (2013) Post-hospital syndrome—An acquired, transient condition of generalized risk. *New England Journal of Medicine 368*:100-102.

Kuetting, D., Feisst, A., Homsi, R., Luetkens, J.A., Thomas, D., Schild, H.H. & Dabir, D. (2016) Short-term sleep deprivation affects heart function. *Radiological Society of North America*. Retrieved from: https//:www.rsna.org/news.aspx?id=20878.

Landrigan, C.P., Barger, L.K., Cade, B.E., Avas, N.T. & Czeisler, C. (2006) Interns' compliance with accreditation council for medical education work-hour limits. *Journal of the American Medical Association 296*(9):1063-70.

Lerner, Barron H. (2006) A case that shook medicine. *Washington Post*.

Leventer-Roberts, M., Zonfrillo, M.R., Sunkyung, Y., Dziura, J.D. & Spiro, D.M. (2013) Overweight physicians during residency: A cross-sectional and longitudinal study. *Journal of Graduate Medical Education. 5*(3): 405-411.

Lindeman, B.M., Sacks, B.C., Hirose, K, & Lipsett, P.A. (2013) Multifaced longitudinal study of surgical resident education, quality of life and patient care before and after July 2011. *Journal of Surgical Education, 70*(6):769-76.

Lobelo, F. & de Quevedo, I.G. (2013) Weighing in on residents' body mass index. A teachable moment for physicians and patients alike? *Journal of Graduate Medical Education. 5*(3): 521-523. Doi: 10.4300/JGME-D-13-00203.1

Lockley, S.W., Cronin, J.W., Evans, E.E., Cade, B.E., Clark, J.L., Landrigan, C.P., Rothschild, J.M., Katz, J.T., Lilly, C.M., Stone, P.H., Aeschbach, D. & Czeisler, C.A. (2004) Effect of reducing interns' weekly work hours on sleep and attentional failures. *New England Journal of Medicine. 351*.1829-1837.

Louwtjie and Christiaan Barnard's Curried Beef: *Master Cook* on the *Internet*.

McCormick, F., Kadzielski, J., Landrigan, C.P., Evans, B., Herndon, J.H. & Rubash, H.E. (2012) Surgeon fatigue: A prospect analysis of the incidence, risk and intervals of predicted fatigue-related impairment in residents. *Archives of Surgery.147*(5):430-5.

Muller, D. (2017) Kathryn. *New England Journal of Medicine. 376*(12):1101-1103.

Olaoye, O. (2016) Sleep time and hospitalist perception of care. *SLEEP,* Vol. 39.

Ornstein, C. (2007) Dennis Quaid files suit over drug mishap. *Los Angeles Times*.

Owen, S. (1993) *The Rice Book*. New York: St. Martin's Press Griffin.

Pear, R. (2000) Interns' long workdays prompt first crackdown. *The New York Times*.

Philibert, I., Chang, B., Flynn, T., Friedman, P. & Minter, E.S. (2009) The 2003 common duty hour limits: Process, outcome and lessons learned. *Journal of Graduate Medical Education. 1*(2):334-337.

President's Commission for the Study of Ethical Problems in Medicine and Biomedical Behavioral Research. (1981) Guidelines for the Determination of Death. *Journal of the American Medical Association 246*:2184-2186.

Report of the Ad Hoc Committee of the Harvard Medical School to Examine the Definition of Brain Death (1968) *Journal of the American Medical Association 205*:337-340.

Roberts, S. (2016) Bertrand M. Bell, who strove to reduce medical trainee's grueling shifts, dies at 86. *New York Times.*

Rosenbaum, L. & Lamas, D. (2012). Residents' duty Hours—Toward an Empirical Narrative. *New England Journal of Medicine 367*:2044-2049.

Rothschild, J.M., Keohane, C.A., Rogers, S., Gardner, R., Lipsitz, S.R., Salzberg, C.A., Yu, T., Yoon, C.S., Williams, D.H. & Wien, M.F. (2009) Risks of complications by attending physicians after performing nighttime procedures, *Journal of the American Medical Association. 302*(14):1565-1572. Doi:10.1001/jama.2009.1423

Ruff, J. (2016) Surgical resident duty hours. *New England Journal of Medicine 374*:2399-2403.

Shanafelt, T.D., Balch, C.M., Bechamps, G.J., Russell, T., Dyrbye, L., Satele, D., Collicott, P., Novotney, P.J., Sloan, J. & Freischlag, J.A. (2009). Burnout and career satisfaction among American surgeons. *Annals of Surgery 250*(3):463-471.

Starr, K. (1997) *The Dream Endures: California Enters the 1940s.* New York. Oxford University Press.

Thomas, E.J., Studdart, D.M., Newhouse, J.P., Zbar, B.I., Howard, K.M., Williams, E.J. & Brennan, T.A. (1999) Costs of medical injuries in Utah and Colorado. *Pub Med 36*(3):255-64.

Thorndike, A.N., Mills, S., Sonnenberg, L., Palakshappa, D., Gao, T., Pau, C.T., & Regan, S. (2014) Activity monitor intervention to promote physical activity of physicians-in-training: Randomized controlled trial. *PLoSOne. 9*(6):e100251. Doi: 10.1371/journal.pone.0100251

Vetter, C., Devore, E.E., Wegrzyn, L.R., Massa, J., Speizer, F., Kawachi, I., Rosner, B., Stampfer, M.J. & Schernhammer, E. (2016) Association between rotating night shift work and risk of coronary heart disease among women. *Journal of the American Medical Association. 315*(16):1725-1734.

Wu, B. (2016) Staying healthy during medical school. Retrieved from https://www.studentdoctor.net
Chapter Fourteen: Sleep and the Military

Alexander, M., Ray, M.A., Hebert, J.R., Youngstedt, S.D., Zhang, H., Steck, S.E., Bogan, R.K. & Burch, J.B. (2016) The National Veteran Sleep Disorder Study: Descriptive Epidemiology and Secular Trends, 2000-2010. *SLEEP, 39*(7):1399-410.

Audie Murphy. Retrieved from Wikipedia Book: https://en.wikipedia.org/wiki/Book:Audie_Murphy

Barton, R. (2010) *Hedy Lamarr: The Most Beautiful Woman in Film.* Lexington, KY: University Press of Kentucky.

Belenky, Col. Gregory. Sleep, sleep deprivation, and human performance in continuous operations. Retrieved from: http://isme.tamu.edu/JSCOPE97/Belenky97/Belenky97.htm

Capener, D.C., Brock, M.S., Walter, R.J., Matsangas, P. & Mysliwiec, V. (2016) Sleep disorders in active duty females. *SLEEP, 39,* Abstract 1016.

Chapman, D.P., Liu, Y., McKnight-Eily, L.R., Croft, J.B., Holt, J.B., Balkin, T.J. & Giles, W.H. (2015) Daily insufficient sleep and active duty status. *Military Medicine 180*(1):68-76.

Conant, J. (2005) *109 East Palace: Robert Oppenheimer and the Secret City of Los Alamos.* NY: Simon and Schuster.

Culver, N.C., McGowan, M.G., Fiorentino, L., Fung, C.H., Song, Y., Dzierewski, J.M., Rodriguez, J., Mitchell, M., Jouldjian, S., Josephson, K.,

Washington, D.L., Yano, E.M., Alessi, C. & Martin, J.L. (2016) Treatment preferences among women veterans with insomnia. *SLEEP,* June 11, 2016 poster session at Denver, CO.

Davidson, M.J. (1999) *A Guide to Military Law.* Anapolis, MD: Naval Institute Press.

Dunn, H. & Ebinkger, V., Eds. (2001) *Savoring the Past: Recipes from Three cultures.* Los Alamos, NM: Los Alamos Historical Society.

Dwight D. Eisenhower Presidential Library, Museum and Boyhood Home in Abilene, Kansas. Retrieved from: www.eisenhower.archives. gov/all_about_ike/favorites.html

Eliasson, A., Kashani, M., Cruz, G.D. & Vernalis, M. (2012) Readiness and associated health behaviors and symptoms in recently deployed Army National Guard soldiers. *Military Medicine,* 177, 11: 1254-1260.

Fink, G. Editor. (2010) *Stress of War, Conflict and Disaster.* San Diego, CA: Elsevier.

Freud, S. (2007) *Living in the Shadow of the Freud Family: Sophie Freud.* Westport, CT: Praeger Publishing.

Holloway, D. & Cheney, B. (2001) *American History in Song.* Lincoln, NE: Authors Choice Press.

Jedick, R. (2014) Tarnak Farm—Reckless Pilots, Speed, or Fog of War? *Go Flight Medicine.* Retrieved from: http://goflightmedicine.com/ tarnak-farm/

Kashani, M., Eliasson, A., Chrosniak, L. & Vernalis, M. (2010) Taking aim at nurse stress. *Military Medicine* 175(2):96.

Killgore, W.D., McBridge, S.A., Killgore, D.B. & Balkin, T.J. (2006) The effects of caffeine. *SLEEP,* 29(6):841-7.

Killgore, W.D.; (2006) The effects of caffeine, dextroamphetamine, and modafinil on humor appreciation during sleep deprivation. *SLEEP, 29* (6):841-847.

Killgore, W.D., Killgore, D.B., Day, L.M., Li, C., Kaminavie, G.H. & Balkin, T.J. (2007) The effects of 53 hours of sleep deprivation on moral judgment. *SLEEP 30*(3):345-352.

Kindleberger, C.P. (2003) Obituary: Economist Helped Design Marshall Plan. *Los Angeles Times.*

Kryger, M.H., Roth, T. & Dement, W.C. (2017) *Principles and Practice of Sleep Medicine.* Philadelphia: Elsevier.

Lamarr, H. (1967) *Ecstasy and Me: My Life as a Woman.* New York: Fawcett.

Marriott, B.M., (1994) Editor: *Food Components to Enhance Performance: An Evaluation of Potential Performance-Enhancing Food Components.* Washington, D.C.: National Academies Press.

Moore, B.A. (2016) Sleep problems persist after PTSD treatment, study of active troops finds. Retrieved from: www.militarytimes.com/sleep-problems-persist-after-PTSD-treatment-study-of-active-troops-find

Ohler, N. (2017) *Blitzed: Drugs in the Third Reich.* New York: Houghton Mifflin Harcourt.

Olsen, O., Pallesen, S. & Eid, J. (2010) Impact of partial sleep deprivation on moral reasoning in military officers. *SLEEP 33*(8):1086-1090.

O'Neal, C.W., Lucier-Greer, M., Mancini, J.A., Ferraro, A.J. & Ross, D.B. (2016) Family relational health, psychological resources, and health behaviors: A dyadic study of military couples. *Military Medicine 181,* 2:152-160.

Osiel, M.J. (1999) *Obeying Orders*. New Brunswick, NJ: Transaction Publishers.

Pappalardo, J. (2017) To Libya and back: Inside a stealth bomber strike against ISIS. Retrieved from: www.popularmechanics.com/military/aviation/a25070/to-libya-and-back

Patton, G. Speech to Third Army. Retrieved from: www.pattonhq.com/speech.html

Peterson, A.L., Goodie, J.L., Sutterfield, W.A. & Brim, W.L. (2008) Sleep disturbance during military deployment. *Military Medicine* *173*(3):230.

Porter, D. (2006) *Brando Unzipped*. New York. Moon Productions Ltd.

Powell, C. (2012) *It Worked For Me: In Life and Leadership*. NY: Harper Perennial.

Rabinowitz, Y.G., Breitbach, J.E. & Warner, C.H. (2009) Managing aviator fatigue in a deployed environment: The relationship between fatigue and neurocognitive functioning. *AMSUS 174*(4):358-362.

Rockswold, P.D. (2016) The importance of sleep in protecting mental health and operational readiness. Retrieved from: Navymedicine. navylive.dodlive.mil/archives/228

Seelig, A.D., Jacobson, I.G., Donoho, C.J., Trone, D.W., Crum-Cianfione, N.F. & Balkin, T.J. (2016) Sleep and health resilience metrics in a large military cohort. *SLEEP 39*(5):1111-1120.

Taylor, M.K., Hilton, S.M., Campbell, J.S., Beckerley, S.E., Shobe, K.K. & Drummond, S.P.A. (2014) Prevalence and mental health correlates of sleep disruption among military members serving in a combat zone. *Military Medicine, 179*(7):744-751.

The Cook Book of the United States Navy. 1945. *Historic Naval Ships Association.* Retrieved from: www.hnsh.org/resources/manuals-documents/single-topic/the-cookbook-of-the-united-states-navy/

Thomas, E. (2012) The brilliant prudence of Dwight Eisenhower. *The Atlantic.*

Thompson, M. (2014) The curse of 'friendly fire'. *Time Magazine.* Retrieved from: http://time.com/2854306/the-curse-of-friendly-fire/

Troxel, W.M., Shih, R.A., Pedersen, E.R., Geyer, L., Fisher, M.P., Griffin, B.A., Haas, A.C., Kurz, J. & Steinberg, P.S. (2015) Sleep in the Military: Promoting Healthy Sleep Among U.S. Servicemembers. Retrieved from: www.rand.org/pubs/research_reports/RR739.html

Troxel, W.M., (2016) Examining the prevalence and correlates of sleep problems among military spouses. *SLEEP* Abstract 1015. Retrieved from: www.aasmnet.org/articles.aspx?id=6313.

Watt, C.G. (2009) *Aircrew Fatigue Management.* Maxwell AFB: Air War College.

Chapter Fifteen

Afaghi, A., O'Connor, H., & Chow, C.M. (2007) High-glycemic index carbohydrate meals shorten sleep onset. *American Journal of Clinical Nutrition 85*(2):426-430.

Coren, S. (1996) *Sleep Thieves: An Eye-opening Exploration into the Science and Mysteries of Sleep.* NY: Free Press Paperbacks.

Howatson, G., Bell, P.G., Tallent, J., Middleton, B., McHugh, M.P. & Ellis, J. (2012) Effect of tart cherry juice on melatonin levels and enhanced sleep quality. *European Journal of Nutrition, 51*(8):909-16.

Lin, H.H., Tsai, P.S., Fang, S.C. & Lie, J.E. (2011) Effect of kiwifruit consumption on sleep quality in adults with sleep problems. *Asia Pacific Journal of Clinical Nutrition, 20*(2):169-74.

O'Connor, A. (2007) The claim: A glass of warm milk will help you get to sleep at night. *New York Times.*

Paredes, S.D., Barriga, C., Reiter, R.J. & Rodriguez, A.B. (2009) Assessment of the potential role of tryptophan as the precursor of serotonin and melatonin for the aged sleep-wake cycle and immune function. *International Journal of Tryptophan Research, 2*:23-36.

Pepper, William. (1911) *The Medical Side of Benjamin Franklin.* Philadelphia: William J. Campbell.

Perkins, D. (2014) Foods that contain melatonin. *Livestrong.com.*

Pigeon, W.R., Carr, M., Gorman, C. & Perlis, M.L. (2010) Effects of a tart cherry juice beverage on the sleep of older adults with insomnia. *Journal of Medicinal Foods, 13*(3): 579-583.

Roizen, M.F. (2013) Take aspirin at night to reap its health and beauty benefits. *US News.* Retrieved from: Health.USNews.com/ health-news/blogs/eat-run/2013/12/17/take-aspirin-at-night-to-reap-its-health-and-beauty-benefits

Thurber, J. (1996) *Thurber Writings and Drawings.* NY: Penguin Books.

Trall, R.T. (1872) "Sleeplessness" in *Health and Diseases of Women.* Pomeroy, WA: Health Research.

INDEX

Printed in the United States
By Bookmasters